An Atlas of Investigation and Diagnosis

LYMPHOID MALIGNANCIES

An Atlas of Investigation and Diagnosis

LYMPHOID MALIGNANCIES

Estella Matutes
MD, PhD, FRCPath
Reader in Haemato-Oncology
Institute of Cancer Research, London, UK
and
Consultant Haematologist
The Royal Marsden NHS Foundation Trust, London, UK

Barbara J Bain
MB BS, FRACP, FRCPath
Professor of Diagnostic Haematology
Faculty of Medicine, Imperial College, London, UK
and
Honorary Consultant Haematologist
St Mary's Hospital NHS Trust, London, UK

Andrew Wotherspoon
MB BCh, MRCPath
Consultant Histopathologist
The Royal Marsden NHS Foundation Trust, London, UK

CLINICAL PUBLISHING
OXFORD

Clinical Publishing
an imprint of Atlas Medical Publishing Ltd
Oxford Centre for Innovation
Mill Street Oxford OX2 0JX UK

Tel: +44 1865 811116
Fax: +44 1865 251550
Email: info@clinicalpublishing.co.uk
Web: www.clinicalpublishing.co.uk

Distributed in USA and Canada by:
Clinical Publishing
30 Amberwood Parkway
Ashland OH 44805 USA

Tel: 800-247-6553 (toll free within US and Canada)
Fax: 419-281-6883
Email: order@bookmasters.com

Distributed in UK and Rest of World by:
Marston Book Services Ltd
PO Box 269
Abingdon
Oxon OX14 4YN UK

Tel: +44 1235 465500
Fax: +44 1235 465555
Email: trade.orders@marston.co.uk

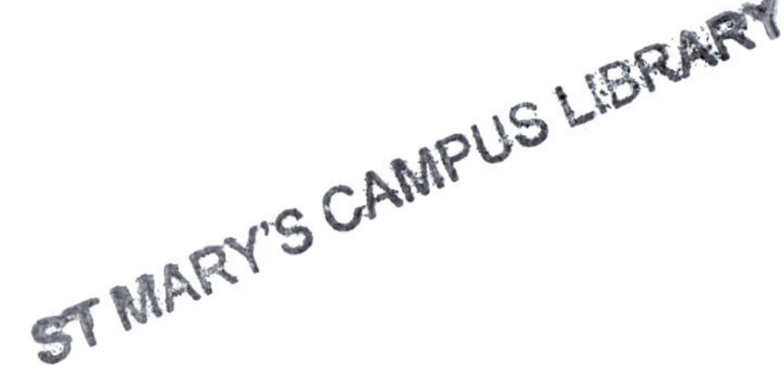

First published 2007

A catalogue record of this book is available from the British Library

ISBN-13 978 1 904392 67 5
ISBN-10 1 904392 67 9

Printed by T G Hostench SA, Barcelona, Spain

Contents

Acknowledgements

We should like to thank Mr Ricardo Morilla, Dr John Swansbury, Dr Julie McCarthy, and other colleagues from the Royal Marsden and St Mary's Hospitals who have generously contributed illustrations or have read sections of the manuscript. They are individually acknowledged in the legends to the figures.

We should also like to thank Professor Daniel Catovsky who contributed a considerable number of figures. His major contribution to the field of lymphoid malignancies over the last 40 years is reflected in these pages and is gratefully acknowledged.

Estella Matutes
Barbara J Bain
Andrew Wotherspoon
September 2007

Abbreviations

ABCM adriamycin (Doxorubicin), BCNU, cyclophosphamide and melphalan
AIDS acquired immune deficiency syndrome
ALCL anaplastic large cell lymphoma
ALL acute lymphoblastic leukaemia
AML acute myeloid leukaemia
APAAP alkaline phosphatase–anti-alkaline phosphatase
ATLL adult T-cell leukaemia/lymphoma
B-PLL B-cell prolymphocytic leukaemia
CHAD cold haemagglutinin disease
CHOP cyclophosphamide, doxorubicin, vincristine and prednisone or prednisolone
CLL chronic lymphocytic leukaemia
CT computed tomography
DLBCL diffuse large B-cell lymphoma
EBER Epstein–Barr virus-encoded RNA
EBV Epstein–Barr virus
EGIL European Group for the Immunological Characterization of Leukemias
EMA epithelial membrane antigen
EORTC European Organization for Research and Treatment of Cancer
FAB French–American–British (classification)
FISH fluorescence *in situ* hybridization
FLIPI Follicular Lymphoma International Prognostic Index
HD Hodgkin's disease
H&E haematoxylin & eosin
HHV8 human herpesvirus 8
HIV human immunodeficiency virus
HTLV-I human T-cell lymphotropic virus I
Ig immunoglobulin
IPSID immunoproliferative small intestinal disease
KIR killer immunoglobulin-like receptor
KSHV Kaposi's sarcoma-associated herpesvirus
L&H lymphocytic and histiocytic Reed–Sternberg variants
LDH lactate dehydrogenase
LGLL large granular lymphocyte leukaemia
LMP1 latent membrane protein 1
MALT mucosa-associated lymphoid tissue
MCL mantle cell lymphoma
MF mycosis fungoides
MGUS monoclonal gammopathy of undetermined significance
MHC major histocompatibility complex
NHL non-Hodgkin's lymphoma
NK natural killer
NLPHD nodular lymphocyte-predominant Hodgkin's disease
PAS periodic acid–Schiff
PCR polymerase chain reaction
PEL primary effusion lymphoma
PET positron emission tomography
PLL prolymphocytic leukaemia
POEMS Polyneuropathy, Organomegaly (hepatomegaly, splenomegaly, lymphadenopathy), Endocrinopathy, M-protein and Skin changes (syndrome)
PUVA psoralen plus ultraviolet light
RT-PCR reverse transcriptase polymerase chain reaction
SLL small lymphocytic lymphoma
SmIg surface membrane immunoglobulin
SMZL splenic marginal zone lymphoma
SS Sézary syndrome
TCR T-cell receptor
TdT terminal deoxynucleotidyl transferase
T-PLL T-cell prolymphocytic leukaemia
VAD vincristine, adriamycin (Doxorubicin) and dexamethasone
WHO World Health Organization

Chapter 1

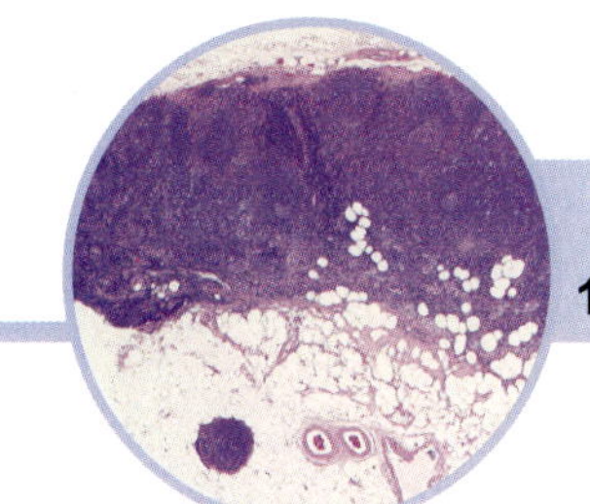

The molecular basis of lymphoma

Lymphomas are neoplasms of T, B or natural killer (NK) lymphoid cells and their precursors. Although having different characteristics from their normal counterparts, the neoplastic cells of many lymphomas have the features of lymphoid cells at a particular stage of differentiation. In addition, lymphoma cells can have the characteristics of lymphocytes that normally reside in a particular organ or tissue. Neoplastic lymphocytes tend to 'home' to the tissues and specific locations where their normal counterparts reside. Lymphomas arise as a result of a series of mutations in a single lymphoid cell. Usually this is a cell already committed to the B, T or NK lineage although rarely the mutation is in a pluripotent myeloid-lymphoid stem cell or in a common lymphoid stem cell. In the former case, exemplified by the 8p11 syndrome, patients can have a B-cell precursor or T-cell precursor leukaemia/lymphoma during one phase of the disease and an acute or chronic myeloid leukaemia during another phase [1]. In the latter instance, exemplified by biphenotypic acute leukaemia, neoplastic cells express various combinations of B-lineage, T-lineage and myeloid markers on cells of the same clone [2]. Lymphomas differ from lymphoid leukaemias in that the predominant disease manifestations are in lymphoid organs or tissues whereas in lymphoid leukaemias the predominant manifestations are in the bone marrow and the blood.

The mutations leading to lymphoma are very variable. Invariably they involve oncogenes and often there is also loss of function of tumour suppressor genes. It is the nature of the molecular events that is the crucial factor determining the nature of the lymphoma. Sometimes these molecular changes are the result of major chromosomal rearrangements, such as a translocation or inversion, and can be predicted by standard cytogenetic analysis [3].

An understanding of the normal immune system necessarily underpins an understanding of the nature of lymphoma.

The normal immune system

The immune system includes lymph nodes, spleen and thymus and, in addition, lymphoid cells in many other organs, including particularly the bone marrow, the liver, the gastrointestinal tract, the upper and lower respiratory tracts and the genitourinary system. Mucosa-associated lymphoid tissue (MALT) includes (i) discrete lymphoid structures such as the appendix, Peyer's patches in the submucosa of the intestine and the tonsils and adenoids (collectively referred to as Waldeyer's ring) in the pharynx and (ii) lymphocytes in the submucosa of various organs that do not form any macroscopically recognizable structure. The various components of the immune system are interconnected by lymphatic channels and by the blood stream. In addition to lymphoid cells and certain plasma proteins, the normal immune system includes other cells with phagocytic and antigen-presenting function, including neutrophils, monocytes, macrophages and dendritic cells [4]. The immune system is both innate and adaptive, and both of these systems have cellular and humoral elements (*Table 1.1*). Innate immunity does not require prior antigen exposure and provides an immediate response; it includes phagocytic cells, natural killer cells and the plasma proteins of the complement system. Adaptive immunity occurs as a response to antigen exposure; it is characterized by specificity and immunological memory with the response being delayed. It is dependent on B cells (which differentiate into antibody-producing plasma cells), CD8-positive T cells

Table 1.1 The normal immune system

	Innate	*Adaptive*
Characteristics	Does not alter with repeat exposure to antigens	Is characterized by specificity and immunological memory; response enhanced by repeat exposure to an antigen
Components	Phagocytic cells (neutrophils, monocytes, macrophages, interdigitating dendritic cells) Cells that release inflammatory mediators (eosinophils, basophils, mast cells) Natural killer cells Complement components and acute phase reactants Cytokines including chemokines Interferons	B cells and plasma cells T cells Antigen-presenting cells (interdigitating dendritic cells including Langerhans cells*, follicular dendritic cells†, macrophages and B lymphocytes*) Immunoglobulins
Main sites	Blood stream and tissues	Lymph nodes, spleen, mucosa-associated lymphoid tissue

* Present antigen to T cells † Present antigen to B cells

(which damage or destroy target cells expressing the relevant antigen) and CD4-positive T cells (which possess effector capability and also enhance and regulate the function of other cells involved in the immune response). Immune responses to self-antigens can also occur. These are maladaptive and often give rise to disease. The bone marrow and thymus, being the sites of B and T lymphocyte development, are referred to as primary lymphoid organs. The lymph nodes and other peripheral lymphoid tissues comprise the secondary lymphoid tissues.

The structure of a normal or reactive lymph node is shown diagrammatically in Figure **1.1** and in histological sections in Figures **1.2**–**1.4**. Lymph nodes are divided into cortex, paracortex and medulla. Within the cortex are primary follicles, which are composed of B lymphocytes and follicular dendritic cells. On antigen exposure, proliferation and maturation of B cells cause the primary follicle to develop into a secondary follicle comprising a germinal centre surrounded by a mantle zone of small B lymphocytes. Outside the mantle zone some lymph node germinal centres (and particularly splenic germinal centres) have a marginal zone, also composed of B lymphocytes. The network of follicular dendritic cells in the germinal centre presents antigen to B cells. T cells occupy the paracortex, which surrounds and underlies the primary and secondary follicles. The paracortex also has abundant dendritic cells. The centre of the lymph node is the medulla, composed of medullary cords and sinuses. The medullary cords are occupied by B and T lymphocytes, plasma cells and macrophages. Lymph, derived from interstitial fluid and containing a variable number of lymphocytes, is brought to the lymph nodes by a number of afferent lymphatics and is transported from the lymph node by an efferent lymphatic, exiting from the hilum of the node. Lymphocytes are also brought to the lymph node by its arterial supply, entering the interstitium of the node through high endothelial venules. Lymphocytes characteristically recirculate, from lymph nodes or other lymphoid tissues through the lymphatics and the blood stream back to lymphoid tissues. Homing of lymphocytes to tissues similar to those from which they originated (e.g. skin or gastrointestinal submucosa) is usual.

Figure 1.1 Diagram showing the structure of a normal lymph node.

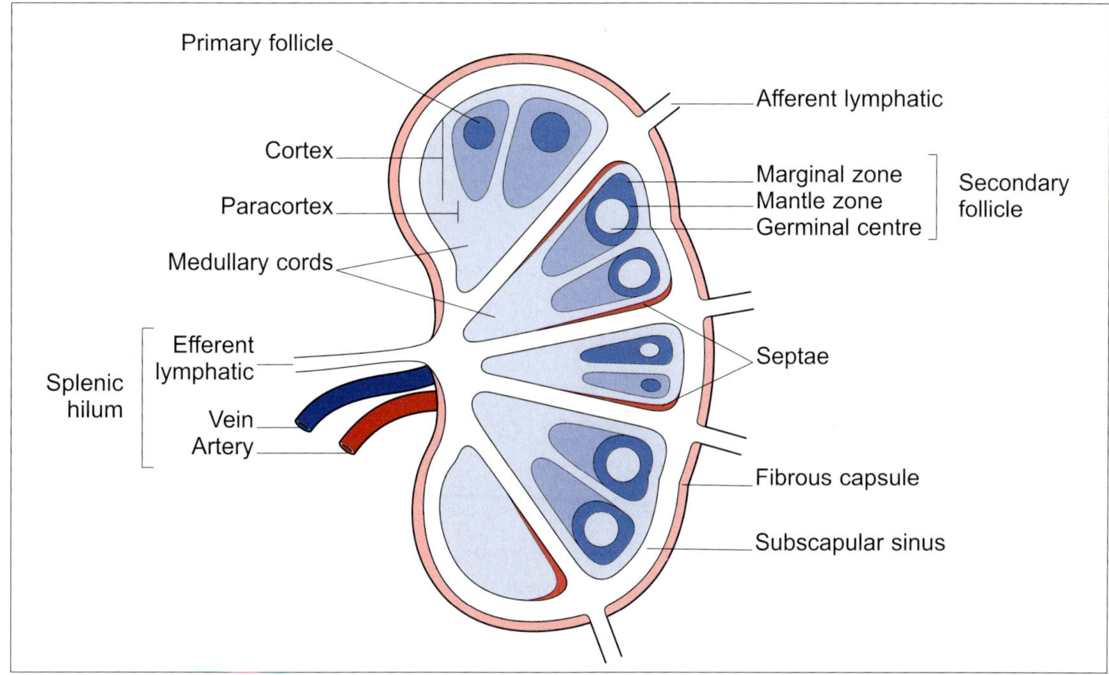

Figure 1.2 Histological section of a lymph node from a patient with reactive lymphadenopathy showing the cortex (containing primary and secondary follicles) and the medulla. H&E, x 4 objective.

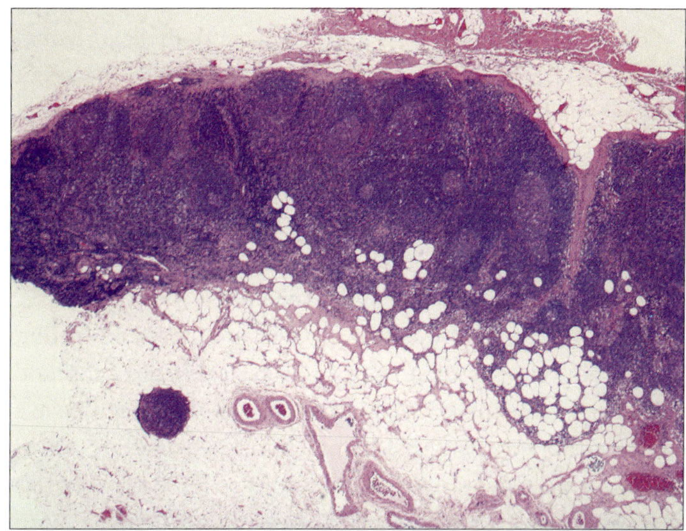

Figure 1.3 Histological section of a lymph node from a patient with reactive lymphadenopathy showing the cortex (containing secondary follicles) and the medulla. H&E, x 10 objective.

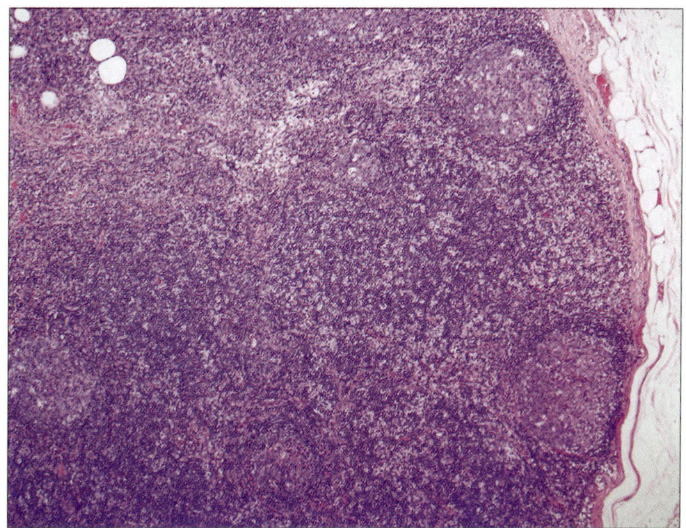

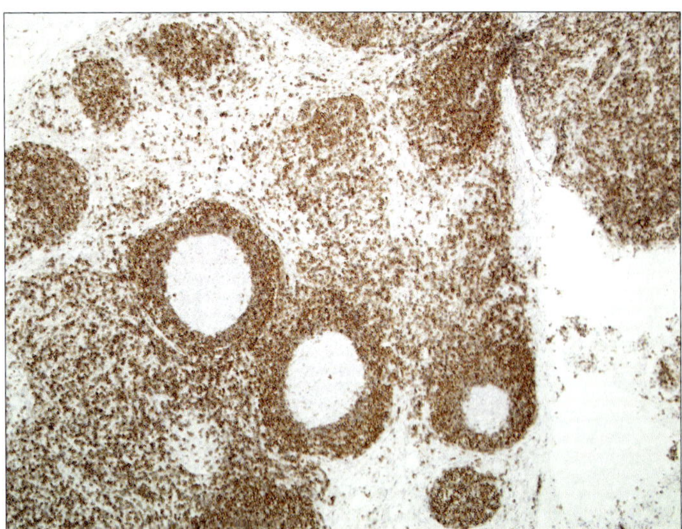

Figure 1.4 Histological section of a lymph node from a patient with reactive lymphadenopathy showing that follicle centres are BCL2 negative. Immunoperoxidase, x 10 objective.

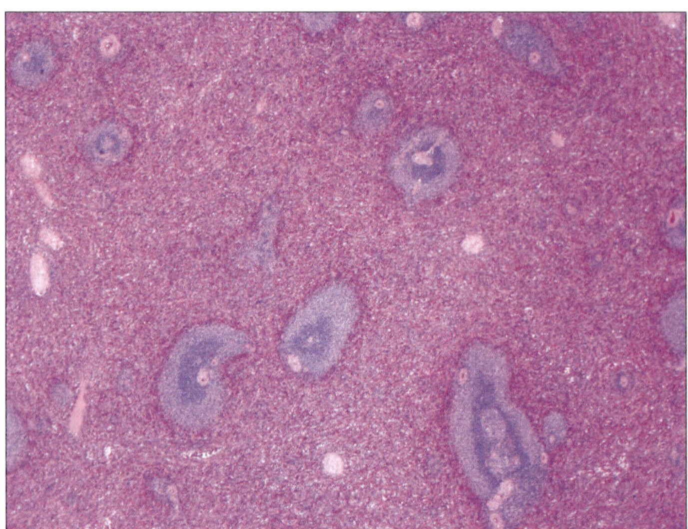

Figure 1.5 Histological section of a normal spleen showing the red pulp and the white pulp. The paler marginal zone is clearly apparent. H&E, x 4 objective.

The spleen is a lymphoid and reticuloendothelial organ of major importance [5]. Its functions include phagocytosis of abnormal circulating cells, 'pitting' of micro-organisms and other inclusions from red cells, phagocytosis of antibody-coated bacteria and antibody production. It is divided into the white pulp and the red pulp (Figure **1.5**). The white pulp surrounds arteries and arterioles, being composed of a peri-arterial and peri-arteriolar sheath of T lymphocytes (among which CD4-positive T cells predominate) within which, between the branching arterioles, there are lymphoid follicles. The primary lymphoid follicles of the spleen have a well developed marginal zone composed mainly of B lymphocytes but also containing T lymphocytes, macrophages, dendritic cells and plasma cells. With antigenic stimulation, germinal centres and a more prominent mantle zone develop. The white pulp is the major site of antigen presentation and antibody production. The red pulp is composed of venous sinuses and splenic cords, the latter containing dendritic cells, macrophages, stromal cells, red cells and a small transitory population of neutrophils, monocytes, lymphocytes (including B cells and CD8-positive T cells) and plasma cells; it is the major site of phagocytosis, and is an important component of the reticuloendothelial system. In addition to lymphoid cells, the spleen contains significant numbers of red cells and about 10% of circulating platelets.

The thymus is a lymphoid organ of major importance in T-cell maturation and in the selection of T cells recognizing peptides derived from foreign rather than self antigens. The thymus is composed of a cortex and a medulla. It contains functionally important epithelial elements, as well as lymphoid cells. Maturation and selection of T cells start in the cortex and continue in the medulla.

The normal development of a B lymphocyte is shown schematically in Figure **1.6** [4, 6, 7]. B lymphocytes originate in the bone marrow from haemopoietic stem cells, which give rise to B-cell precursors (B lymphoblasts or 'haematogones'), which in turn give rise to naïve B lymphocytes. These travel to the primary follicle of the lymph node or other secondary lymphoid tissue. There they either meet a cognate antigen (presented by a follicular dendritic cell), and proliferate and differentiate further, or die by apoptosis. B cells that encounter antigen are thought to migrate to the mantle zone surrounding the primary follicle. Interaction with antigen-specific T cells results in proliferation followed by migration of the activated lymphocytes to form a primary focus of clonal expansion within the follicle centre. These B lymphocytes develop into centroblasts and centrocytes, leading to formation of the germinal centre of the secondary follicle. Immunoglobulin class switching (idiotype switching) and somatic hypermutation occur in the germinal centre. Further maturation can occur in the marginal zone where the lymphoid cell may assume a monocytoid appearance. Thereafter the cell either becomes a long-lived circulating memory B cell or develops into a plasma cell in the bone

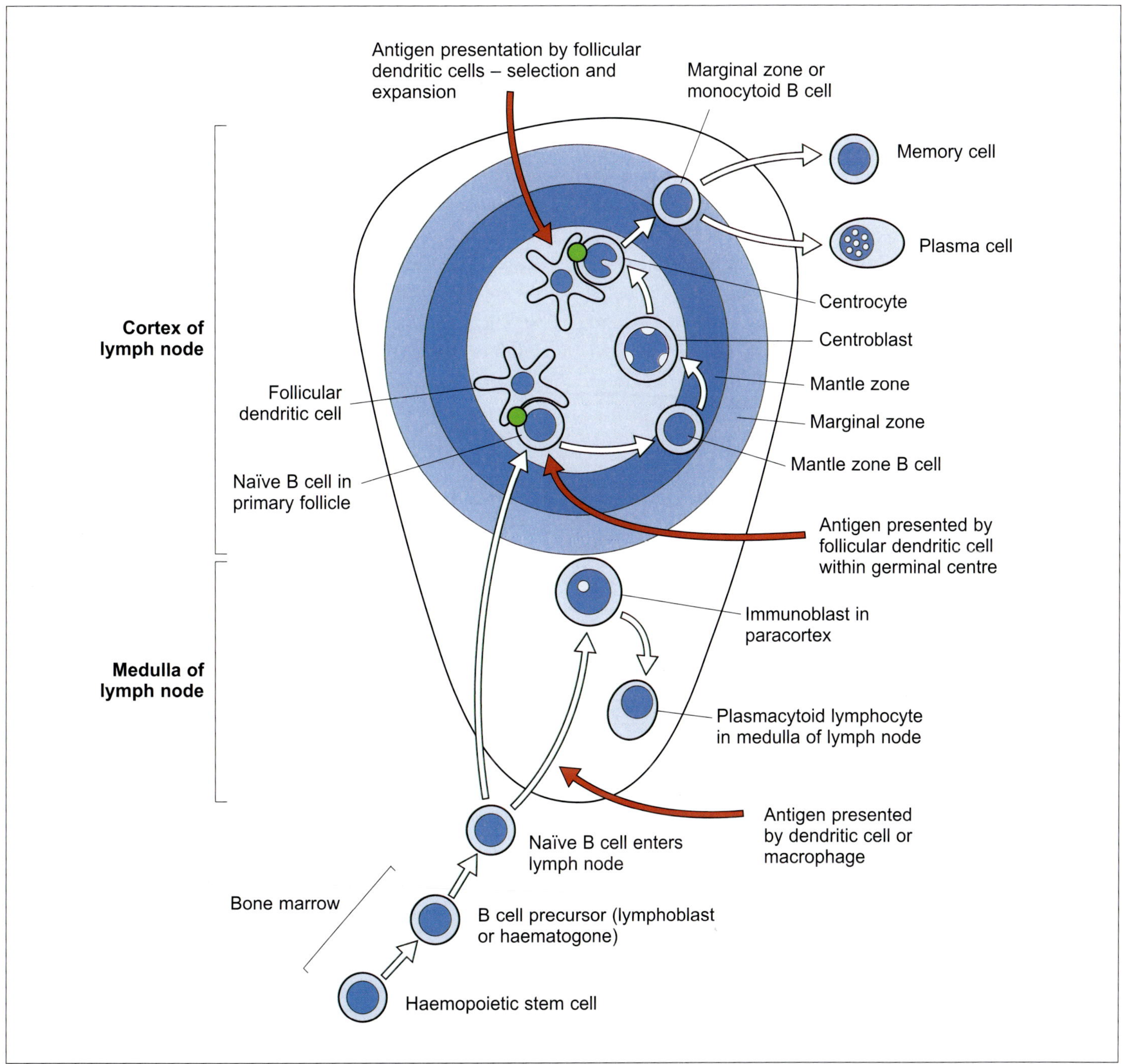

Figure 1.6 Diagram showing the normal development of a B lymphocyte. A haemopoietic stem cell in the bone marrow gives rise to a B-cell precursor and then to a naïve B cell, which migrates either to secondary lymphoid tissues such as a lymph node primary follicle or medulla. If the B cell is presented with antigen by a dendritic cell or macrophage, further development occurs. A naïve (IgM- or IgD-expressing) B cell in the primary follicle responds to antigen by class switching and migration to the mantle zone. The mantle zone B cell then migrates back into the germinal centre and transforms to a centroblast and then a centrocyte within what is now a secondary follicle containing a germinal centre. These germinal centre cells undergo somatic hypermutation before migrating to the marginal zone and then the blood stream. Post-germinal centre B cells become memory cells in blood or tissues or plasma cells in tissues.

marrow or other tissue. During this process of differentiation there are genetic, immunophenotypic and functional changes occurring in the B cell.

The normal development of a T cell is shown in Figure **1.7**. A haemopoietic stem cell of bone marrow origin migrates to the corticomedullary junction of the thymus where development into a T-cell precursor occurs. At this stage the cell, now known as a thymocyte, does not express either CD4 or CD8, i.e. is 'double negative'. It migrates into the cortex where rearrangement of T-cell receptor genes (*TCRA*, *TCRB*) commences and expression of CD4 and CD8 occurs, producing a 'double positive' cortical thymocyte. CD3 is expressed and the thymocyte migrates towards the thymic medulla, encountering cortical thymic epithelium expressing MHC class I or class II molecules, which present peptides. Cells that are not actively selected through encounter with a compatible peptide-presenting MHC molecule die by apoptosis. This is the fate of more than 98% of the initial thymocyte population. Those that do encounter a matching peptide-presenting MHC class I molecule develop into CD8-positive medullary thymocytes. Those that encounter a matching peptide-presenting MHC class II molecule develop into CD4-positive medullary thymocytes. Self-reactive T cells are deleted, probably in the thymic medulla. Mature CD4- or CD8-positive T cells migrate from the thymus to lymph nodes and other lymphoid organs where they are located preferentially in the paracortex and the medulla.

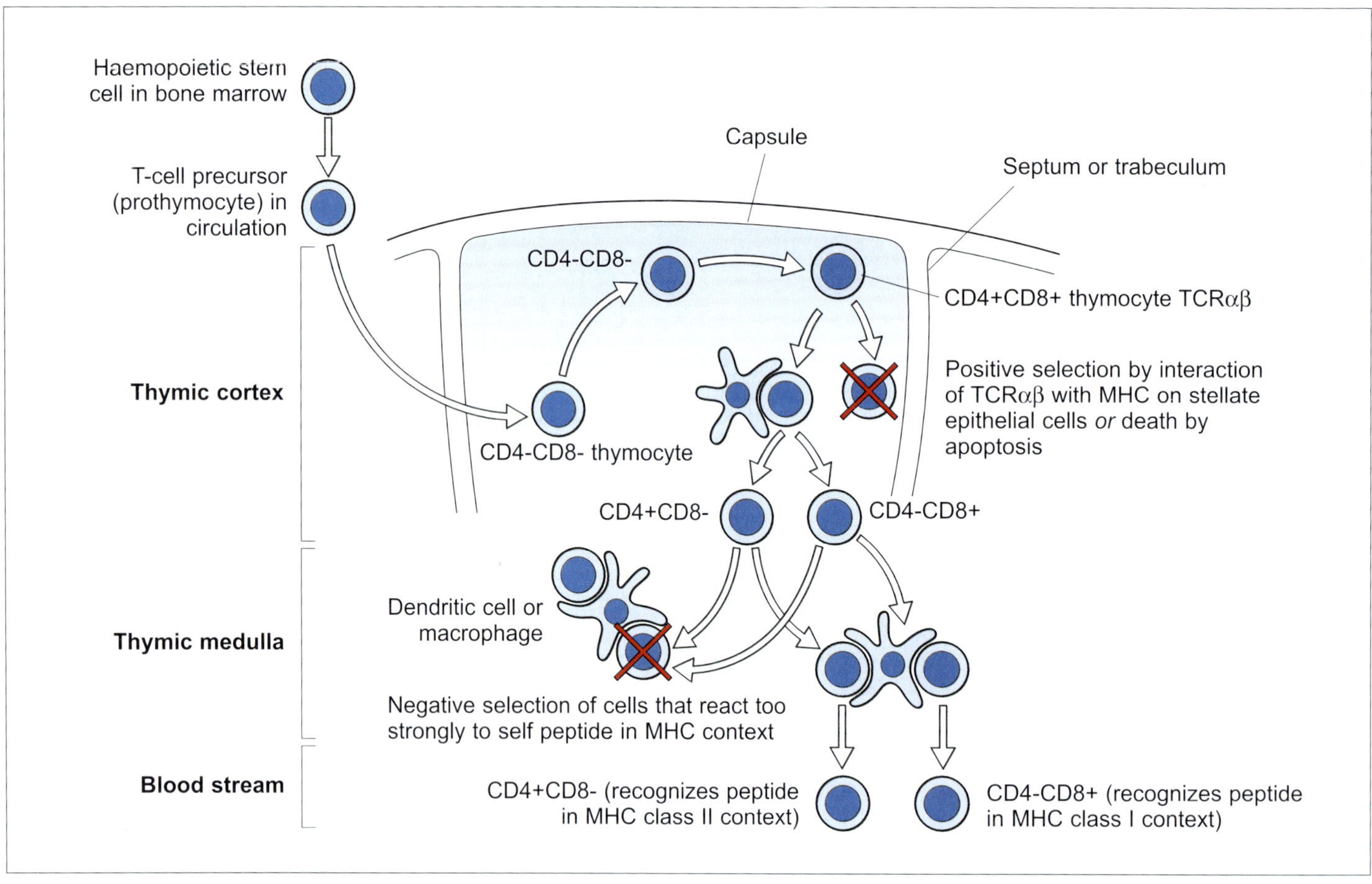

Figure 1.7 Diagram showing the normal development of a T lymphocyte in the thymus. Haemopoietic stem cells in the bone marrow give rise to T-cell precursors, which enter the thymic medulla and then migrate from the medulla to the cortex. Cortical thymocytes undergo positive selection. If they recognize a specific foreign peptide presented in an MHC I or II context by a thymic epithelial cell they survive; if not, they undergo apoptosis. Surviving cells develop into either CD4+CD8- or CD4-CD8+ cells which migrate to the thymic medulla. Medullary thymocytes undergo negative selection. Cells with a strong affinity for a self peptide presented by a dendritic cell or a macrophage in an MHC context undergo apoptosis and are thus deleted. Surviving cells leave the thymus as T cells, which migrate to secondary lymphoid tissues where they undergo clonal expansion if they recognize a peptide presented by a dendritic cell in an MHC context.

NK cells originate in the bone marrow, probably being derived from a lymphoid precursor that is shared with B and T lymphocytes and being ultimately derived from a haemopoietic stem cell.

T and B lymphocyte precursors have germline genes that are unusual in that they are divided into segments. These must be assembled into functional genes by a process of deletion and rearrangement of gene segments to form the genes that encode the various chains of immunoglobulin (Ig) molecules (*IGH*, *IGK* and *IGL*) and, similarly, the T-cell receptor genes (*TCRA*, *TCRB*, *TCRG*, *TCRD*); surface membrane immunoglobulin molecules (SmIg) are part of a complex that functions as a B-cell receptor. The segments that comprise a heavy chain gene are a variable region segment (V_H), a diversity segment (D), a joining segment (J_H) and a constant region segment (C); the latter is specific for each heavy chain class (Cμ, Cδ, $C\gamma_3$, $C\gamma_1$, $C\alpha_1$, $C\gamma_2$, $C\gamma_4$, Cε and $C\alpha_2$). These gene segments are assembled as shown in Figure **1.8**. The process of VDJ recombination occurs in the bone marrow leading to a μ-expressing pre-B cell. The *RAG1* and *RAG2* genes are then reactivated leading to rearrangement of an *IGK* gene, or if this fails, an *IGL* gene. The rearranged light chain-encoding *IGK* and *IGL* genes are composed of a variable region and a joining region only,

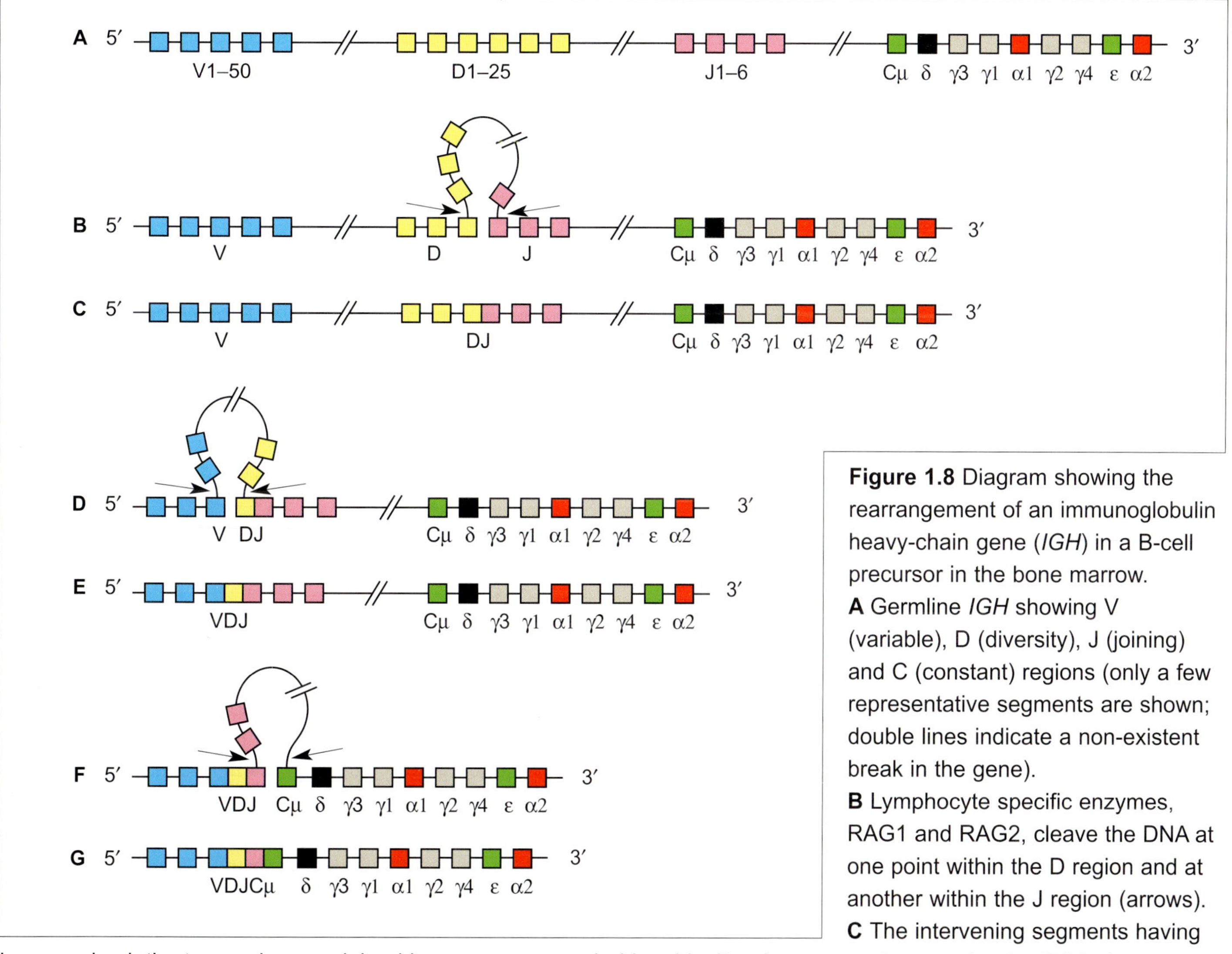

Figure 1.8 Diagram showing the rearrangement of an immunoglobulin heavy-chain gene (*IGH*) in a B-cell precursor in the bone marrow. **A** Germline *IGH* showing V (variable), D (diversity), J (joining) and C (constant) regions (only a few representative segments are shown; double lines indicate a non-existent break in the gene). **B** Lymphocyte specific enzymes, RAG1 and RAG2, cleave the DNA at one point within the D region and at another within the J region (arrows). **C** The intervening segments having been excised, the two ends are rejoined by enzymes encoded by ubiquitously expressed genes, to give DJ fusion. **D** *RAG1* and *RAG2* are reactivated and cleavage occurs within the V and D regions. **E** Rejoining occurs to give VDJ fusion. **F** Cleavage occurs within the J region and between the final J segment and the first (μ) exon of the C region. **G** Rejoining results in a *VDJCμ* gene, encoding μ heavy chain (a switch region, Sμ, upstream of Cμ, is also included in the sequence so that the sequence can also be represented as *VDJSμCμ* – see Figure **1.9**).

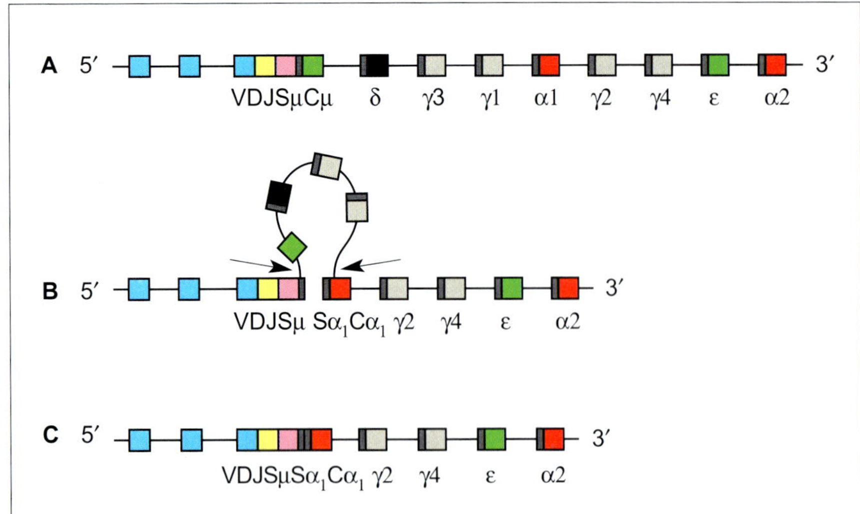

Figure 1.9 Class or isotype switching of a B cell, which occurs within a germinal centre. **A** Gene that has undergone VDJ recombination and is expressing IgM (*IGK* or *IGL* having also been effectively rearranged); the sequence is *VDJSμCμ*; the switch region of each gene segment is represented in grey. **B** As a result of activation-induced deamination, DNA cleavage occurs between the switch region and the coding region of Cμ and also upstream of the switch region of one of the other C segments, in the case illustrated $C\alpha_1$. **C** The intervening sequence having been excised, there is rejoining of two switch regions, in this case Sμ and $S\alpha_1$ resulting in the sequence $VDJS\mu S\alpha_1 C\alpha_1$; the cell is now able to express IgA_1.

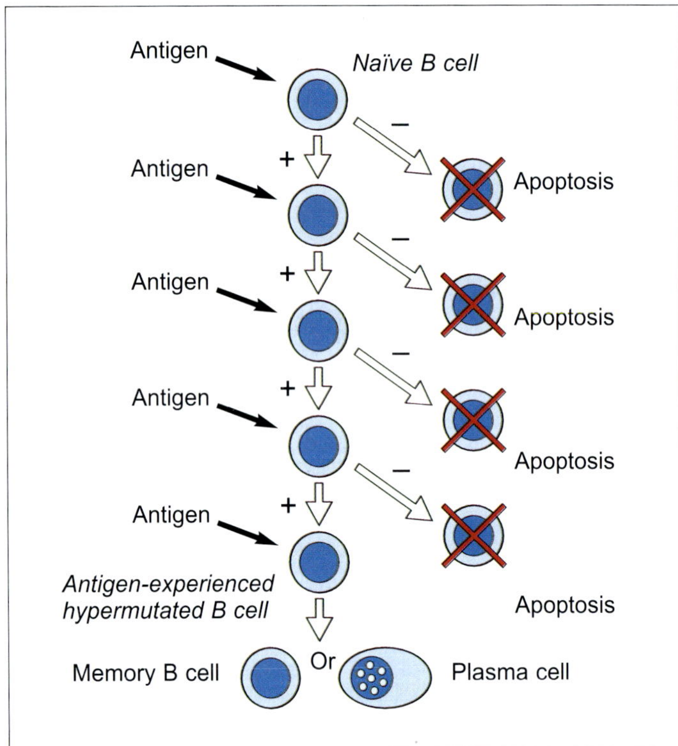

Figure 1.10 The process of somatic hypermutation, which occurs within the germinal centre on exposure to antigen. Cells that are capable of binding to that antigen are selected for survival (+) and cells that are not (–) die by apoptosis; cells that undergo mutation of V_H and V_L segments that lead to a higher binding affinity for the antigen are selected for survival (+) rather than those with a lower affinity (–); this leads to progressive expansion of a clone of antigen-experienced cells that have a high affinity for the antigen.

Vκ + Jκ or Vλ + Jλ. Once a light chain gene has been effectively rearranged, immunoglobulin is expressed on the surface of the cell and the pre-B cell becomes an IgM-expressing B cell. The next stage of B-cell differentiation, class or isotype switching (Figure **1.9**), occurs within a germinal centre, leading to a cell that expresses IgG, IgA or IgE rather than IgM with or without IgD. The final event in the genetic development of a B cell is somatic hypermutation, a process of multiple point mutations and, to a lesser extent, deletions and duplications, occurring in the variable region of the gene. Somatic hypermutation occurs in germinal centres, e.g. in lymph nodes, spleen and tonsils, when a naïve B lymphocyte recognizes antigen presented in an MHC context by an antigen-presenting cell such as a dendritic cell. The result of this process is that the immunoglobulin expressed on the surface membrane of the B cell more closely matches the antigen that has been presented and binding affinity is thereby increased. Naïve B cells that reach germinal centres but do not find a matching antigen die by apoptosis (Figure **1.10**). Each mutation that increases affinity for antigen selects for cell survival rather than cell death. Continuing cycles of selection and mutation produce cells with a high affinity for the antigen. It is these high-affinity B cells that differentiate into plasma cells and give rise to memory B cells. Plasma cells home to the bone marrow, spleen, lymph nodes and gastrointestinal tract. Memory cells comprise about 40% of circulating B cells, the other 60% being naïve B cells.

The process of rearrangement of gene segments also occurs in T cells, which rearrange V, D and J segments in genes encoding α, β, γ and δ chains. Somatic hypermutation

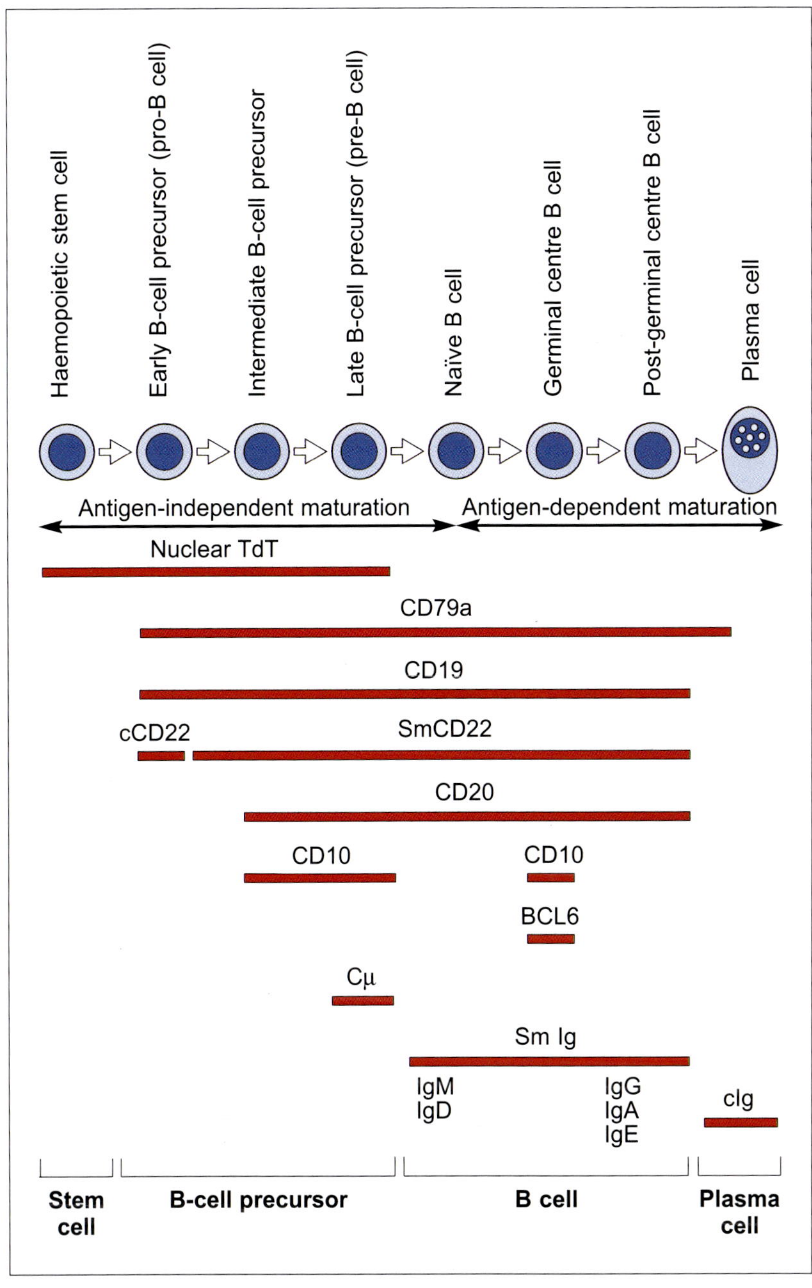

Figure 1.11 Alterations in expression of surface membrane and cytoplasmic antigens that occur with B-cell maturation. Abbreviations: c, cytoplasmic; Ig, immunoglobulin; Sm, surface membrane; TdT, terminal deoxynucleotidyl transferase.

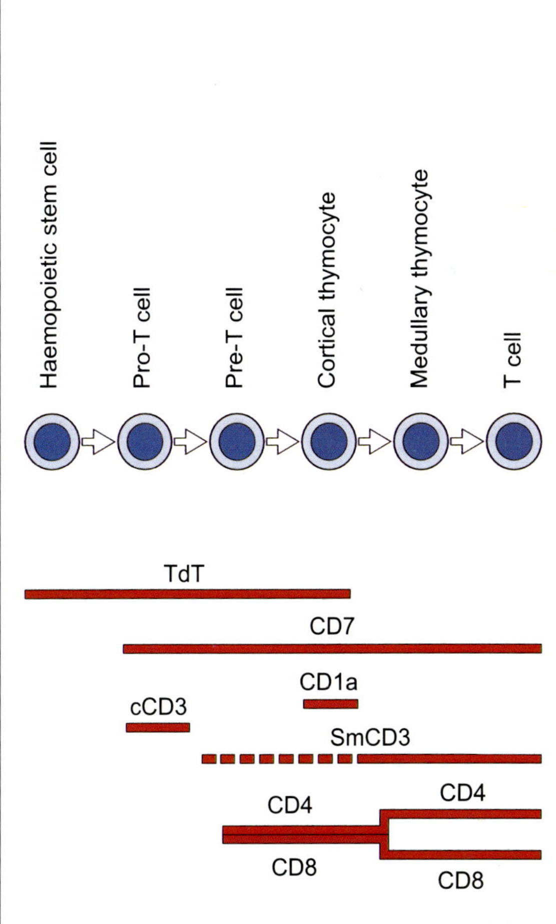

Figure 1.12 Alterations in expression of surface membrane and cytoplasmic antigens that occur with T-cell maturation. Abbreviations: c, cytoplasmic; Sm, surface membrane; TdT, terminal deoxynucleotidyl transferase.

and class switching do not occur and it has been hypothesized that it is the greater degree of genetic rearrangement occurring in B cells that make B-cell lymphomas far more common than T-cell lymphomas. Most mature T cells have a surface membrane complex composed of α and β chains of the T-cell receptor together with CD3 and either CD4 or CD8, which recognize specific peptides in an MHC context, MHC class I in the case of CD8-positive cells and MHC class II in the case of CD4-positive cells [4].

NK cells, being part of the innate rather than the adaptive immune system, appear not to undergo any gene rearrangement.

The genetic rearrangement that occurs in B and T cells is paralleled by alterations in expression of surface membrane and cytoplasmic antigens [7, 8]. These changes are illustrated in Figures **1.11** and **1.12**.

Relationship of lymphomas to putative normal homologues

The putative relationship between the normal stages of B-cell and T-cell differentiation and B- and T-lineage neoplasms is shown in Figures **1.13** and **1.14**.

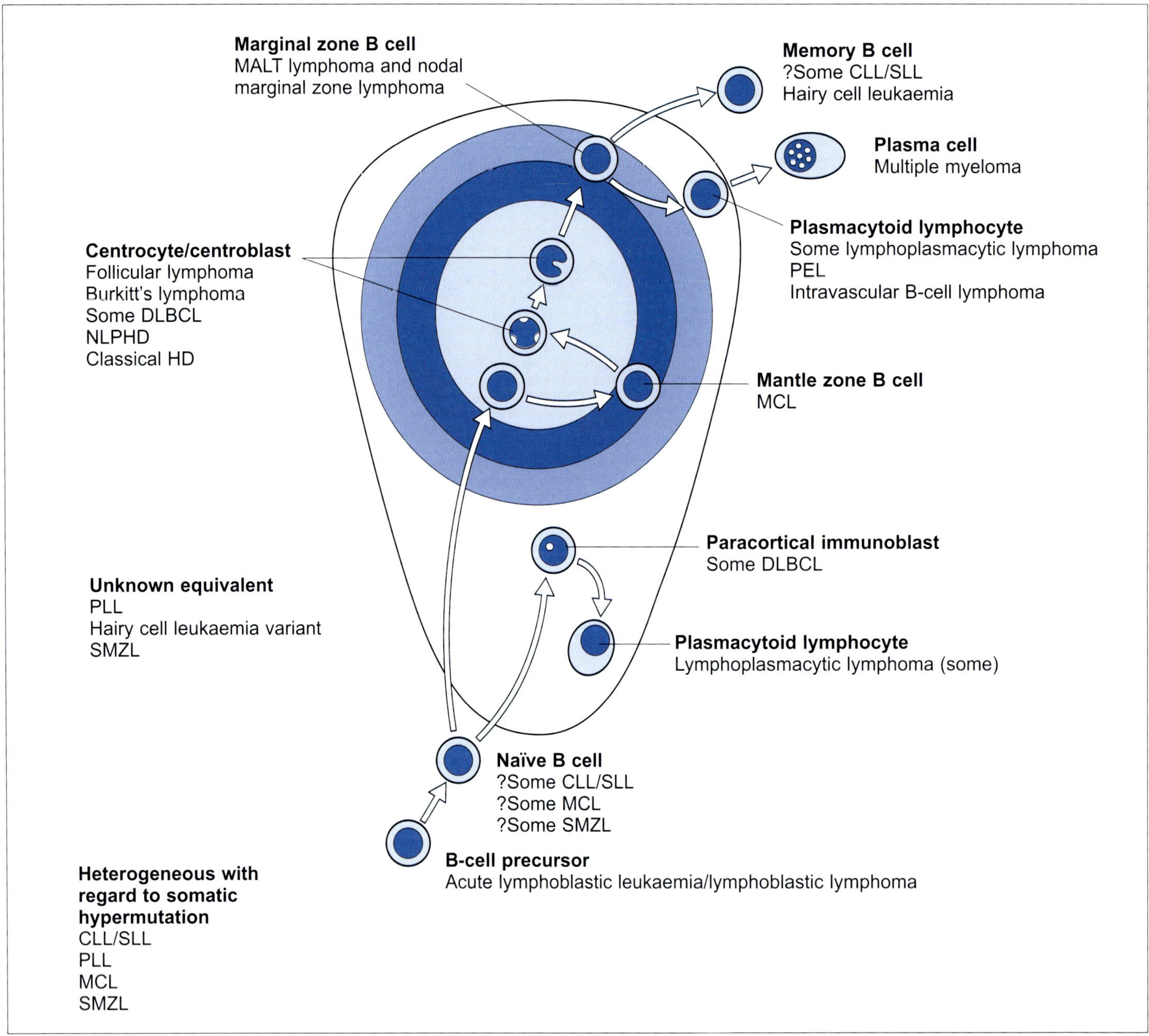

Figure 1.13 Putative relationship between normal B-cell differentiation and B-lineage neoplasms. Abbreviations: CLL, chronic lymphocytic leukaemia; DLBCL, diffuse large B-cell lymphoma; classical HD, classical Hodgkin's disease; MALT, mucosa-associated lymphoid tissue; MCL, mantle cell lymphoma; NLPHD, nodular lymphocyte-predominant Hodgkin's disease; PEL, primary effusion lymphoma; PLL, prolymphocytic leukaemia; SLL, small lymphocytic lymphoma; SMZL, splenic marginal zone lymphoma.

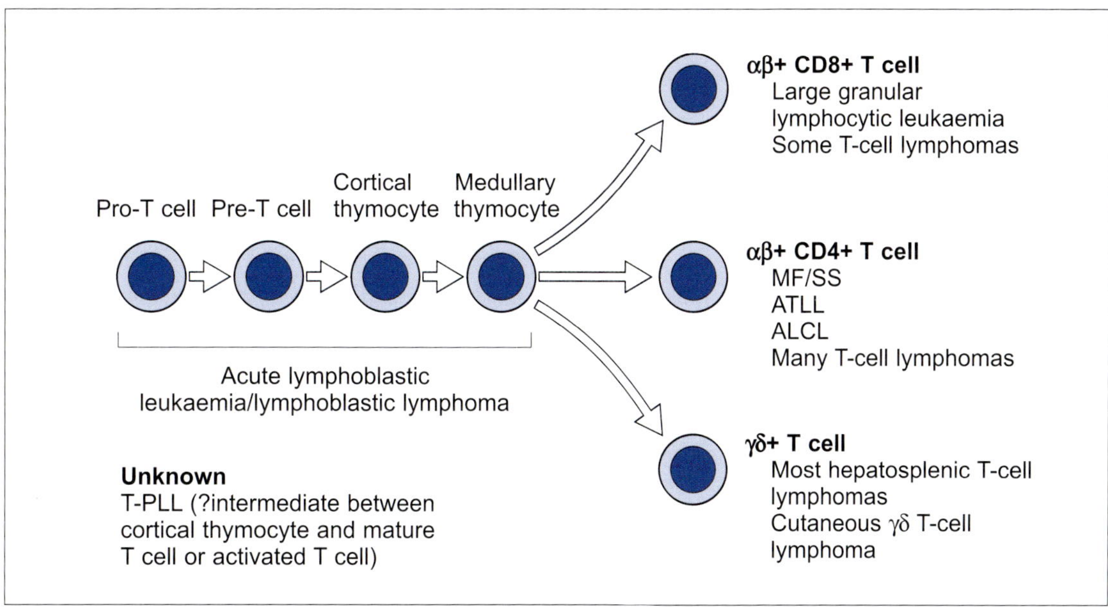

Figure 1.14 Putative relationship between normal T-cell differentiation and T-lineage neoplasms. Abbreviations: ALCL, anaplastic large cell lymphoma; ATLL, adult T-cell leukaemia/lymphoma; MF, mycosis fungoides; SS, Sézary syndrome; T-PLL, T-cell prolymphocytic leukaemia.

The molecular basis of acute lymphoblastic leukaemia/lymphoblastic lymphoma

The molecular basis of acute lymphoblastic leukaemia (ALL) and the related lymphoblastic lymphomas varies between T- and B-lineage cases and also between different subtypes. Often there is a mutation that leads to either dysregulated expression of a normal transcription factor gene or to expression of a gene encoding an abnormal transcription factor. More than one mutation is needed in order to give rise to an acute leukaemia. One mutation may interfere with transcription factor function and another with intracellular signalling so that cells continue to proliferate but differentiation does not occur.

The two most common subtypes of B-lineage ALL are those associated with hyperdiploidy and with a cryptic reciprocal translocation, t(12;21)(p13;q22). The molecular mechanism of leukaemogenesis of the former is unknown while the latter is associated with fusion of two transcription factor genes to give an *ETV6-RUNX1* (previously known as *TEL-AML1*) fusion gene. Several other less common subtypes of ALL are also associated with formation of a fusion gene. The subtype associated with t(4;11)(q21;q23) has an *AF4-MLL* fusion gene whereas the subtype associated with t(1;19)(q23;p13) has an *E2A-PBX1* fusion gene. In adults, about one-quarter of cases of B-lineage ALL are associated with t(9;22)(q34;q11) and a *BCR-ABL* fusion gene; it is likely that there are other undiscovered molecular events in this subtype, explaining why the phenotype is that of acute lymphoblastic leukaemia since the dysregulated tyrosine kinase activity of *BCR-ABL* usually leads to chronic myeloid leukaemia.

In T-lineage ALL the two abnormalities most often observed are t(5;14)(q35;q32), in about 20% of cases, and *TAL*^{d} in about one-third of cases. The mechanism of leukaemogenesis in the former is dysregulation of *HOX11L2*, probably by proximity to the transcription regulatory elements of *BCL11B* (*CTIP2*) at 14q32.1. In the case of *TAL*^{d}, there is a cryptic deletion that results in most of the sequences of *TAL1*, a transcription factor gene on chromosome 1, being fused with the promoter of an upstream gene, *SIL*. This leads to dysregulation of *TAL1*, which is not normally expressed in T cells. Another frequent mechanism of leukaemogenesis in T-lineage ALL is dysregulation of a transcription factor gene by proximity to a T-cell receptor gene (*TCRA*, *TCRB*, *TCRG* or *TCRD*); genes that can be dysregulated in this manner include *TAL1*, *TAL2*, *HOX11*, *LMO1*, *LMO2*, *LCK* and *LYL1*.

Second mutations occurring in the cell that gives rise to the leukaemic clone may or may not be specific to a cytogenetic/molecular genetic subtype. For example, in B-lineage ALL associated with *ETV6-RUNX1* there has often also been deletion of the second *ETV6* allele whereas in T-lineage ALL an activating mutation of *NOTCH1* has been found as a second event in all major cytogenetic/molecular genetic subtypes. *NOTCH1* encodes a membrane receptor that regulates normal T-cell development.

The molecular basis of B-lineage non-Hodgkin's lymphoma, chronic B-lineage leukaemias and multiple myeloma

The molecular basis of B-lineage non-Hodgkin's lymphoma (NHL) often involves dysregulation of an oncogene as the result of a translocation that brings it under the influence of an enhancer of the immunoglobulin heavy chain gene (*IGH*) at 14q32 or of the kappa (κ) and lambda (λ) genes (*IGK* and *IGL*) at 2p12 and 22q11 respectively. Examples of this mechanism include the three translocations that can underlie follicular lymphoma, dysregulating *BCL2*, and the three that can underlie Burkitt's lymphoma, dysregulating *MYC*. An alternative mechanism is formation of a fusion gene as the result of a translocation, such as the *AP12-MALT* fusion gene in gastric MALT-type lymphoma with t(11;18)(q21;q21). Sometimes different molecular abnormalities affect a common signalling mechanism, e.g. dysregulation of *MALT* by proximity to *IGH* is an alternative to formation of an *AP12-MALT* fusion gene. In some B-lineage lymphomas and leukaemias the molecular mechanisms of oncogenesis are largely unknown. This is so for small lymphocytic lymphoma/chronic lymphocytic leukaemia (SLL/CLL), in which many cytogenetic and molecular abnormalities have been described (mainly deletions or gene amplification rather than translocations) without a primary oncogenic event yet being identified. In some leukaemias and lymphomas characteristic chromosomal abnormalities have similarly been recognized without an associated oncogenic molecular change yet being identified. This is so for trisomy 3 in splenic marginal zone lymphoma and for trisomy 12 in CLL.

Cytogenetic and molecular analysis can be very important in diagnosis, e.g. in confirming a diagnosis of Burkitt's lymphoma so that specific treatment regimes can be used or confirming a diagnosis of follicular lymphoma or mantle cell lymphoma if other features are not diagnostic.

The molecular basis of multiple myeloma often involves translocations that bring oncogenes under the influence of enhancers of *IGH*, e.g. t(4;14)(p16.3;q32), t(6;14)(p21;q32), t(11;14)(q13;q32), t(14;16)(q32;q23) and t(14;20)(q32;q11). Cytogenetic analysis has demonstrated the same chromosomal rearrangements in cases of monoclonal gammopathy of undetermined significance. The mechanism of oncogenesis in plasma cell tumours differs somewhat from that in other B-cell neoplasms since translocations usually involve the switch region and thus separate an intronic and a 3′ enhancer; there can therefore be an oncogene under the influence of an enhancer on both of the derivative chromosomes rather than on one. This is the case, for example in t(4;14)(p16.3;q32) when both *FGFR3* on chromosome 14 and *MMSET* on chromosome 4 are dysregulated. Other unknown oncogenic mechanisms relate to loss of 13, 13q or 13q14, any of which is associated with a worse prognosis (at least when detected in metaphases).

Cytogenetic and molecular analysis in NHL can reveal not only initial or early events in oncogenesis but also genetic alterations that are of prognostic significance or correlate with disease progression, such as loss or inactivation of the tumour suppressor gene, *TP53*. Cytogenetic/molecular analysis also gives information as to the nature of apparent high-grade transformation. It has been found, for example, that transformation of follicular lymphoma to diffuse high-grade B-cell lymphoma does indeed represent transforming events in a cell of the neoplastic clone whereas in CLL many examples of 'Richter's transformation' (about 40%) actually represent an independent neoplasm, sometimes EBV-related, resulting from immunosuppression.

In addition to the putative oncogenic events, molecular analysis will show whether or not somatic hypermutation has occurred. This gives information as to the nature of the cell in which the oncogenic mutations occurred, i.e. whether pre-germinal centre or post-germinal centre, and may throw some light on possible aetiology. Such information can also be of prognostic significance, e.g. in CLL somatic hypermutation correlates with a better prognosis.

Cytogenetic and molecular genetic analysis often yield information of prognostic significance, e.g. in CLL and multiple myeloma. Sometimes specific abnormalities indicate likely refractoriness to treatment, e.g. cases of gastric MALT lymphoma with t(11;18) do not usually respond to elimination of *Helicobacter pylori* infection.

Some genetic abnormalities observed in B-lineage NHL are summarized in *Table 1.2*.

Table 1.2 Cytogenetic and molecular genetic abnormalities observed in different subtypes of B-lineage non-Hodgkin's lymphoma

Lymphoma	*Cytogenetic abnormality*	*Molecular abnormality*
Follicular lymphoma	t(14;18)(q32;q21) t(2;18)(p12;q21) t(18;22)(q21;q11)	Dysregulation of *BCL2* by proximity to *IGH* Dysregulation of *BCL2* by proximity to *IGK* at 2p12 Dysregulation of *BCL2* by proximity to *IGL* at 22q11
Mantle cell lymphoma	t(11;14)(q13;q32)	Dysregulation of *CCND1* (*BCL1*, *PRAD1*), the gene encoding cyclin D1, by proximity to *IGH*
Diffuse high-grade B-cell lymphoma	t(14;18)(q32;q21) t(3;14)(q27;q32)	Dysregulation of *BCL2* by proximity to *IGH* Dysregulation of *BCL6* by proximity to *IGH*
Burkitt's lymphoma	t(8;14)(q24;q32) t(2;8)(p12;q24) t(8;22)(q24;q11)	Dysregulation of *MYC* by proximity to *IGH* at 14q32 Dysregulation of *MYC* by proximity to *IGK* at 2p12 Dysregulation of *MYC* by proximity to *IGL* at 22q11
Lymphoplasmacytic lymphoma	t(9;14)(p13;q32)	Dysregulation of *PAX5* by proximity to *IGH* at 14q32
Gastric and sometimes pulmonary or intestinal MALT-type lymphoma	t(11;18)(q21;q21) t(1;14)(p22;q32)	*AP12-MALT* fusion Dysregulation of *BCL10* by proximity to *IGH*
MALT lymphoma of ocular adnexae, skin or thyroid	t(3;14)(p14.1;q32)	Dysregulation of *FOXP1* by proximity to *IGH*
MALT-type lymphoma of salivary gland	t(14;18)(q32;p21)	Dysregulation of *MALT1* by proximity to *IGH*

The molecular basis of T-lineage and NK-lineage non-Hodgkin's lymphoma and leukaemia

The molecular basis of T-lineage non-Hodgkin's lymphoma (NHL) is less well established than that of B-lineage neoplasms.

Recurring cytogenetic/molecular genetic abnormalities have been observed in association with T-cell prolymphocytic leukaemia (T-PLL). About three-quarters of cases show either inv(14)(q11q32) or t(14;14)(q11;q32). These chromosomal rearrangements involve the *TCRAD* locus at 14q11 and two oncogenes, *TCL1* and *TCL1b*, at 14q32.1. *TCL1* and *TCL1b* are dysregulated and, when over-expressed, inhibit apoptosis.

Anaplastic large cell lymphoma is also associated with several recurring cytogenetic abnormalities, of which t(2;5)(p23;q35) is the most frequent, with known oncogenic mechanisms (Figurc **1.15**).

However, for the majority of T-cell and NK cell disorders no recurring abnormality has been discovered and in those instances when recurring cytogenetic abnormalities have been detected the molecular basis is not yet known.

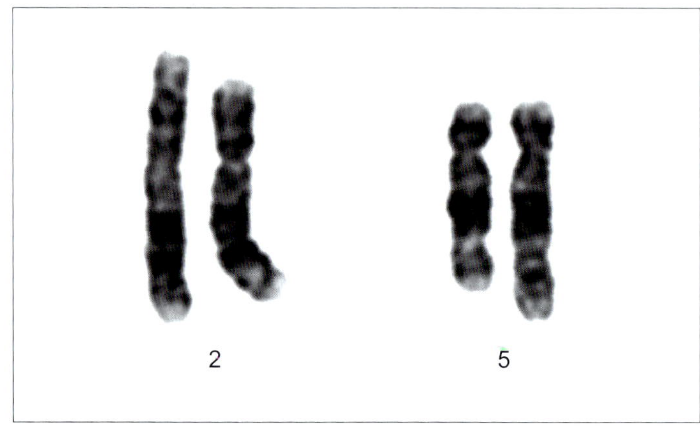

Figure 1.15 Karyogram showing t(2;5)(p23;q35) in a patient with anaplastic large T-cell lymphoma. With thanks to Dr John Swansbury.

References

1. Inhorn RC, Aster JC, Roach SA, Slapak CA, Soiffer R, Tantravahi R and Stone RM (1995). A syndrome of lymphoblastic lymphoma, eosinophilia and myeloid hyperplasia/malignancy associated with t(8;13)(p11;q11): description of a distinctive clinicopathologic entity. *Blood*, **85**, 1881–1887.
2. Beer P, Abdalla SH, Matutes E and Bain BJ (2005). Teaching cases from the Royal Marsden and St Mary's Hospital Case 29: Striking generalized lymphadenopathy in 'acute myeloid leukaemia'. *Leukemia & Lymphoma*, **46**, 155–156.
3. Bain BJ (2001). The role of cytogenetics in the diagnosis and classification of haematological neoplasms. *In* Rooney D. *Human Cytogenetics: Malignancy and Acquired Abnormalities: a Practical Approach*, 3rd edn, Oxford University Press, Oxford, pp. 111–128.
4. Delves PJ and Roitt IM (2000). The immune system. *N Engl J Med*, **343**, 37–49, 108–117.
5. Wilkins BS and Wright DH (2000). *Illustrated Pathology of the Spleen*. Cambridge University Press, Cambridge.
6. Küppers R, Klein U, Hansmann ML and Rajewsky K (1999). Cellular origin of human B-cell lymphomas. *N Engl J Med*, **341**, 1520–1539.
7. Harris NL (2001). Mature B-cell neoplasms: introduction. *In* Jaffe ES, Harris NL, Stein H and Vardiman JW (Eds). *World Health Organization Classification of Tumours of Haematopoietic and Lymphoid Tissues*, IARC Press, Lyon, pp. 121–126.
8. Jaffe ES and Ralfkiaer E (2001). Mature T-cell and NK-cell neoplasms: introduction. *In* Jaffe ES, Harris NL, Stein H and Vardiman JW (Eds). *World Health Organization Classification of Tumours of Haematopoietic and Lymphoid Tissues*, IARC Press, Lyon, pp. 191–194.

Chapter 2

Acute lymphoblastic leukaemia

Acute lymphoblastic leukaemia (ALL) and lymphoblastic lymphoma are two closely related conditions. In the French–American–British (FAB) classification, which largely predated immunophenotyping, ALL was categorized according to morphology, as L1, L2 and L3. In the World Health Organization (WHO) classification ALL and lymphoblastic lymphoma are grouped together as precursor B-cell and precursor T-cell neoplasms.

In cases of ALL occurring in infants the leukaemia often has its origin in intra-uterine life and in childhood cases there may be a pre-leukaemic clone already present at the time of birth [1, 2].

Clinical features

The more common cases of B-lineage ALL show a peak incidence between the ages of 2 and 10 years. This childhood peak is particularly characteristic of developed countries. T-lineage cases tend to be older and show a male predominance.

Clinical features differ between lymphoblastic lymphoma and ALL and differ somewhat between B- and T-lineage cases. Overall, presentation as lymphoma is much less common than presentation as leukaemia. T-lineage cases are more likely than B-lineage to present as lymphoma. About three-quarters of cases are B-lineage and about one-quarter T-lineage.

Patients with ALL present either with clinical features of bone marrow failure (pallor and bruising) or with clinical features resulting more directly from proliferation of leukaemic cells (lymphadenopathy, splenomegaly, hepatomegaly, bone pain, testicular enlargement and, in the case of T-ALL, respiratory difficulty resulting from thymic enlargement). Occasional patients present with abdominal masses resulting from massive renal infiltration.

In patients presenting with lymphoma rather than leukaemia, there may be thymic disease without involvement of the bone marrow and blood (T lymphoblastic lymphoma) or soft tissue involvement (T or B lymphoblastic lymphoma).

Haematological and pathological features

The peripheral blood usually shows anaemia, thrombocytopenia and leucocytosis, the latter as a result of the presence of leukaemic blast cells in the circulation (Figure **2.1**). Less often there is anaemia and thrombocytopenia with few if any circulating blast cells.

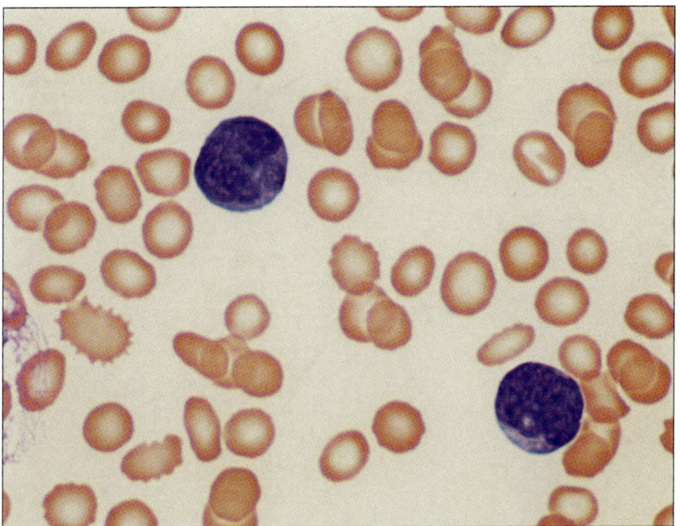

Figure 2.1 Peripheral blood film from a patient with T-lineage ALL showing severe thrombocytopenia and two blast cells. Romanowsky stain, x 100 objective.

Some patients have reactive eosinophilia and occasionally eosinophils are very numerous. The blast cells are usually small to medium sized with a high nucleocytoplasmic ratio and sometimes nucleoli. Smaller blast cells can show some chromatin condensation. Cells are regular in shape in the majority of cases and much more pleomorphic in a minority. Cytoplasm is weakly to moderately basophilic; it may contain vacuoles and, less often, peroxidase-negative granules. In occasional patients there is a polar cytoplasmic projection, cells being described as 'hand-mirror cells'. Blast cells are negative for myeloperoxidase and chloroacetate esterase. They may be negative with Sudan black B or stain very weakly; when a counter-stain is used, the weak staining is usually not apparent. They may show block positivity with a periodic acid–Schiff (PAS) stain (more likely in B-lineage ALL) (Figure **2.2**) and in T-lineage ALL there may be focal acid phosphatase activity (Figure **2.3**). Non-specific esterase stains can also show focal positivity. PAS, acid phosphatase and non-specific esterase stains are redundant for diagnosis if immunophenotyping is available.

In the case of ALL, a bone marrow aspirate shows almost complete replacement by lymphoblasts; there may be some

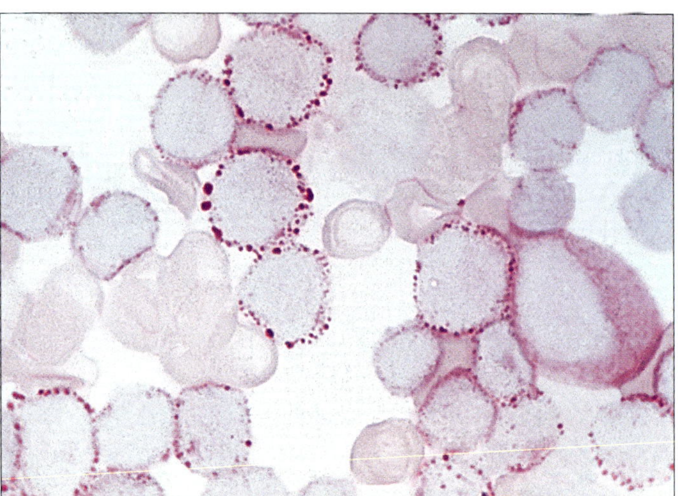

Figure 2.2 Blast cells of a patient with B-lineage ALL showing PAS block positivity. PAS, x 100 objective.

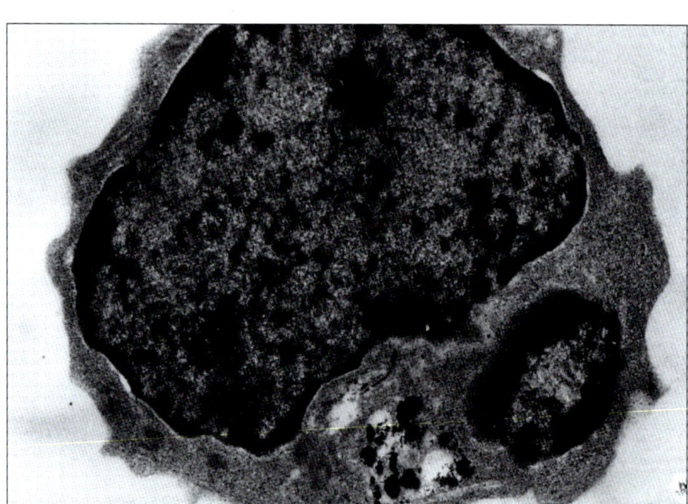

Figure 2.3 Ultrastructure of a blast cell of a patient with T-lineage ALL showing focal acid phosphatase positivity. Lead nitrate and uranyl acetate stain, acid phosphatase reaction.

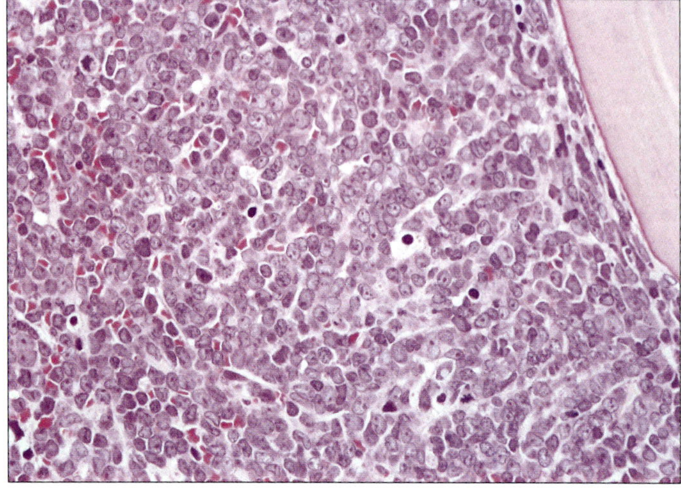

Figure 2.4 Trephine biopsy section from a patient with ALL showing diffuse infiltration by blast cells. H&E, x 60 objective.

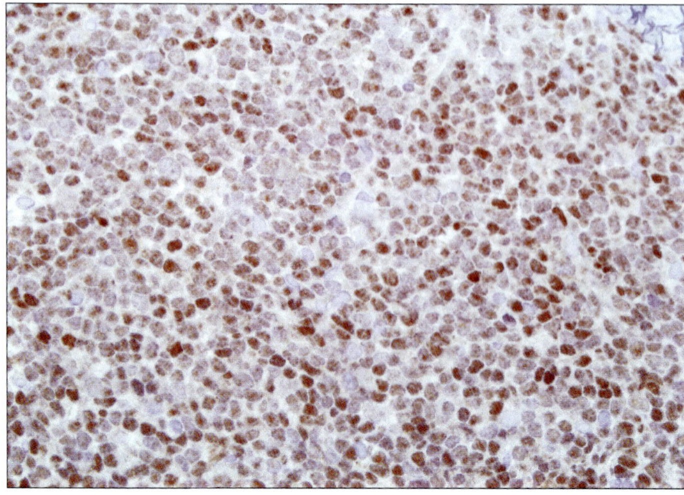

Figure 2.5 Trephine biopsy section from a patient with ALL (same patient as Figure **2.4**) showing that blast cells express nuclear terminal deoxynucleotidyl transferase (TdT). Immunoperoxidase, x 60 objective.

degree of bone marrow infiltration in lymphoblastic lymphoma but blast cells are less than 20–30%. Bone marrow and lymph node infiltration is diffuse (Figures **2.4** and **2.5**). Good quality sections are essential to avoid ALL being misdiagnosed as lymphoma on trephine biopsy sections. The delicate chromatin structure and the relatively high mitotic rate are important in making the distinction.

A significant minority of patients with ALL present initially with pancytopenia with a hypocellular bone marrow. Following remission, either spontaneous or occurring following corticosteroid therapy, there is an interval of several months followed by the emergence of typical ALL.

Cases of ALL were categorized in the FAB classification as L1, L2 and L3. L1 describes typical childhood ALL with small to medium sized blast cells that are cytologically fairly uniform (Figures **2.6** and **2.7**). The cells of L2 ALL are more pleomorphic and tend to be larger (Figures **2.8** and **2.9**). Cases categorized as L3 in the FAB classification (Figure **2.10**) mainly represent a leukaemic phase of Burkitt's lymphoma, being immunophenotypically mature B cells (see Chapter 13); they are categorized in the WHO classification as non-Hodgkin's lymphoma rather than as ALL.

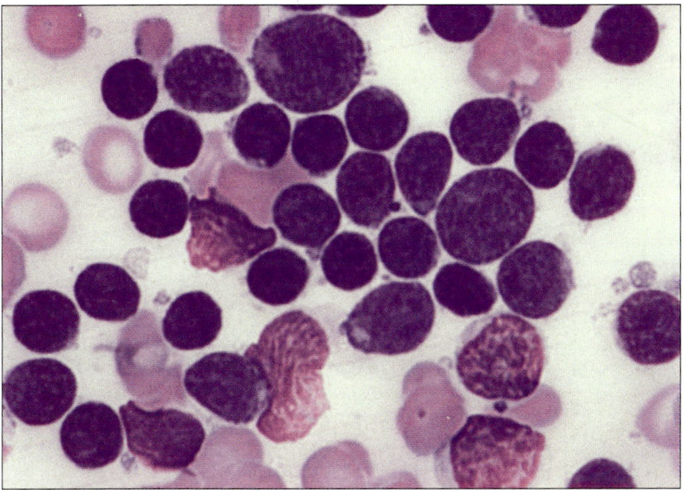

Figure 2.6 Bone marrow aspirate from a patient with FAB L1 type ALL. Romanowsky stain, x 100 objective.

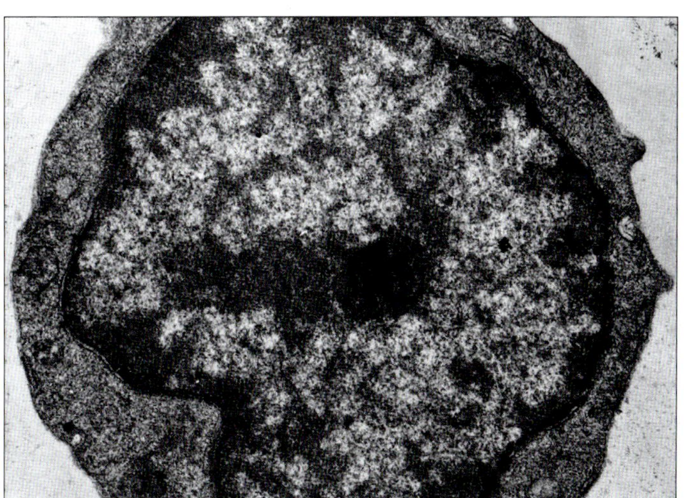

Figure 2.7 Ultrastructure of a blast cell from a patient with FAB L1 type ALL. Lead nitrate and uranyl acetate stain.

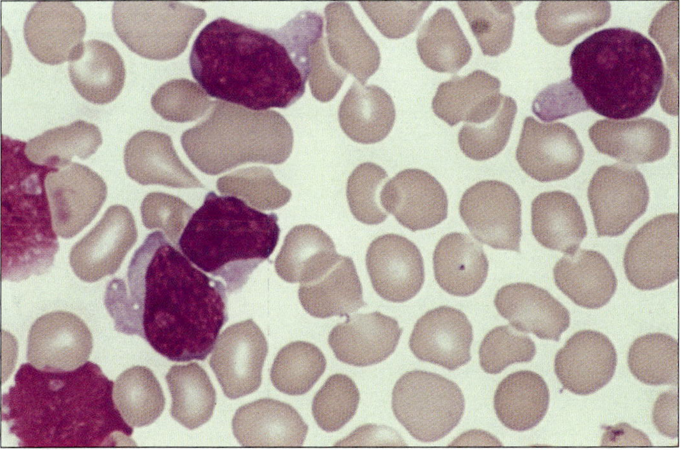

Figure 2.8 Peripheral blood film from a patient with T-lineage ALL of FAB L2 type. Romanowsky stain, x 100 objective.

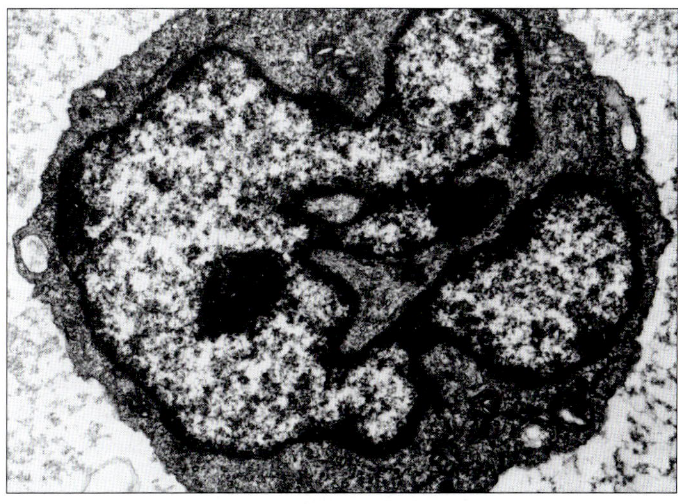

Figure 2.9 Ultrastructure of a blast cell from a patient with FAB L2 type ALL. Lead nitrate and uranyl acetate stain.

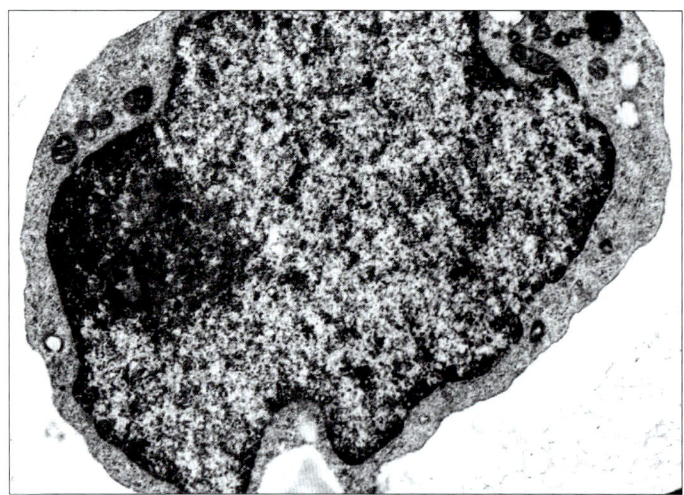

Figure 2.10 Ultrastructure of a blast cell from a patient with FAB L3 type ALL. Lead nitrate and uranyl acetate stain.

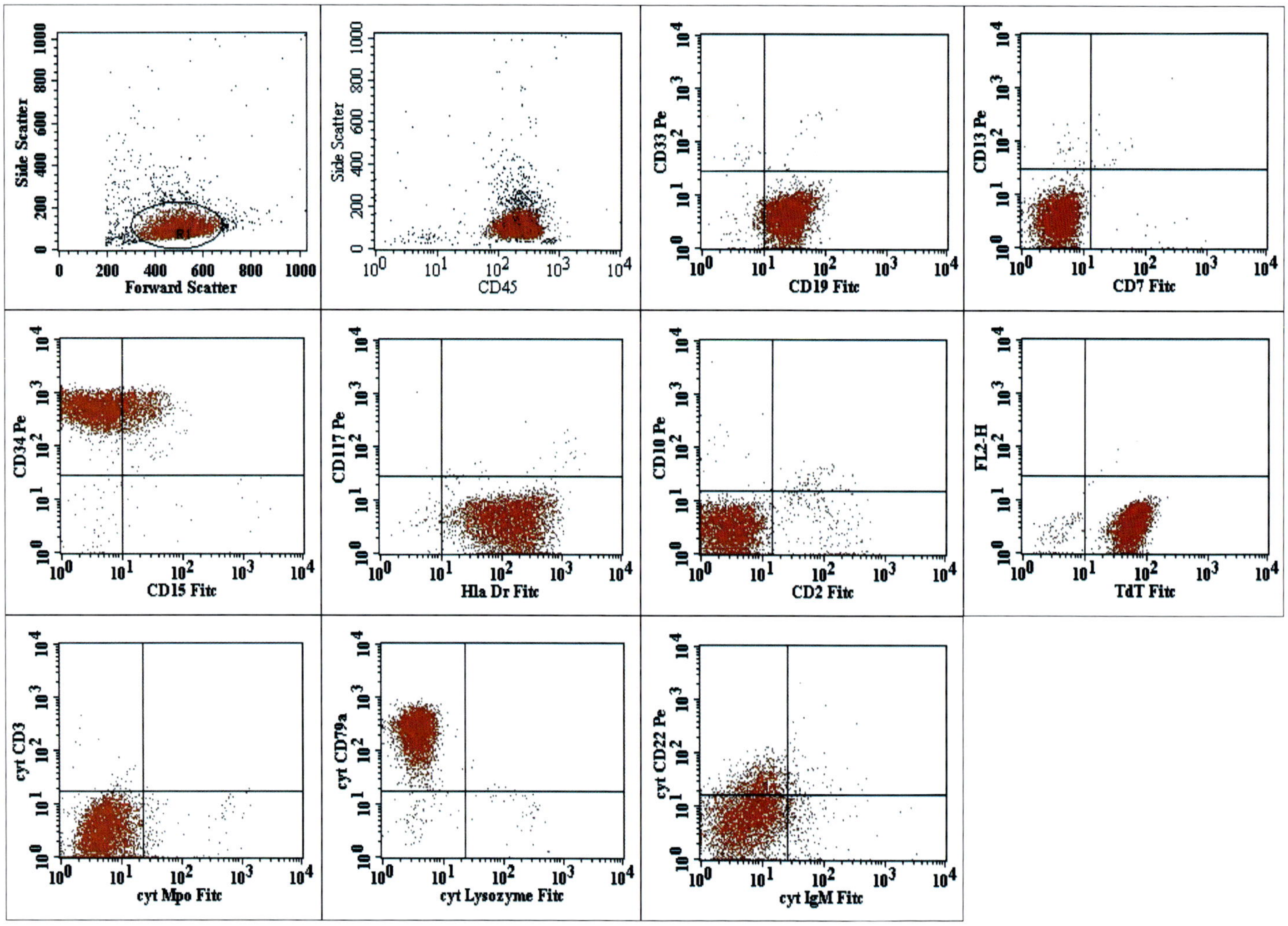

Figure 2.11 Flow cytometry immunophenotyping of a case of pro-B ALL. Cells express CD45, CD19, cytoplasmic CD79a, CD34, HLA-DR and TdT. A minority of cells show weak expression of cytoplasmic CD22 and some show weak expression of CD15. There is no expression of other myeloid markers or T-lineage markers. CD10 and cytoplasmic μ chain are not expressed. With thanks to Mr Ricardo Morilla.

Immunophenotype

The immunophenotype reflects to some extent normal maturation of precursors of B and T cells [3, 4]. In the case of B-lineage disease, the different stages of maturation are indicative of prognosis because they correlate with different cytogenetic and molecular genetic abnormalities. They can be categorized as early B-cell ALL (Figure **2.11**), common ALL (Figure **2.12**), pre-B ALL (Figure **2.13**) and mature B-cell ALL (= non-Hodgkin's lymphoma of Burkitt type) (*Table 2.1* and Chapter 13). A similar categorization of T-lineage cases into four stages of maturation (*Table 2.2*) (Figures **2.14–2.16**) is of less clinical significance since the correlation with prognosis is weak. Some T-lineage cases are CD10 positive (weaker expression than B lineage) and some are weakly positive for CD79a [5, 6]. The great majority of

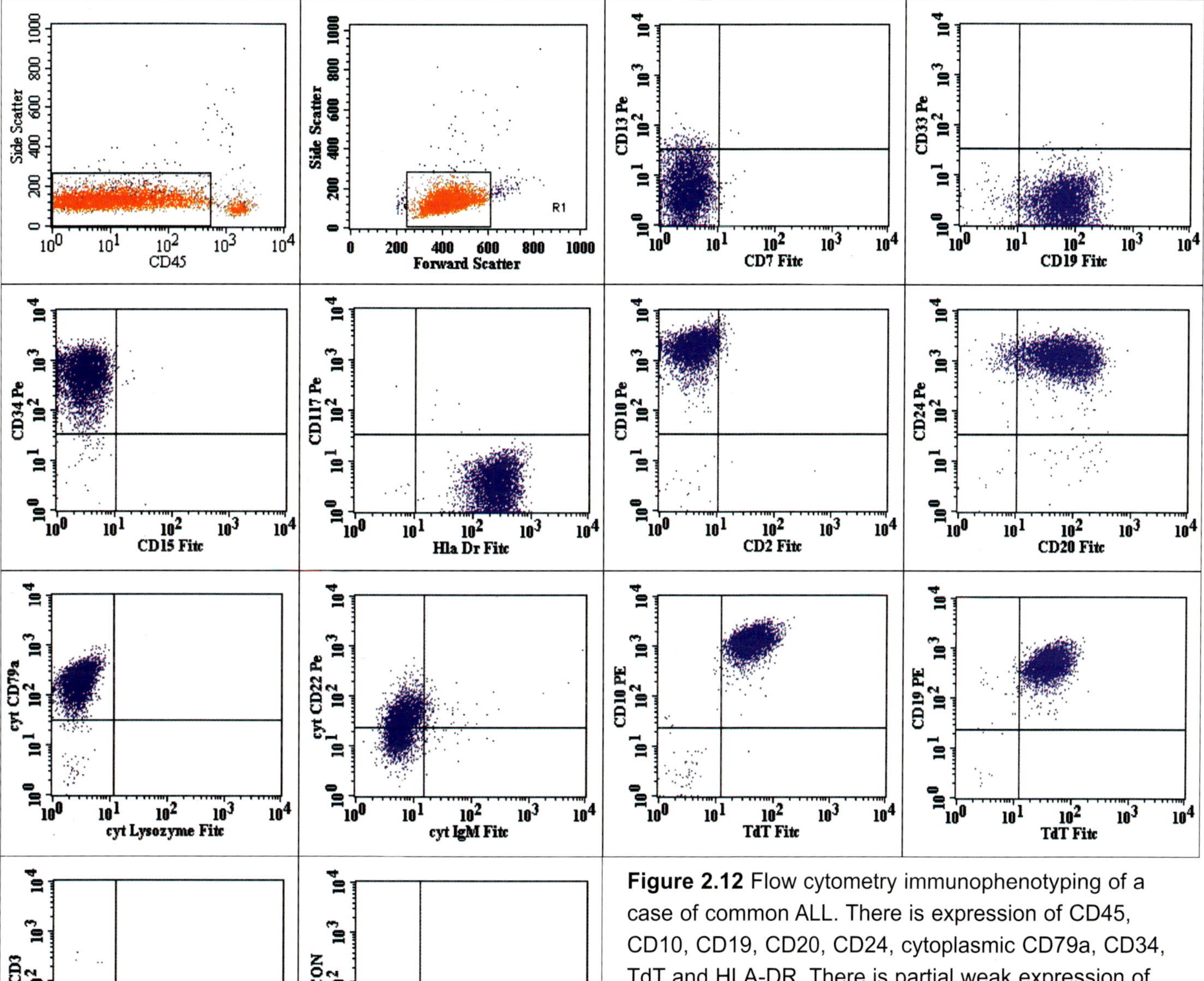

Figure 2.12 Flow cytometry immunophenotyping of a case of common ALL. There is expression of CD45, CD10, CD19, CD20, CD24, cytoplasmic CD79a, CD34, TdT and HLA-DR. There is partial weak expression of cytoplasmic CD22. Cytoplasmic μ chain, myeloid markers and T-lineage markers are not expressed. With thanks to Mr Ricardo Morilla.

cases express nuclear terminal deoxynucleotidyl transferase, expression being stronger in B-lineage than T-lineage cases; overall about 5% of cases are negative, these being mainly T-lineage cases. The stem cell marker, CD34, is often expressed in B-lineage cases (about 50% of cases) but is rarely expressed in T-lineage cases. Around a third of cases show aberrant expression of one or more myeloid-associated antigens, particularly CD13 or CD33; this is more common in Philadelphia-positive cases and in cases associated with t(4;11) (see below).

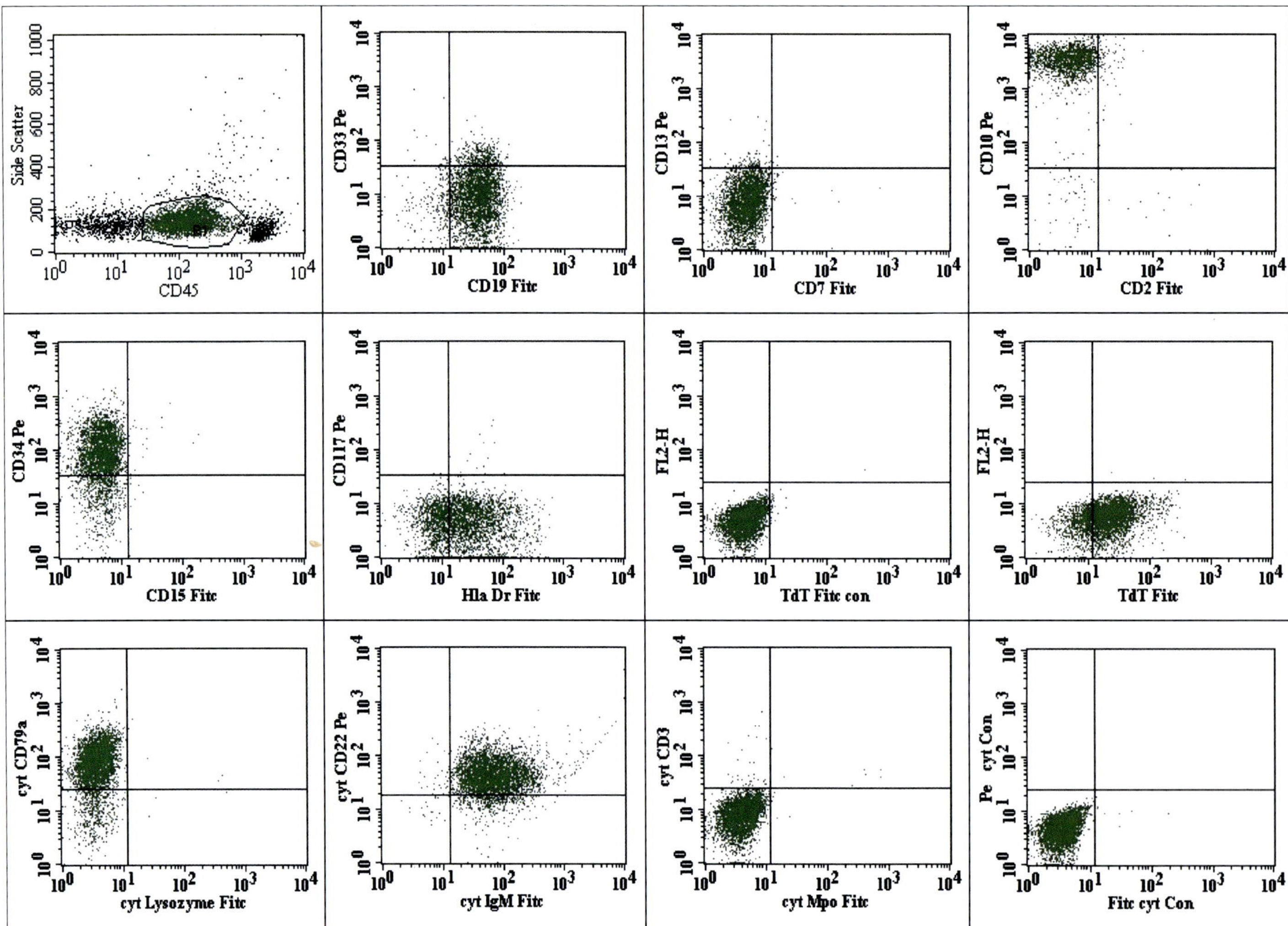

Figure 2.13 Flow cytometry immunophenotyping of a case of pre-B ALL. There is expression of CD45, CD10, CD19, cytoplasmic CD22, cytoplasmic CD79a, CD34, TdT (weak), HLA-DR (weak) and cytoplasmic μ chain. With thanks to Mr Ricardo Morilla.

Table 2.1 Classification of B-lineage acute lymphoblastic leukaemia according to the European Group for the Immunological Characterization of Leukemias (EGIL)

Category	*Immunophenotype*	*Possible cytogenetic abnormality*
Pro-B or early B	CD10–, cμ–, SmIg–	t(4;11)(q21;q23)
Common ALL	CD10+, SmIg–, cμ–	High hyperdiploidy or t(12;21)(p13;q22)
Pre-B ALL	cμ+	t(1;19)(q23;p13)
B-ALL*	c or Sm κ or λ+	t(8;14)(q24;q32)

Positive for CD19 and/or CD79a and/or CD22; most cases, except B-ALL, are TdT positive

* Classified as non-Hodgkin's lymphoma in the WHO classification; c, cytoplasmic; CD, cluster of differentiation; Ig, immunoglobulin; Sm, surface membrane; TdT, terminal deoxynucleotidyl transferase

Table 2.2 Classification of T-lineage acute lymphoblastic leukaemia according to the European Group for the Immunological Characterization of Leukemias (EGIL)

Category	*Immunophenotype**
Pro-T	CD7+, CD2–, CD5–, CD8–, CD1a–
Pre-T	CD2+ and/or CD5+ and/or CD8+, CD1a–
Cortical T	CD1a+, membrane CD3+ or –
Mature T	Membrane CD3+, CD1a–
Group a	Anti-TCR αβ+
Group b	Anti-TCR γδ+

* All cases are positive for c or Sm CD3; some cases are CD10 positive; c, cytoplasmic; CD, cluster of differentiation; Sm, surface membrane; TCR, T-cell receptor

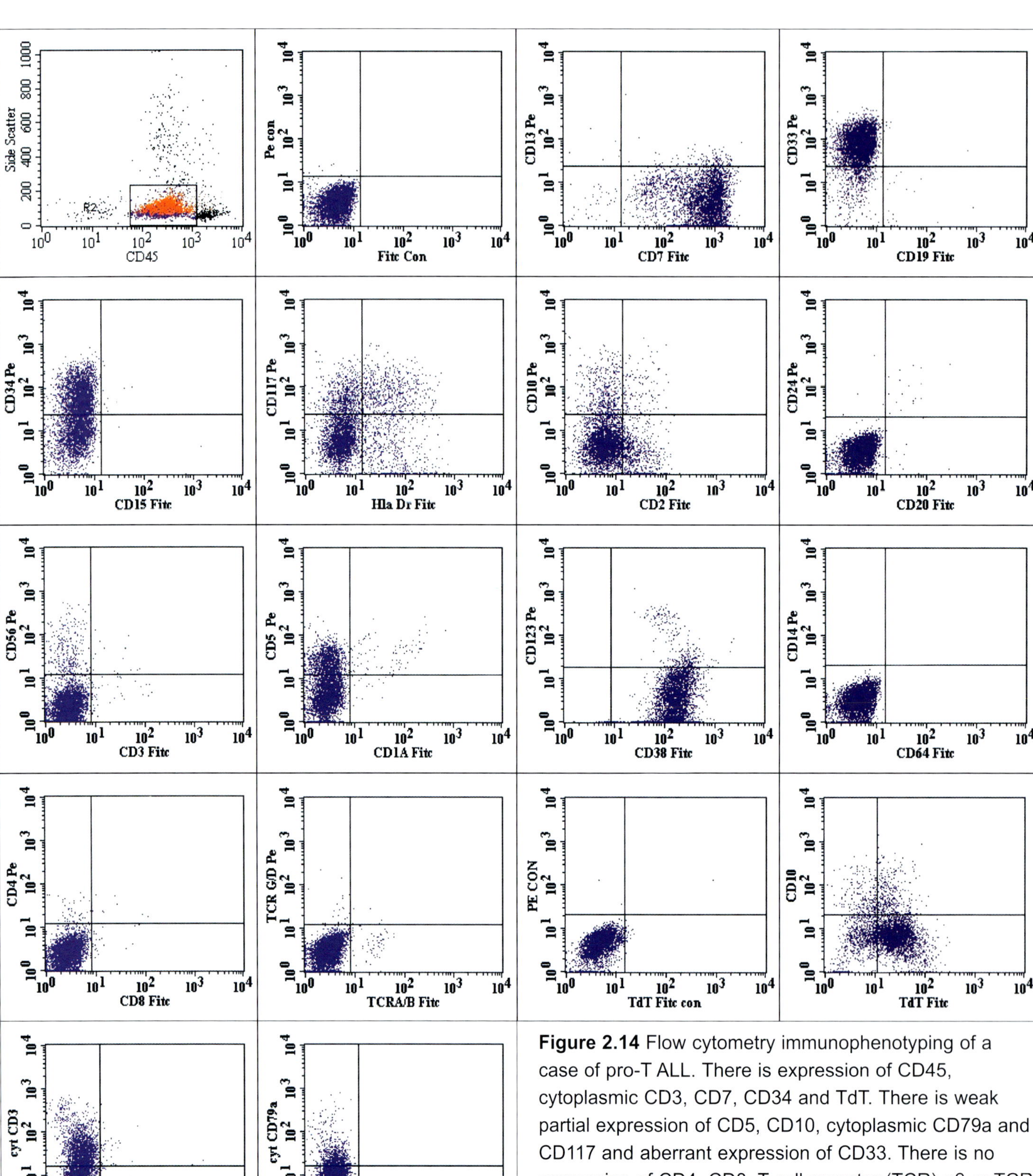

Figure 2.14 Flow cytometry immunophenotyping of a case of pro-T ALL. There is expression of CD45, cytoplasmic CD3, CD7, CD34 and TdT. There is weak partial expression of CD5, CD10, cytoplasmic CD79a and CD117 and aberrant expression of CD33. There is no expression of CD4, CD8, T-cell receptor (TCR) αβ or TCR γδ. With thanks to Mr Ricardo Morilla.

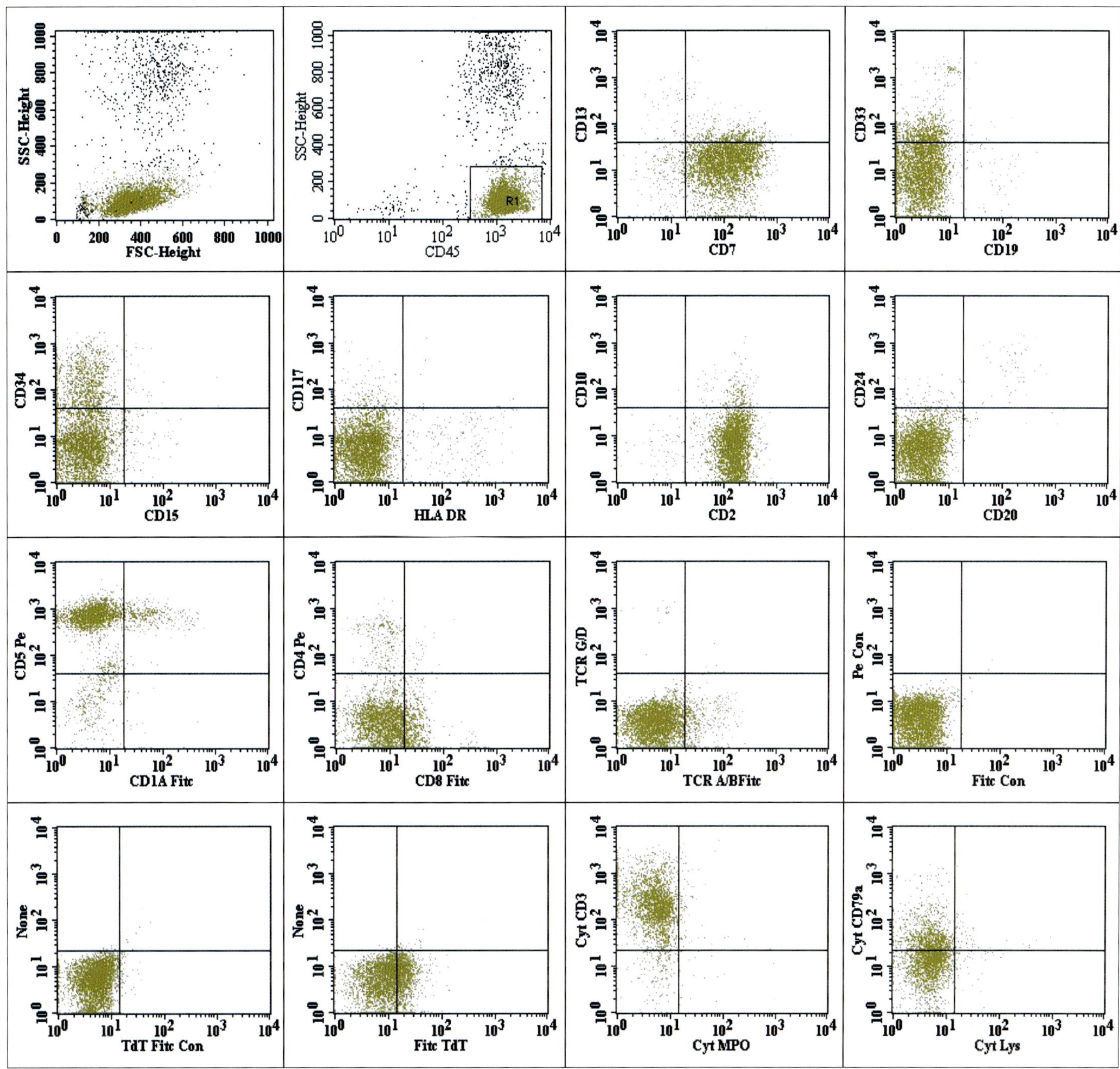

Figure 2.15 Flow cytometry immunophenotyping of a case of pre-T ALL. There is expression of CD45, CD2, cytoplasmic CD3, CD5 and CD7 and partial expression of CD34. There is no expression of CD1a, CD4, CD8, TCR αβ, TCR γδ or TdT. There is weak partial expression of CD79a. With thanks to Mr Ricardo Morilla.

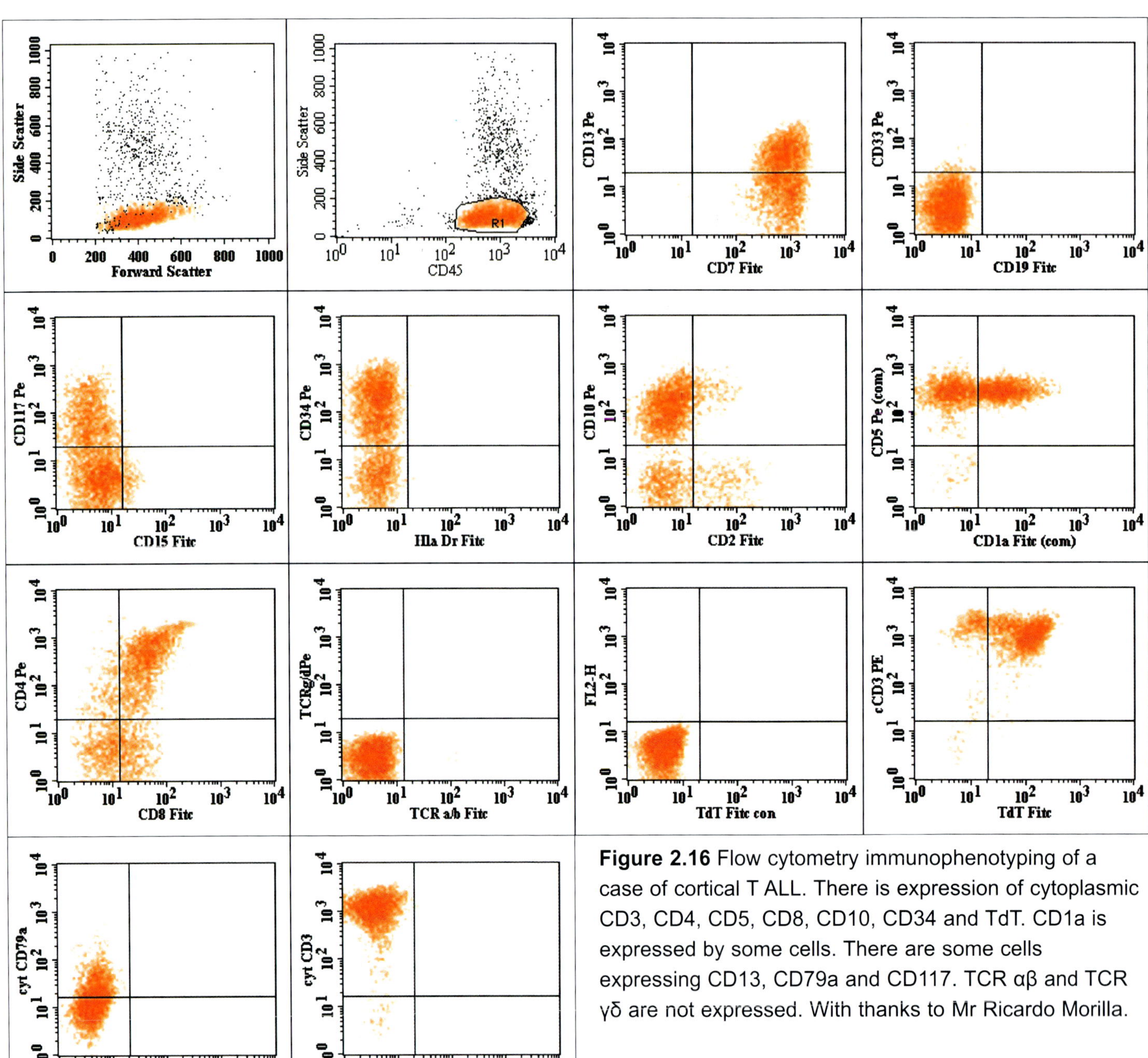

Figure 2.16 Flow cytometry immunophenotyping of a case of cortical T ALL. There is expression of cytoplasmic CD3, CD4, CD5, CD8, CD10, CD34 and TdT. CD1a is expressed by some cells. There are some cells expressing CD13, CD79a and CD117. TCR αβ and TCR γδ are not expressed. With thanks to Mr Ricardo Morilla.

Cytogenetic and molecular genetic abnormalities

In ALL/lymphoblastic lymphoma, both cytogenetic and molecular genetic analyses give information relevant to prognosis and management [7, 8].

Common cytogenetic and molecular genetic abnormalities in B-lineage ALL are summarized in relation to immunophenotype in *Table 2.1*. Cytogenetic/molecular subgroups differ significantly in their clinical and haematological features and their prognosis. The two most common abnormalities, a cryptic t(12;21)(p13;q22) and high hyperdiploidy (more than 50 but fewer than 66 chromosomes) (Figure **2.17**) are associated with the typical childhood peak of ALL and with a common ALL immunophenotype. They are both associated with a relatively good prognosis although, in the case of t(12;21), late relapses (perhaps arising in a cell of a preleukaemic clone) can occur. The molecular mechanism associated with t(12;21) is formation of an *ETV6-RUNX1* fusion gene (previously known as *TEL-AML1*). In high hyperdiploidy the acquisition of extra chromosomes is not random. Those most often duplicated are 4, 5, 6, 8, 10, 14, 17, 18 and 21; the molecular mechanism of leukaemogenesis in this subtype is unknown. ALL associated with t(4;11)(q21;q23) (Figure **2.18**) has distinctive characteristics. It most often occurs in infants, is associated with a high white cell count and prominent organomegaly and has a poor prognosis. Older children and adults occasionally also have t(4;11). The immunophenotype in this subset is that of an early B cell (pro-B ALL) with co-expression of the myeloid antigen, CD15, being common, and with chondroitin sulphate proteoglycan (detected by monoclonal antibody NG2) often being expressed. This translocation, which leads to formation of an *AF4-MLL* fusion gene, occurs in a pluripotent stem cell and relapse as acute monoblastic leukaemia can occur. ALL associated with t(1;19)(q23;p13) (Figure **2.19**) is often associated with a pre-B immunophenotype. Prognosis with earlier treatment regimes was adverse but this is no longer so. A further important subgroup of B-lineage ALL in adults is Philadelphia (Ph)-positive ALL, associated with t(9;22)(q34;q11) and a *BCR-ABL* fusion gene. It is found in a quarter to a third of adult cases with its prevalence increasing steadily with age. It is quite uncommon among childhood cases. It has no specific immunophenotype and is associated with a very adverse prognosis.

The two most frequent cytogenetic/molecular genetic abnormalities in T-lineage ALL are TAL^{d} (present in about a third of cases) and t(5;14)(q35;q32), present in about a fifth of cases. Both are cryptic rearrangements. In TAL^{d}, there is a small deletion at 1q32, which leads to the fusion of most of the sequences of *TAL1* (which encodes a transcription factor normally expressed in haemopoietic precursors and endothelial cells but not T cells) to the promoter of the upstream *SIL* gene. This leads to dysregulation of *TAL1*. The cryptic translocation, t(5;14)(q35;q32), leads to upregulation of *HOX11L2* at 5q35, probably by proximity to the transcription regulatory elements of *BCL11B* (*CTIP2*) at 14q32.1.

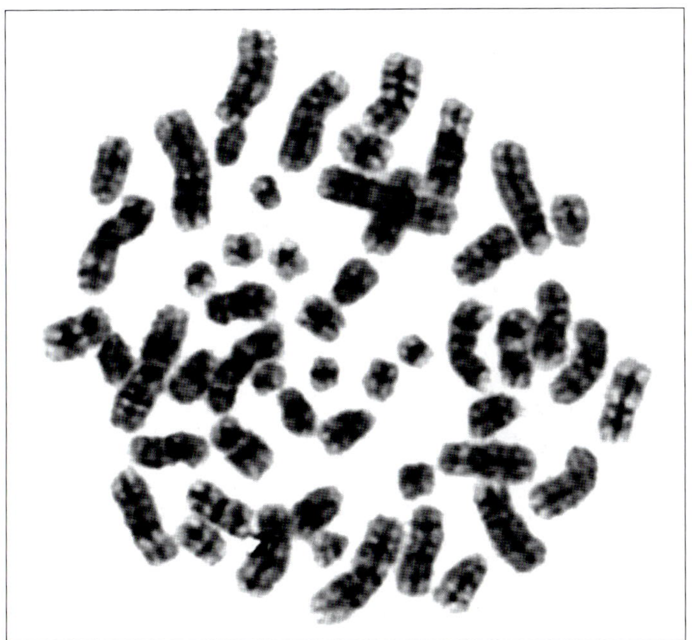

Figure 2.17 A metaphase spread from a patient with B-lineage ALL and hyperdiploidy. With thanks to Dr John Swansbury.

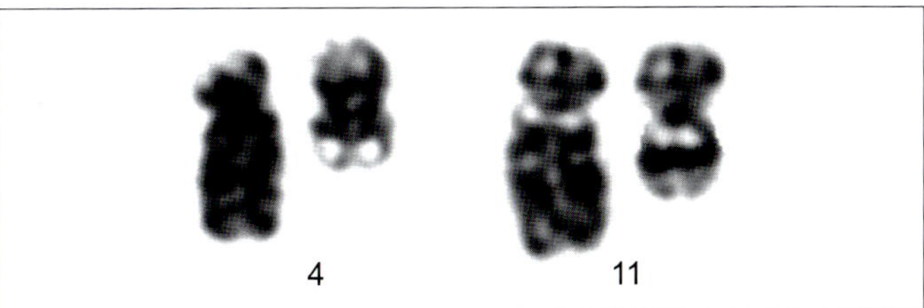

Figure 2.18 A partial karyogram from a patient with t(4;11)(q21;q23). With thanks to Dr John Swansbury.

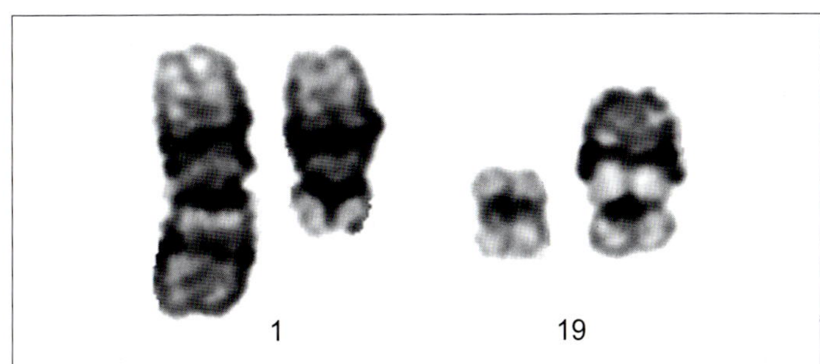

Figure 2.19 A partial karyogram from a patient with t(1;19)(q23;p13). With thanks to Dr John Swansbury.

Diagnosis and differential diagnosis

The diagnosis of ALL is usually straightforward, on the basis of cytology and immunophenotyping. It is important, however, to distinguish normal immature B-lineage cells, known as haematogones (Figure **2.20**), from leukaemic blasts. The former may express CD10 and terminal deoxynucleotidyl transferase but, in contrast to leukaemic blasts, they are cytologically and immunophenotypically heterogeneous. In the absence of immunophenotyping, misidentification of acute myeloid leukaemia (AML) with very immature blast cells (FAB M0 AML) and acute megakaryoblastic leukaemia (FAB M7 AML) as ALL can occur.

Diagnosis is more difficult in the case of presentation with an aplastic marrow but, if immunophenotyping is performed, an abnormal lymphoid population may be detected during the aplastic phase.

Prognosis

Prognosis is very variable, being related to age and more specifically to the cytogenetic/molecular genetic subtype. Overall about 80% of childhood cases are curable as are about 40% of adult cases [9]. Prognosis is best in children between the ages of 1 and 10 years. It is adverse in adults and in infants less than a year of age. A good prognosis is associated with high hyperdiploidy and t(12;21)and a particularly adverse prognosis with t(4;11), t(9;22) and hypodiploidy. A high white cell count is associated with a worse prognosis. There are conflicting data as to whether or not T-lineage ALL is associated with a worse prognosis than B-lineage but with modern treatment regimes no adverse effect is seen [9]. The adverse effect of male gender has also disappeared [9].

Treatment

Treatment of ALL requires intensive combination chemotherapy followed by a period of maintenance therapy. Prophylactic treatment of the central nervous system is also required. In the case of Ph-positive ALL, it is possible that the prognosis will be improved if imatinib, an inhibitor of the BCR-ABL tyrosine kinase, is added to conventional chemotherapy.

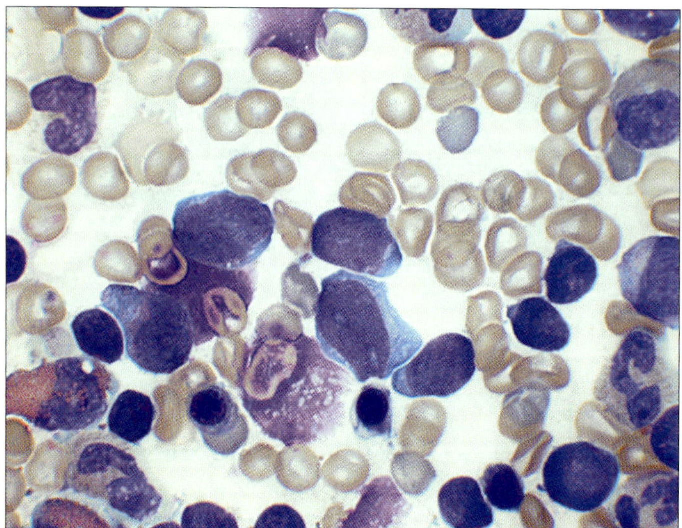

Figure 2.20 A bone marrow aspirate film from a three-week-old baby showing haematogones. Romanowsky stain, x 100 objective.

References

1. Greaves M (2003). Pre-natal origins of childhood leukemia. *Rev Clin Exp Hematol*, 7, 233–245.
2. Greaves M (2005). *In utero* origins of childhood leukaemia. *Early Hum Dev*, **81**, 123–129.
3. Bene MC, Castoldi G, Knapp W, Ludwig WD, Matutes E, Orfao A and van't Veer MB; European Group for the Immunological Characterization of Leukemias (EGIL) (1995). Proposals for the immunological classification of acute leukemias. *Leukemia*, **9**, 1783–1786.
4. De Zen L, Orfao A, Cazzaniga G, Masiero L, Cocito MG, Spinelli M *et al.* (2000). Quantitative multiparametric immunophenotyping in acute lymphoblastic leukemia: correlation with specific genotype. I. ETV6/AML1 ALLs identification. *Leukemia*, **14**, 1225–1231.
5. Pilozzi E, Pulford K, Jones M, Muller-Hermelink HK, Falini B, Ralfkiaer E *et al.* (1998). Co-expression of CD79a (JCB117) and CD3 by lymphoblastic lymphoma. *J Pathol*, **186**, 140–143.
6. Hashimoto M, Yamashita Y and Mori N (2002). Immunohistochemical detection of CD79a expression in precursor T cell lymphoblastic lymphoma/leukaemias. *J Pathol*, **197**, 341–347.
7. Okuda T, Fisher R and Downing JR (1996). Molecular diagnostics in pediatric acute lymphoblastic leukemia. *Mol Diagn*, **1**, 139–151.
8. Pilozzi E, Muller-Hermelink HK, Falini B, Wolf-Peeters C, Fidler C, Gatter K and Wainscoat J (1999). Gene rearrangements in T-cell lymphoblastic lymphoma. *J Pathol*, **188**, 267–270.
9. Pui C-H and Evans WE (2006). Treatment of acute lymphoblastic leukemia. *N Engl J Med*, **354**, 166–178.

Chapter 3

Chronic lymphocytic leukaemia/small lymphocytic lymphoma

In Western countries, chronic lymphocytic leukaemia (CLL) is by far the most common lymphoid malignancy [1–3]. It is a disease predominantly of the middle aged and elderly with the incidence being considerably higher in men than in women. In some instances a familial tendency to develop CLL can be demonstrated [4] and family members may have monoclonal B-cell lymphocytosis [5]. Diagnosis requires the presence of significant lymphocytosis, often arbitrarily defined as a lymphocyte count exceeding either 5 or 10×10^9/l. The lymphocytes are clonal B cells with a very characteristic immunophenotype. There is often a long asymptomatic phase in CLL so that incidental diagnosis is common and many patients subsequently die with the disease rather than of the disease.

Small lymphocytic lymphoma is a lymphoma in which the neoplastic cells have the same cytological and immunophenotypic features as those of chronic lymphocytic leukaemia but without there being significant lymphocytosis at diagnosis. In some patients with small lymphocytic lymphoma a leukaemic phase subsequently occurs.

Clinical features

In patients in whom the diagnosis of CLL is incidental there may be no symptoms and no abnormal physical findings. In other patients with more advanced disease, presentation may be with lymphadenopathy, with or without splenomegaly or hepatomegaly, or with infection, bruising or symptoms of anaemia (Figures **3.1** and **3.2**). Infections

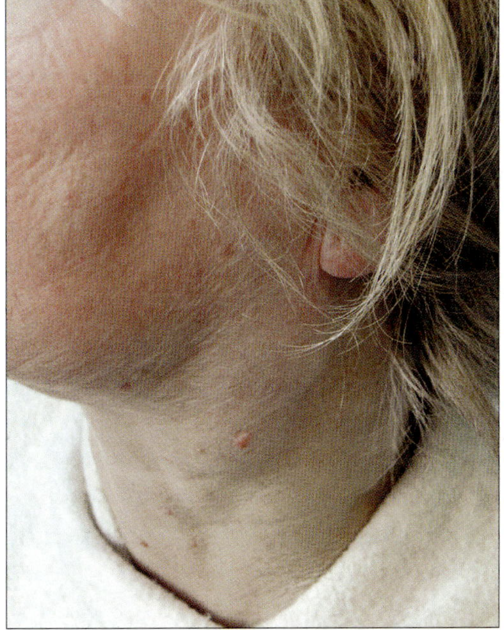

Figure 3.1 Clinical photograph showing cervical lymphadenopathy in a patient with CLL.

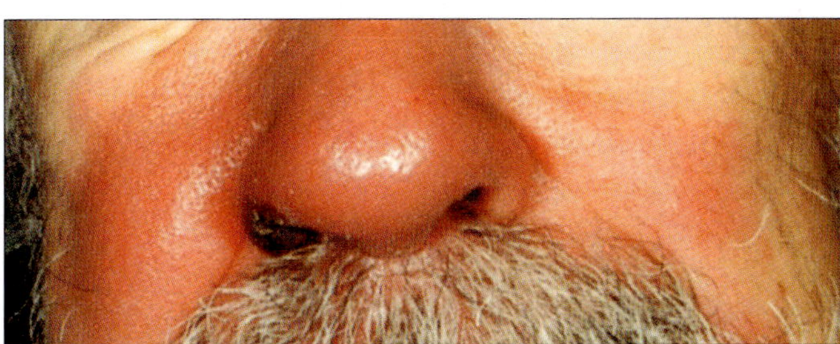

Figure 3.2 Clinical photograph showing skin infiltration in a patient with CLL.

that are particularly prevalent among these patients are herpes zoster (Figure **3.3**) and pneumococcal pneumonia. Autoimmune complications, specifically autoimmune haemolytic anaemia, autoimmune thrombocytopenic purpura and pure red cell aplasia, may be present at diagnosis and are common during the course of the disease. Small lymphocytic lymphoma usually presents with lymphadenopathy, with or without splenomegaly or hepatomegaly.

CLL can undergo transformation to a large cell lymphoma. In addition, diffuse large B-cell lymphoma can arise in a B cell that does not belong to the neoplastic CLL population, this being found in around half of cases [6]. Epstein Barr virus (EBV) is an aetiological factor in some cases of large cell lymphoma arising from a cell of the CLL clone and also in some cases arising in an unrelated non-clonal B cell; this occurrence reflects the immune deficiency of CLL. All these types of transformation are encompassed by the term 'Richter's syndrome'. Richter's syndrome can arise in a lymph node or at an extra-nodal site including bone marrow. It should be suspected when there is a sudden disproportionate increase in size of a single lymph node or cluster of lymph nodes, unexplained cytopenia or B symptoms. Small lymphocytic lymphoma can undergo similar transformation.

Several staging systems for CLL have been devised, based on both clinical and other characteristics. Of these, the Binet classification (*Table 3.1*) [7] is most used.

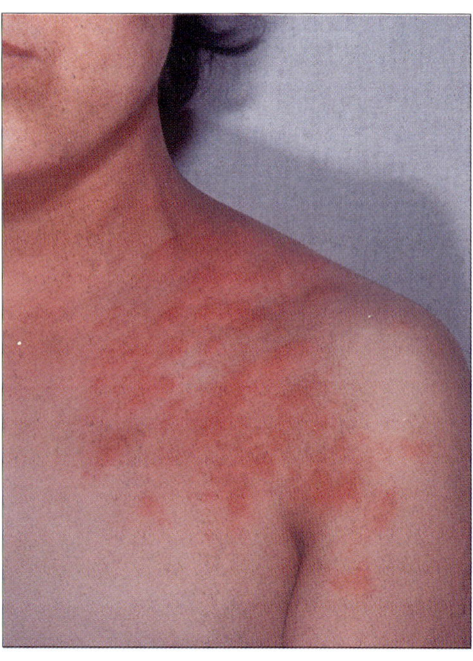

Figure 3.3 Clinical photograph showing herpes zoster in a patient with CLL.

Haematological and pathological features

In patients with early disease, lymphocytosis is the only abnormality detected in the blood count. In those with more advanced disease there may also be anaemia or thrombocytopenia but neutropenia is unusual in the untreated patient.

The blood film shows an increase of mature small lymphocytes with condensed chromatin [8] (Figures **3.4** and **3.5**). Sometimes the chromatin condensation produces a mosaic pattern and sometimes it is more uniform. Nucleoli may be present but they are usually small and inconspicuous. The nuclear outline is usually regular. The cytoplasm is weakly basophilic and occasionally contains crystals (Figure **3.6**) or small vacuoles. The cells of CLL show increased mechanical fragility and this leads to formation of 'smear cells' (see Figure **3.4**), which are the

Table 3.1 The Binet staging system for chronic lymphocytic leukaemia [7]

Stage	*Criteria*
A	Lymphocytosis with no more than two regions* having enlarged lymph nodes or other lymphoid organ; haemoglobin concentration greater than 10 g/dl and platelet count greater than 100 x 10^9/l
B	Lymphocytosis with three or more regions having enlarged lymph nodes or other lymphoid organ; haemoglobin concentration greater than 10 g/dl and platelet count greater than 100 x 10^9/l†
C	Haemoglobin concentration less than 10 g/dl, platelet count less than 100 x 10^9/l or both†

* A region being cervical, axillary, inguinal, liver or spleen (regardless of whether lymph node involvement is unilateral or bilateral)

† Although not specified by Binet and colleagues, the appropriateness of classifying patients with anaemia or thrombocytopenia with an immune basis as stage C could be questioned

result of damage to cells during the spreading of the blood film; this feature is useful in diagnosis, although not pathognomonic. In the mixed cell type of CLL the leukaemic cells are more pleomorphic. There may be some larger cells with more abundant cytoplasm or cells may have irregular or cleft nuclei or be plasmacytoid. Nucleoli may be more prominent than in typical CLL. Sometimes a proportion of cells resemble prolymphocytes, being larger than typical CLL cells with a vesicular nucleolus (Figure **3.7**); it has been suggested that the designation CLL/PL be used if there are more than 10% prolymphocytes and atypical CLL/mixed cell type if there are more than 15% of lymphoplasmacytic or cleft cells.

If anaemia is present it is usually normocytic or normochromic without any specific blood film features. However, when there is complicating autoimmune haemolytic anaemia there will be spherocytes and polychromatic cells, an increased reticulocyte count and a positive direct antiglobulin test (Figure **3.8**). In pure red cell aplasia, the anaemia is normocytic and normochromic, there

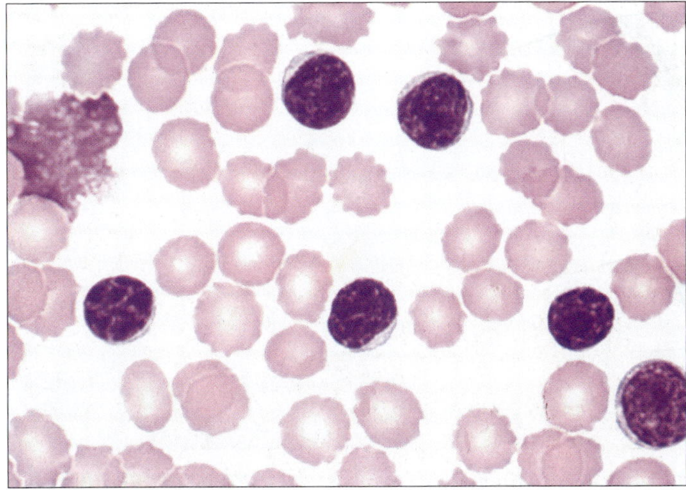

Figure 3.4 Blood film showing mature small lymphocytes with clumped chromatin and one smear cell. Romanowsky stain, x 100 objective.

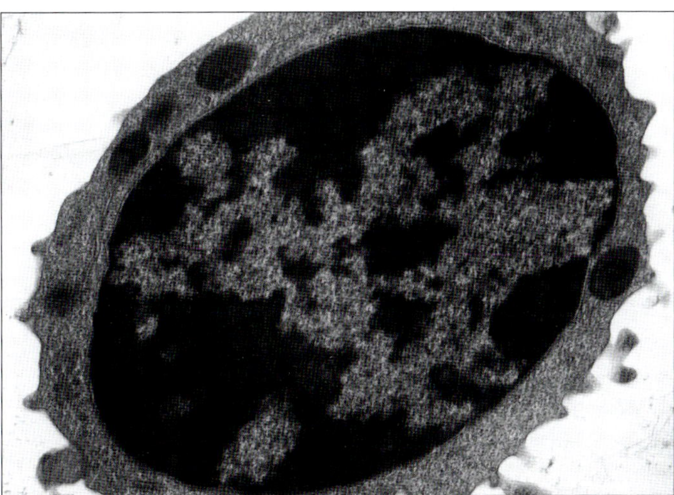

Figure 3.5 Ultrastructure of a CLL lymphocyte. Electron microscopy. Lead nitrate and uranyl acetate stain.

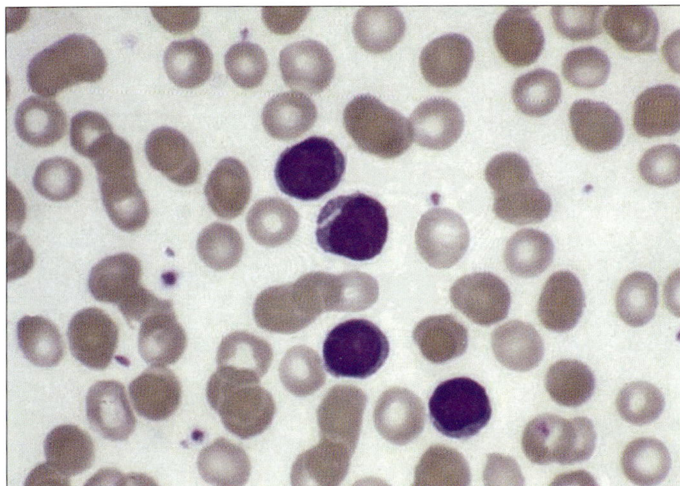

Figure 3.6 Blood film showing mature small lymphocytes, one of which contains a crystal. Romanowsky stain, x 100 objective.

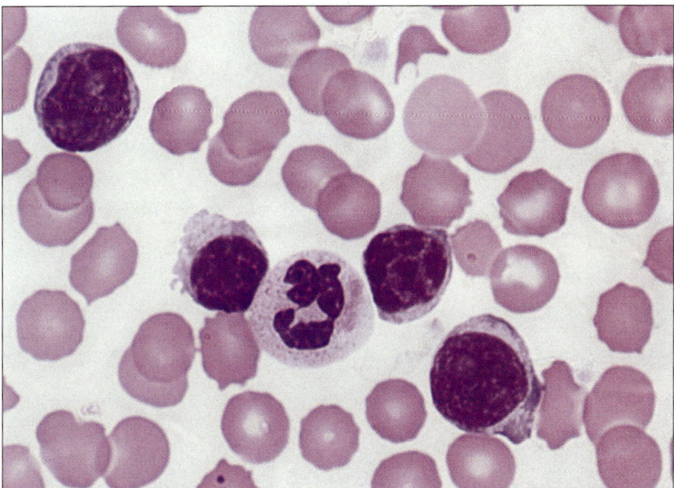

Figure 3.7 Blood film from a patient with mixed cell type of CLL (CLL/PL) showing two mature small lymphocytes, one prolymphocyte (bottom right) and one intermediate cell. Romanowsky stain, x 100 objective.

is a lack of polychromasia despite anaemia and the reticulocyte count is inappropriately low. There are no blood film features that reliably distinguish immune thrombocytopenia from thrombocytopenia as a result of heavy bone marrow infiltration, although large platelets are more likely in the former condition. An inappropriate reduction of cells of a single lineage, out of proportion to what is expected for the stage of the disease, should lead to the suspicion of an autoimmune complication.

Biochemical tests show hypogammaglobulinaemia in patients with advanced disease. A paraprotein (IgM) is present in a low concentration in a minority of patients. Hypercalcaemia is seen only with very advanced disease. Hyperuricaemia is common.

The bone marrow is infiltrated by cells with similar cytological features to those in the blood. The presence of

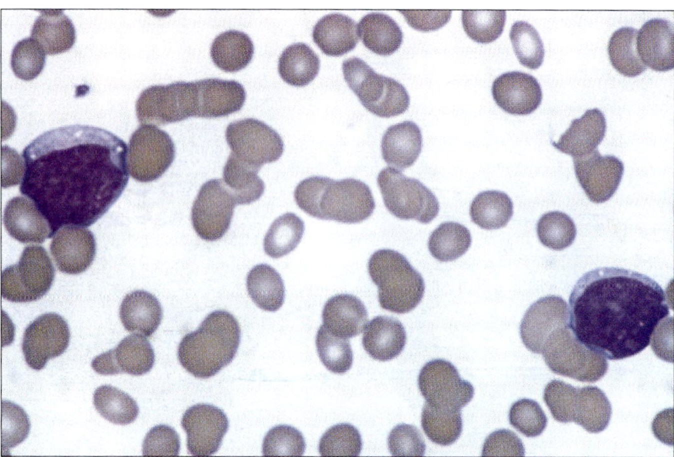

Figure 3.8 Blood film from a patient with autoimmune haemolytic anaemia complicating CLL, showing two leukaemic lymphocytes, spherocytes and polychromasia. The lymphocytes are slightly immature with visible nucleoli and small vacuoles. Romanowsky stain, x 100 objective.

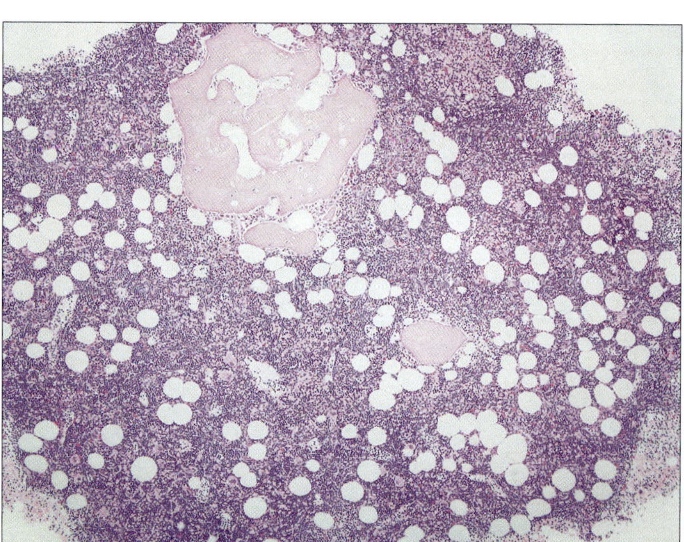

Figure 3.9 Trephine biopsy section from a patient with CLL showing heavy interstitial infiltration. H&E, x 10 objective.

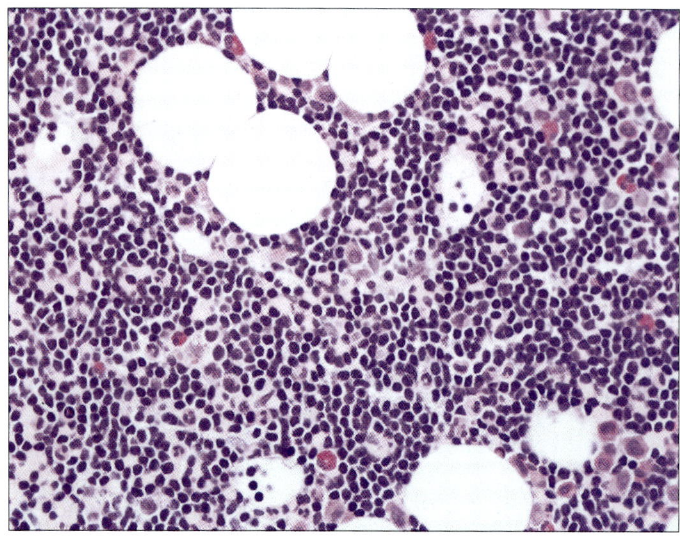

Figure 3.10 Trephine biopsy section from a patient with CLL (same patient as Figure **3.9**), showing heavy interstitial infiltration. Residual neutrophil and eosinophil precursors are also apparent. H&E, x 60 objective.

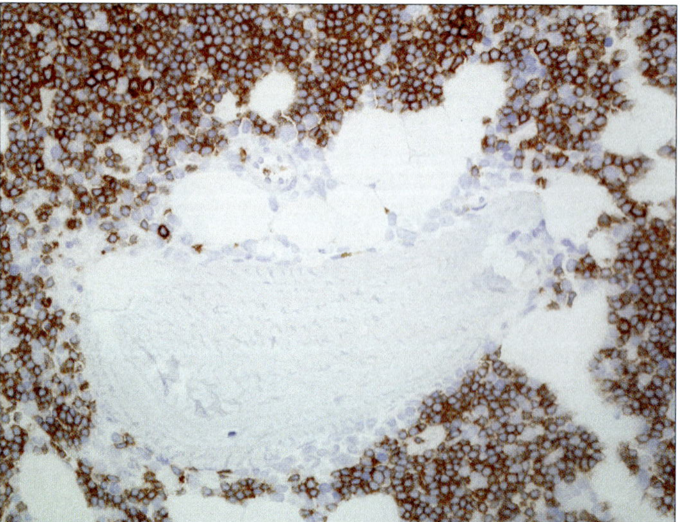

Figure 3.11 Trephine biopsy section from a patient with CLL (same patient as Figure **3.9**), showing that the leukaemic cells express CD5. Immunoperoxidase, x 40 objective.

40% of lymphocytes in the bone marrow is sometimes taken as a criterion for a diagnosis of CLL. Otherwise an aspirate gives little useful information, except in patients being investigated for suspected pure red cell aplasia or autoimmune thrombocytopenic purpura. A trephine biopsy is much more useful, giving information relevant both to diagnosis and to prognosis. The pattern of infiltration may be interstitial, nodular or mixed or there may be a 'packed marrow' pattern, often referred to as 'diffuse infiltration' (Figures **3.9**–**3.13**). Proliferation centres are often seen (Figures **3.14** and **3.15**). Paratrabecular infiltration is not a feature of CLL.

The pattern of infiltration in lymph nodes is diffuse, although there may be proliferation centres of slightly larger nucleolated cells referred to as paraimmunoblasts (Figure **3.16**); these 'pseudo-follicles' need to be distinguished from

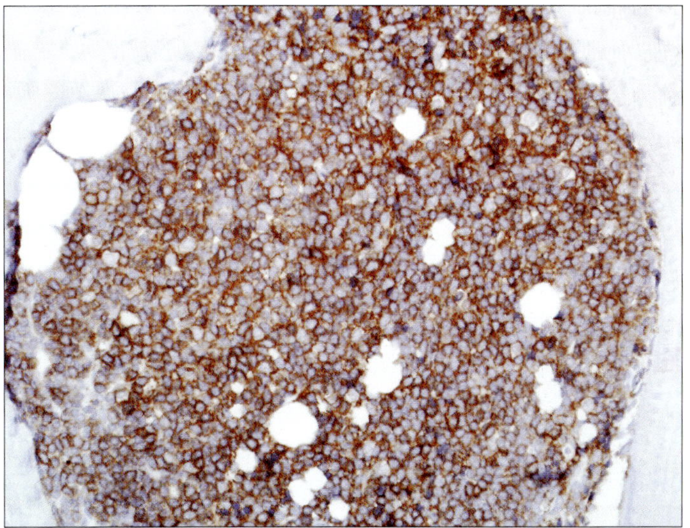

Figure 3.12 Trephine biopsy section from a patient with CLL (same patient as Figure **3.9**), showing that the leukaemic cells express CD23. Immunoperoxidase, x 40 objective.

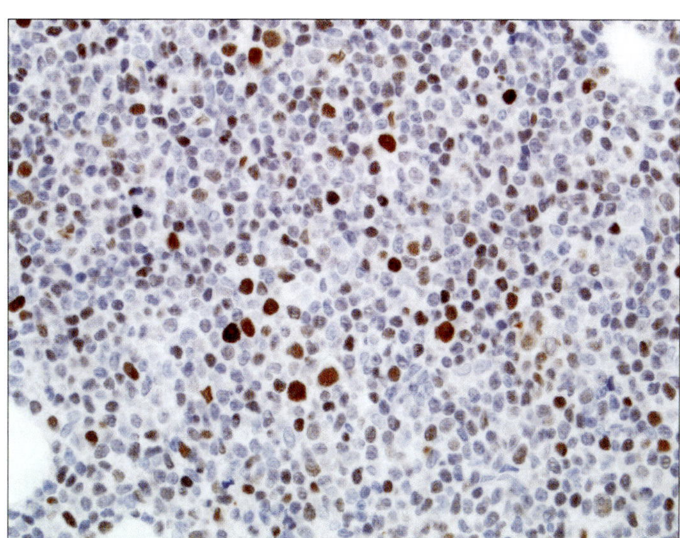

Figure 3.13 Trephine biopsy section from a patient with CLL (same patient as Figure **3.9**), showing that the leukaemic cells express p53; this is indicative of mutation in the *TP53* gene. Immunoperoxidase, x 60 objective.

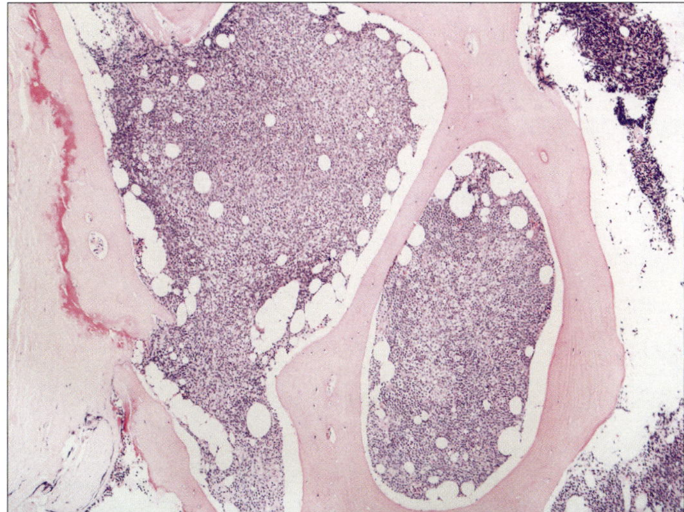

Figure 3.14 Trephine biopsy section from a patient with CLL showing mixed heavy interstitial/diffuse infiltration and several proliferation centres. H&E, x 10 objective.

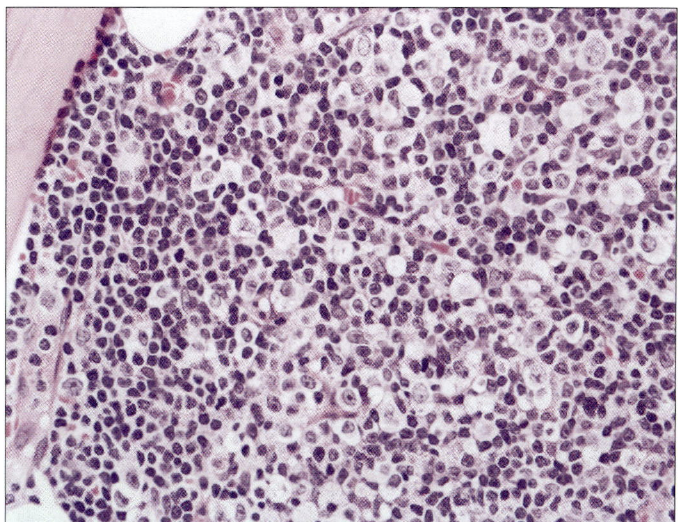

Figure 3.15 Trephine biopsy section from a patient with CLL (same patient as Figure **3.14**) showing nucleolated paraimmunoblasts within a proliferation centre. H&E, x 60 objective.

the follicles of follicular lymphoma. Lymph node biopsy is not necessary for the diagnosis of CLL and is only indicated if transformation is suspected. However, it is usually required for the diagnosis of small lymphocytic lymphoma.

Splenic infiltration is predominantly in the red pulp but the white pulp is also involved; proliferation centres may be present.

In small lymphocytic lymphoma either there is a normal lymphocyte count or there are small numbers of clonal lymphocytes in the blood but insufficient for a diagnosis of CLL. The bone marrow and other tissue manifestations are the same as those of CLL.

When Richter's transformation occurs, large transformed B cells may be seen in the peripheral blood (Figures **3.17** and **3.18**), bone marrow (Figures **3.19**–**3.21**) or other tissues. The large cells have a high proliferating fraction, as demonstrated by expression of Ki67 (Figure **3.22**). Immunohistochemistry and *in situ* hybridization can be used to demonstrate the EBV in cases where the transformation is attributed to this virus (Figures **3.23** and **3.24**).

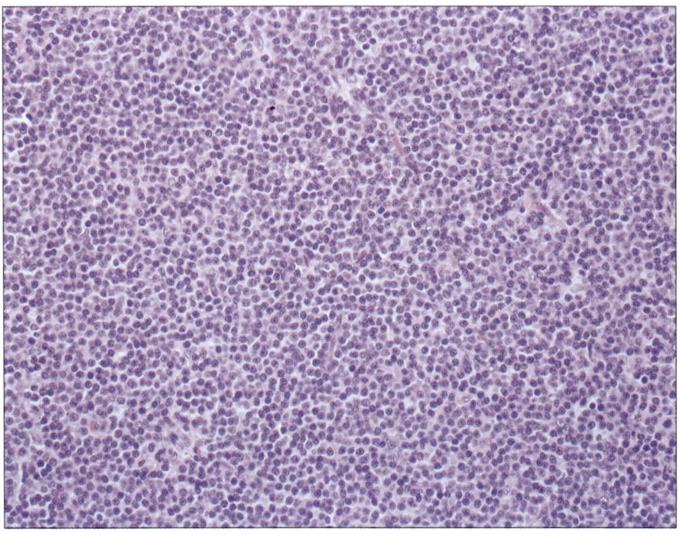

Figure 3.16 Lymph node biopsy from a patient with CLL showing diffuse infiltration by mature small lymphocytes. H&E, x 40 objective.

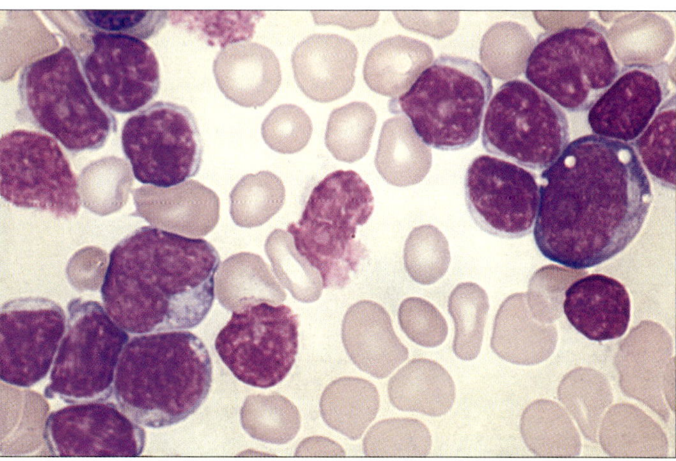

Figure 3.17 Blood film of a patient with Richter's transformation of CLL showing a large nucleolated transformed cell (middle right) on a background of mainly mature small lymphocytes and smear cells. Romanowsky stain, x 100 objective.

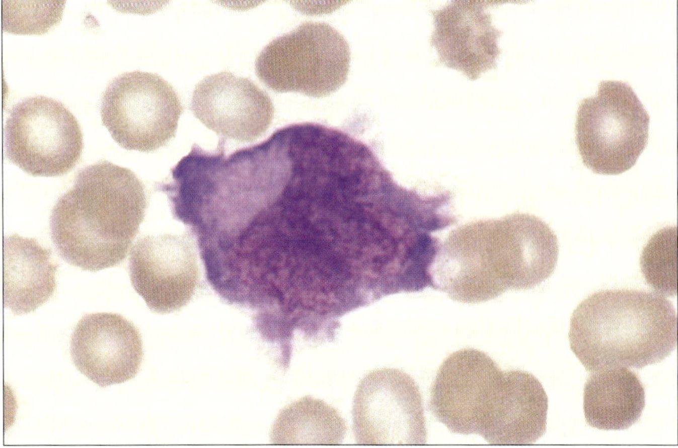

Figure 3.18 Blood film of a patient with Richter's transformation of CLL showing a very large transformed cell with an irregular nucleus and strongly basophilic cytoplasm in which the Golgi zone is apparent. Romanowsky stain, x 100 objective.

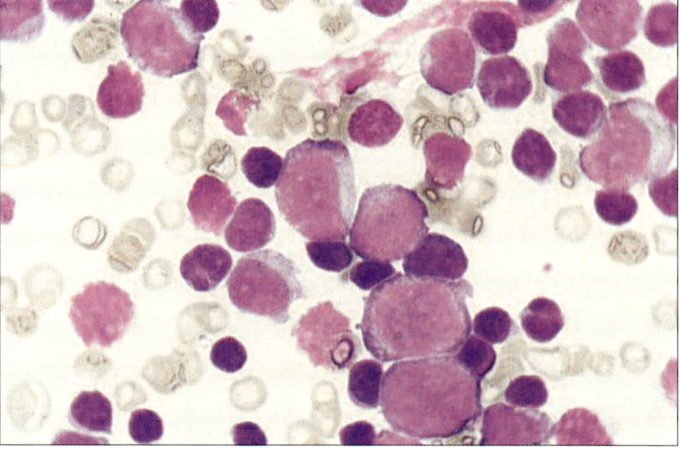

Figure 3.19 Bone marrow aspirate from a patient with Richter's transformation of CLL showing a mixture of large lymphoma cells and background of small lymphocytes. Romanowsky stain, x 100 objective.

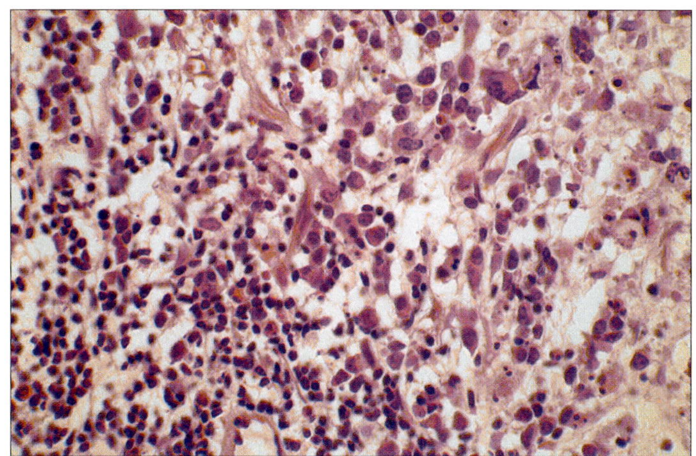

Figure 3.20 Bone marrow trephine biopsy section from a patient with Richter's transformation of CLL showing diffuse large B-cell lymphoma cells (right) and residual CLL infiltrate (left). H&E, x 60 objective.

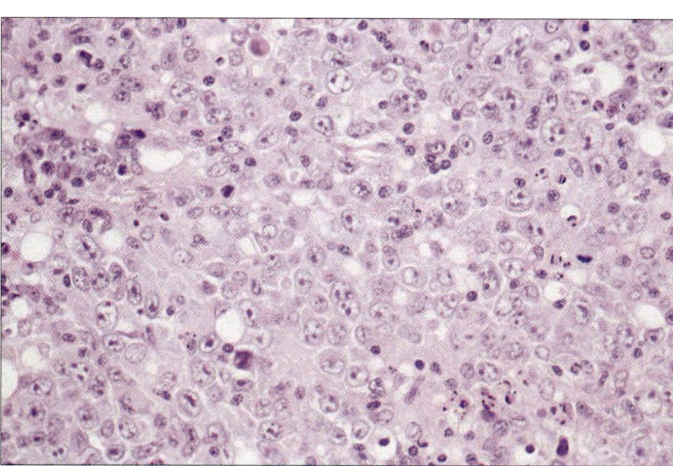

Figure 3.21 Bone marrow trephine biopsy section from a patient with Richter's transformation of CLL showing effacement of bone marrow by diffuse large B-cell lymphoma cells. H&E, x 60 objective.

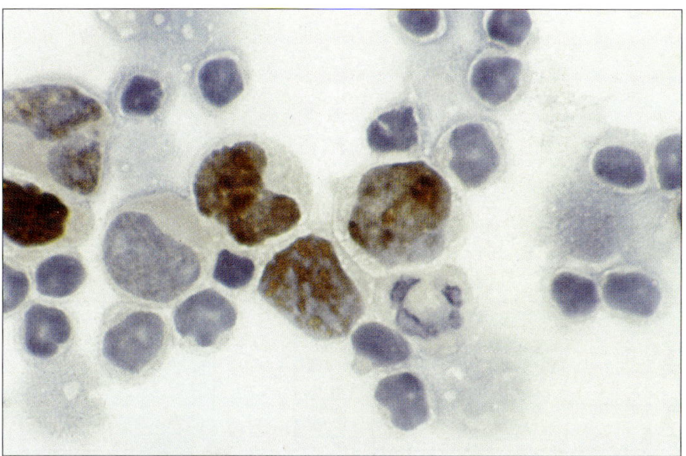

Figure 3.22 Cytological preparation in Richter's syndrome showing expression of Ki67 by the large transformed cells but not by the residual small lymphocytes. Immunoperoxidase, x 100 objective.

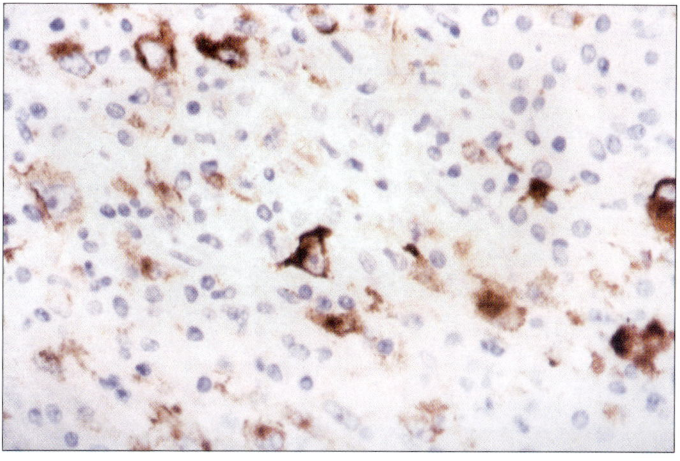

Figure 3.23 Bone marrow trephine biopsy section from a patient with Richter's transformation of CLL showing expression of EBV LMP1 (Epstein–Barr virus latent membrane protein 1) in the large lymphoma cells (but not in the background small lymphocytes). Immunoperoxidase, x 60 objective.

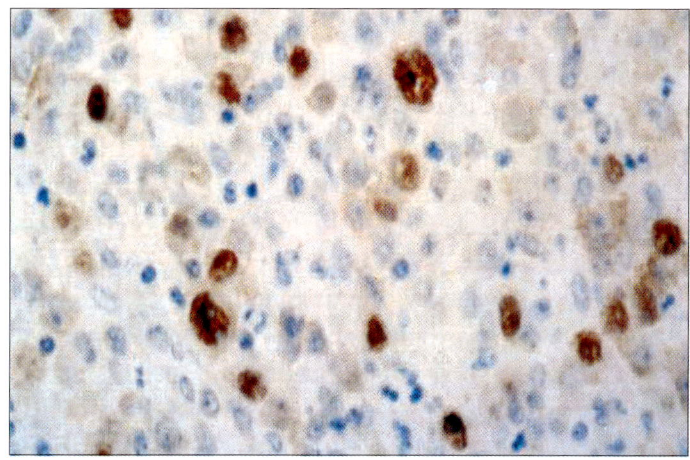

Figure 3.24 Bone marrow trephine biopsy section from a patient with Richter's transformation of CLL showing expression of EBER (Epstein–Barr virus early RNA) in the large lymphoma cells (but not in the background small lymphocytes). *In situ* hybridization, x 60 objective.

Immunophenotype

Observation of the characteristic immunophenotype (Figure **3.25**) is essential for the diagnosis of CLL [8, 9]. Cells are mature, monoclonal B cells with expression of light-chain-restricted surface membrane immunoglobulin, IgM or IgM and IgD; immunoglobulin expression is usually weak and occasionally is almost undetectable. There is also weak expression of the B-cell markers CD20, CD22 and CD79b, whereas other B-cell markers, such as CD19, show moderate expression. CD23 and CD5 (the latter more characteristic of T cells than of B cells) are usually expressed. FMC7, which is characteristically expressed in non-Hodgkin's lymphoma, is usually not expressed in CLL. CD11c, CD25, CD103 and CD123 are usually not expressed. CD38 [10, 11] (Figure **3.26**) and ZAP70 [12, 13] (Figure **3.27**) may be expressed and expression of either is of adverse prognostic significance. The characteristic immunophenotype of CLL and its differences from the immunophenotype of non-Hodgkin's lymphoma have been exploited in a scoring system that helps to establish the diagnosis (*Table 3.2*). A score of 4 or 5 is seen in a large majority of patients with CLL whereas a score of 3 may be seen in either CLL or non-Hodgkin's lymphoma and a score of 0, 1 or 2 means that a diagnosis of CLL is rather unlikely [8]. On immunohistochemistry, there is positivity for CD20, CD79a, CD23 and CD5.

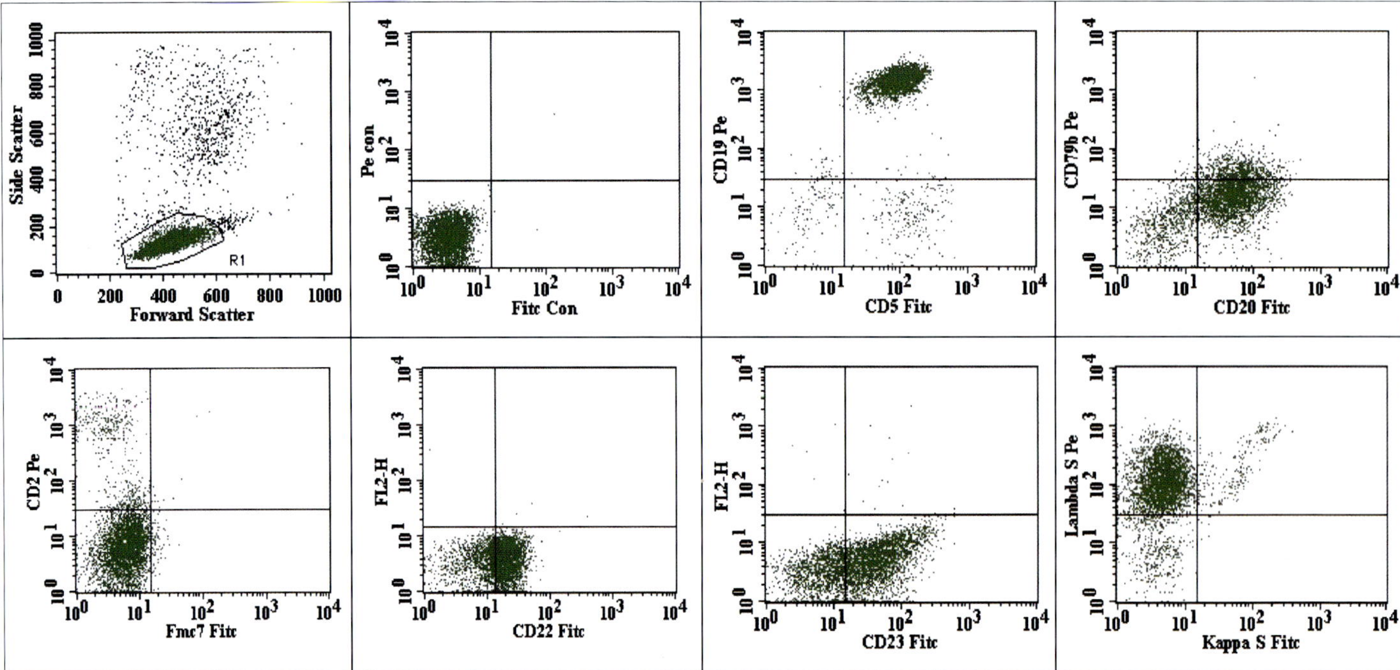

Figure 3.25 Flow cytometry immunophenotyping in a patient with CLL. Forward scatter and sideways scatter have been used to gate on the lymphocytes. The cells express CD5, CD19, CD23 and weak lambda light chain. They show weak expression of CD20 and CD22 and very weak expression of CD79b. FMC7 is not expressed. The CLL score is 5. With thanks to Mr Ricardo Morilla.

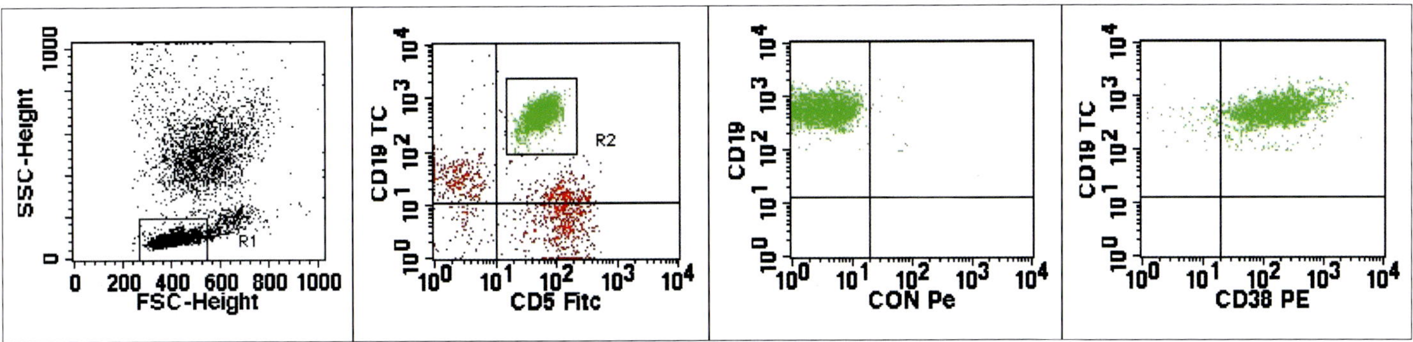

Figure 3.26 Flow cytometry immunophenotyping in a patient with CD38-positive CLL. Sequential gating has been used. Forward scatter and sideways scatter have been used to gate on the lymphocytes (R1) and subsequently gating of CD19/CD5-positive lymphocyte has been used (R2). 97% of cells in the R2 gate express CD38. With thanks to Mr Ricardo Morilla.

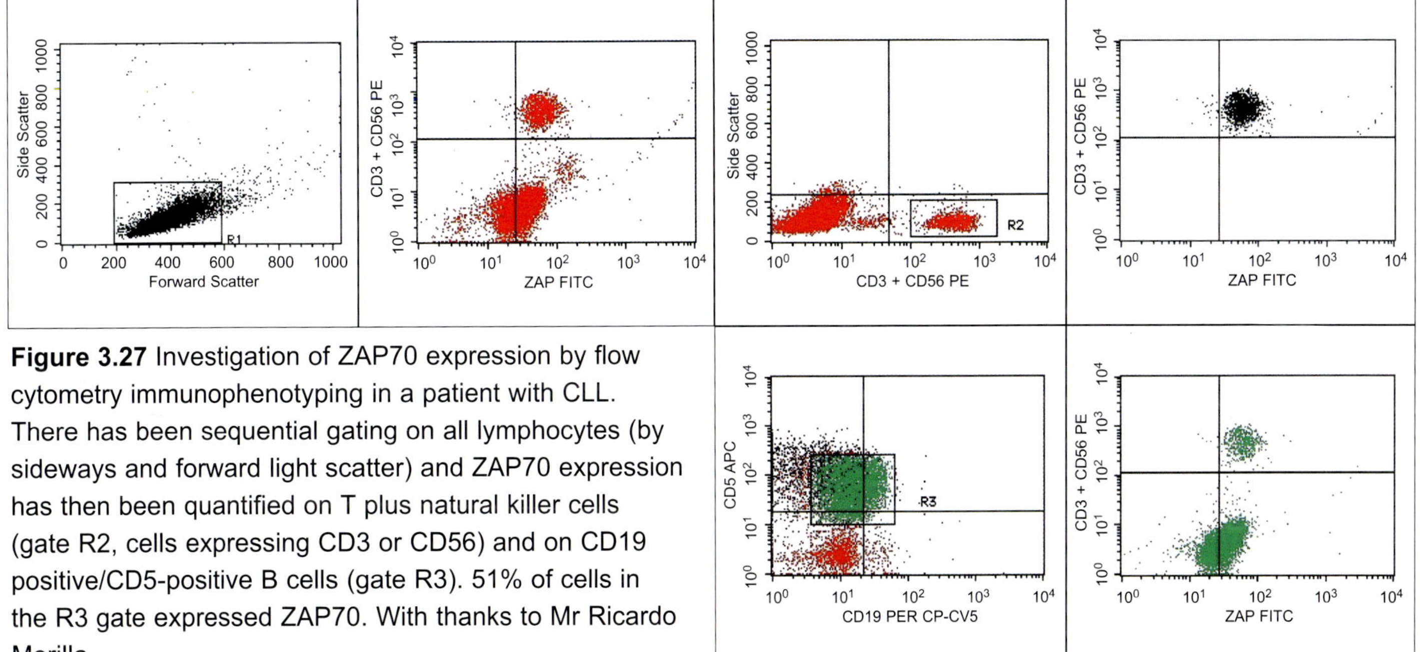

Figure 3.27 Investigation of ZAP70 expression by flow cytometry immunophenotyping in a patient with CLL. There has been sequential gating on all lymphocytes (by sideways and forward light scatter) and ZAP70 expression has then been quantified on T plus natural killer cells (gate R2, cells expressing CD3 or CD56) and on CD19 positive/CD5-positive B cells (gate R3). 51% of cells in the R3 gate expressed ZAP70. With thanks to Mr Ricardo Morilla.

Table 3.2 A scoring system for the immunophenotypic diagnosis of chronic lymphocytic leukaemia [8]

Score 1 for each of the following:

- Weak expression of SmIg
- Expression of CD5
- Expression of CD23
- No expression of FMC7
- Absent or weak expression of CD79b (or CD22)

A score of ≥4 is confirmatory of CLL

CLL, chronic lymphocytic leukaemia; SmIg, surface membrane immunoglobulin

Cytogenetic and molecular genetic abnormalities

There is no single cytogenetic abnormality characteristic of CLL. Fluorescence *in situ* hybridization (FISH) analysis is much more informative than standard cytogenetic analysis since the leukaemic cells often do not enter mitosis. Recurrent abnormalities observed include del(6)(q21), del(13)(q14), del(11)(q23), trisomy 12 and del(17)(p21) [14, 15]. Advanced disease can be associated with deletion or increased expression of *TP53* at 17p13 (increased expression being indicative of mutation) and both deletion and mutation of *ATM* at 11q23 [16–18]. Cells from close to one-half of CLL cases show somatic hypermutation of the variable region of the immunoglobulin heavy chain gene, this correlating with a better prognosis [19–21] and correlating inversely with CD38 and ZAP70 expression.

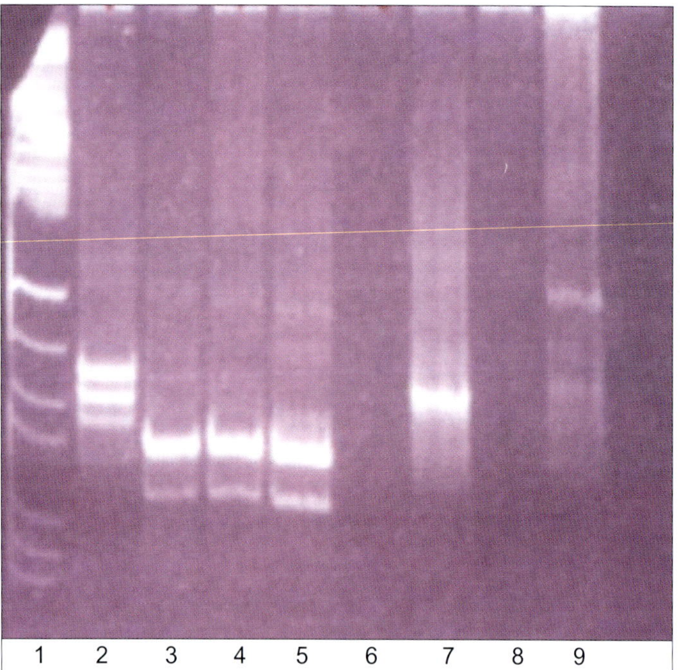

Figure **3.28** Polymerase chain reaction on DNA of two patients with EBV-positive Richter's syndrome. Lanes 3 and 4 represent a pre-transformation sample of a patient whose post-transformation sample in lane 5 shows an identical band, indicating that transformation of a clonal CLL B cell has occurred. Lane 7 is a pre-transformation sample of another patient whose post-transformation sample (lane 9) shows a second different band indicating a second clone and therefore transformation of a non-CLL B cell.

Nevertheless, cases of CLL showing and not showing hypermutation have a homogeneous gene expression profile [22], similar to that of a normal memory B-cell rather than a naïve B-cell.

In Richter's syndrome, investigation of rearrangement of immunoglobulin genes can be used to show whether a transformation event occurred in the original clone or in a 'bystander' lymphocyte (Figure **3.28**).

Diagnosis and differential diagnosis

The diagnosis of CLL requires immunophenotyping as well as cytological assessment. The differential diagnosis includes non-Hodgkin's lymphoma, particularly splenic marginal zone lymphoma, follicular lymphoma, mantle cell lymphoma, large granular lymphocyte leukaemia and the small cell variant of T-lineage prolymphocytic leukaemia. Although cytological features can sometimes be confusing, particularly in the case of the mixed cell type of CLL, the distinction is usually readily made by immunophenotyping. However, if the CLL score is 3 rather than 4 or 5 it is important to carry out further tests to exclude non-Hodgkin's lymphoma. CLL also needs to be distinguished from monoclonal B-cell lymphocytosis of undetermined significance in which the peripheral blood contains clonal B cells with a similar immunophenotype to that of CLL but the number is insufficient for a diagnosis of CLL and the tissue manifestations of small lymphocytic lymphoma are also absent. Some such individuals subsequently show progression to CLL but long term studies are needed to assess the frequency with which this occurs.

Prognosis

The prognosis of CLL depends on the stage of the disease and on a number of biological variables, which are summarized in *Table 3.3*. Loss or mutation of *TP53* correlates with lack of response to alkylating agents and purine analogues.

Table 3.3 Prognostic factors in chronic lymphocytic leukaemia

Variable	*Better prognosis*	*Worse prognosis*
Gender	Female	Male
Stage	Non-progressive stage A	Progressive stage A, stage B or stage C
Doubling time of lymphocyte count	Greater than 12 months	Less than 12 months
Lymphocyte count in Binet stage A patients	Less than 30 x 10^9/l	Greater than 30 x 10^9/l
Prolymphocytes in blood	Absent	Present
Bone marrow pattern of infiltration	Interstitial, nodular or mixed	'Packed marrow' pattern
Serum CD23, serum CD138, β2-microglobulin, lactate dehydrogenase	Lower levels	Higher levels
ZAP70 expression*	Not expressed	Expressed
CD38*	Not expressed	Expressed
Somatic hypermutation of IG_VH genes*	Mutated (post-germinal centre memory B-cell genotype) or use of VH3.21	Unmutated (naïve pre-germinal centre genotype) or use of VH3.21 whether mutated or unmutated
Cytogenetic abnormalities	Del(6)(q21), del(13)(q14), no abnormality detected. Del(11)(q23) and trisomy 12 intermediate	Del(17)(p13)
Molecular genetic abnormalities		*TP53* or *ATM* mutation

* Inter-related but independent prognostic factors

Treatment

In non-progressive stage A disease no treatment is indicated. Treatment is usually considered indicated in progressive stage A disease and in stage B and C disease [23]. Standard first line treatment is chlorambucil, although fludarabine, which is associated with a faster and more complete response, is increasingly being used as first line rather than second line treatment either as single agent or in combination with cyclophosphamide. Despite the weak expression of CD20, treatment with rituximab is of some benefit, particularly in combination with chemotherapy. Alemtuzumab (anti-CD52) therapy may be useful but not in those with bulky lymphadenopathy. Splenectomy is sometimes useful for cytopenia in patients with significant splenomegaly. More experimental treatments applicable to younger patients include autologous and allogeneic stem cell transplantation, the latter with a non-myeloablative conditioning regime. Autoimmune complications require treatment in their own right with corticosteroids and other immunosuppressive agents.

References

1. Bennett JM, Catovsky D, Daniel M-T, Flandrin G, Galton DAG, Gralnick HR and Sultan C (1989). Proposals for the classification of chronic (mature) B and T lymphoid leukaemias. *J Clin Pathol*, **42**, 567–584.
2. Caligaris-Cappio F (1996). B-chronic lymphocytic leukemia: a malignancy of anti-self B cells. *Blood*, **87**, 2615–2620.

3. Müller-Hermelink HK, Catovsky D, Montserrat E and Harris NL (2001). Chronic lymphocytic leukaemia/small lymphocytic lymphoma. *In* Jaffe ES, Harris NL, Stein H and Vardiman JW (Eds). *World Health Organization Classification of Tumours: Pathology and Genetics of Tumours of Haematopoietic and Lymphoid Tissues*, IARC Press, Lyon, pp. 127–130.
4. Yuille MR, Matutes E, Marossy A, Hilditch B, Catovsky D and Houlston RS (2000). Familial chronic lymphocytic leukaemia: A survey and review of published studies. *Br J Haematol*, **109**, 794–799.
5. Rawstron AC, Yuille MR, Fuller J, Cullen M, Kennedy B, Richards SJ *et al.* (2002). Inherited predisposition to CLL is detectable as subclinical monoclonal B-lymphocyte expansion. *Blood*, **100**, 2289–2290.
6. Thornton PD, Bellas C, Santon A, Shah G, Pocock C, Wotherspoon AC, Matutes E and Catovsky D (2005). Richter's transformation of chronic lymphocytic leukemia. The possible role of fludarabine and the Epstein–Barr virus in its pathogenesis. *Leuk Res*, **29**, 389–395.
7. Binet JL, Auquier A, Dighiero G, Chastang C, Piguet H, Goasguen J *et al.* (1981). A new prognostic classification of chronic lymphocytic leukemia derived from multivariate survival analysis. *Cancer*, **48**, 198–206.
8. Matutes E and Polliack A (2000). Morphological and immunophenotypic features of chronic lymphocytic leukemia. *Rev Clin Exp Haematol*, **4**, 22–47.
9. Delgado J, Matutes E, Morilla AM, Morilla RM, Owusu-Ankomah KA, Rafiq-Mohammed F, del Giudice I and Catovsky D (2003). Diagnostic significance of CD20 and FMC7 expression in B-cell disorders. *Am J Clin Pathol*, **120**, 754–759.
10. Damle RN, Wasil T, Fais F, Ghiotto F, Valetto A, Allen SL *et al.* (1999). Ig V gene mutation status and CD38 expression as novel prognostic indicators in chronic lymphocytic leukemia. *Blood*, **94**, 1840–1847.
11. Ibrahim S, Keating M, Do K-A, O'Brien S, Huh YO, Jilani I *et al.* (2001). CD38 expression as an important prognostic factor in B-cell chronic lymphocytic leukemia. *Blood*, **98**,181–186.
12. Chen L, Widhopf G, Huynh L, Rassenti L, Rai KR, Weiss A and Kipps TJ (2002). Expression of ZAP-70 is associated with increased B-cell receptor signaling in chronic lymphocytic leukemia. *Blood*, **100**, 4609–4614.
13. Crespo M, Bosch F, Villamor N, Bellosillo B, Colomer D, Rozman M *et al.* (2003). ZAP-70 expression as a surrogate for immunoglobulin-variable-region mutations in chronic lymphocytic leukemia. *N Engl J Med*, **348**, 1764–1775.
14. Juliusson G, Oscier DG, Fitchett M, Ross FM, Stockdill G, Mackie MJ *et al.* (1990). Prognostic subgroups in B-cell chronic lymphocytic leukemia defined by specific chromosomal abnormalities. *N Engl J Med*, **323**, 720–724.
15. Matutes E, Oscier D, Garcia-Marco J, Ellis J, Copplestone A, Gillingham R *et al.* (1996). Trisomy 12 defines a group of CLL with atypical morphology: correlation between cytogenetic, clinical and laboratory features in 544 patients. *Br J Haematol*, **92**, 382–388.
16. Dohner H, Fischer K, Bentz M, Hansen K, Benner A, Cabot G *et al.* (1995). p53 gene deletion predicts poor survival and non-response to therapy with purine analogs in chronic B-cell leukemias. *Blood*, **85**, 1580–1589.
17. Lens D, Dyer MJ, Garcia-Marco JM, de Schouwer PJ, Hamoudi RA, Jones D *et al.* (1997). p53 abnormalities in CLL are associated with excess of prolymphocytes and poor prognosis. *Br J Haematol*, **99**, 848–857.
18. Dohner H, Stilgenbauer S, Benner A, Leupolt E, Krober A, Bullinger L *et al.* (2000). Genomic aberrations and survival in chronic lymphocytic leukemia. *New Engl J Med*, **343**,1910–1916.
19. Hamblin TJ, Davis Z, Gardiner A, Oscier DG and Stevenson FK (1999). Unmutated Ig V(H) genes are associated with a more aggressive form of chronic lymphocytic leukemia. *Blood*, **94**, 1848–1854.
20. Matrai Z, Lin K, Dennis M, Sherrington P, Zuzel M, Pettitt AR and Cawley JC (2001). CD38 expression and Ig VH gene mutation in B-cell chronic lymphocytic leukemia. *Blood*, **97**, 1902–1903.
21. Rassenti LZ, Huynh L, Toy TL, Chen L, Keating MJ, Gribben JG *et al.* (2004). ZAP-70 compared with immunoglobulin heavy-chain gene mutation status as a predictor of disease progression in chronic lymphocytic leukemia. *New Engl J Med*, **351**, 893–901.
22. Klein U, Tu Y, Stolovitzky GA, Mattiolo M, Cattoretti G, Husson H, Freedman A *et al.* (2001). Gene expression profiling of B cell chronic lymphocytic leukemia reveals a homogeneous phenotype related to memory B cells. *J Exp Med*, **194**, 1625–1638.
23. Oscier D, Fegan C, Hillmen P, Illidge T, Johnson S, Maguire P, Matutes E and Milligan D; Guidelines Working group of the UK CLL Forum. British Committee for Standards in Haematology (2004). Guidelines on the diagnosis and management of chronic lymphocytic leukaemia. *Br J Haematol*, **125**, 294–317.

Chapter 4

Prolymphocytic leukaemia

Prolymphocytic leukaemia (PLL) is a rare lymphoproliferative disorder resulting from a clonal proliferation of mature B lymphocytes with specific cytological features [1]. Prognosis is generally poor but a more indolent form of the disease has also been recognized [2].

Clinical features

The disease affects mainly the elderly and is more common in men than in women. Splenomegaly is characteristic with lymphadenopathy usually being minor.

Haematological and pathological features

The white cell count is often high and about half of patients have anaemia and thrombocytopenia. In one study prolymphocytes constituted more than 55% of circulating cells and this was suggested as a diagnostic cut-off point [3]. However, it should be noted that a large proportion of prolymphocytes is also occasionally observed in advanced chronic lymphocytic leukaemia (CLL) and this cut-off point is therefore arbitrary. Prolymphocytes are medium to large lymphoid cells with a single prominent nucleolus (Figures **4.1**–**4.3**); perinucleolar chromatin condensation gives the

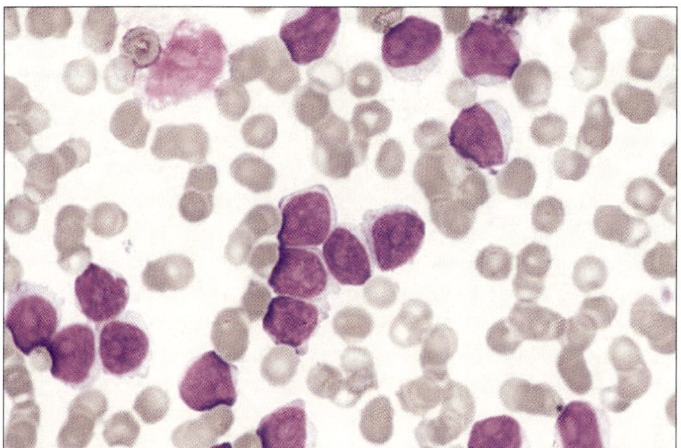

Figure 4.1 Peripheral blood film from a patient with PLL showing one smear cell and a fairly uniform population of medium sized lymphoid cells with large prominent nucleoli. Romanowsky stain, x 60 objective.

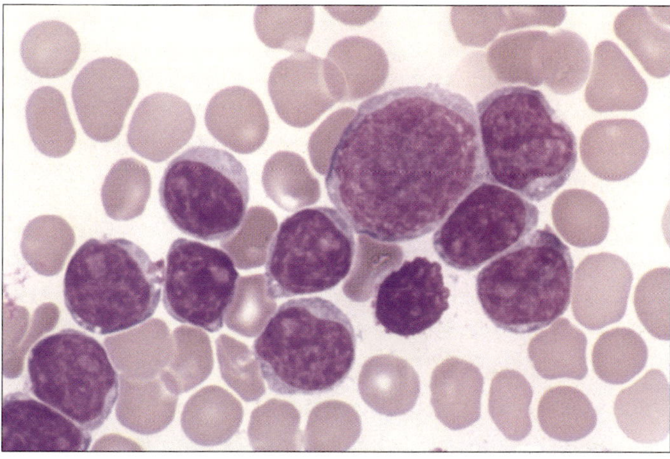

Figure 4.2 Peripheral blood film from a patient with PLL showing mainly medium sized prolymphocytes and one very large cell. Romanowsky stain, x 100 objective.

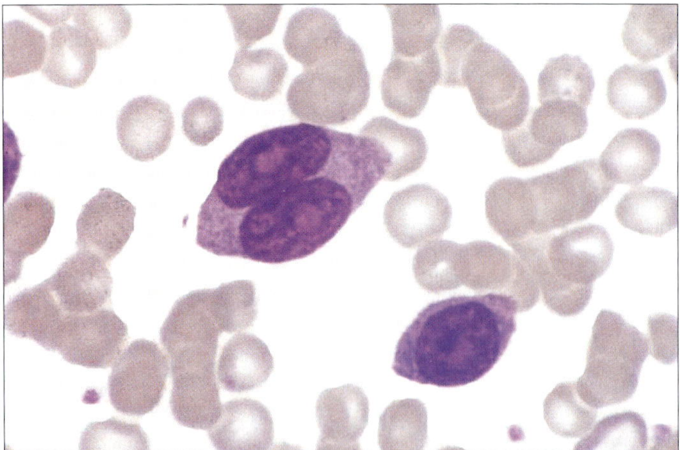

Figure 4.3 Peripheral blood film from a patient with PLL showing two prolymphocytes, one of which is binucleated. Romanowsky stain, x 100 objective.

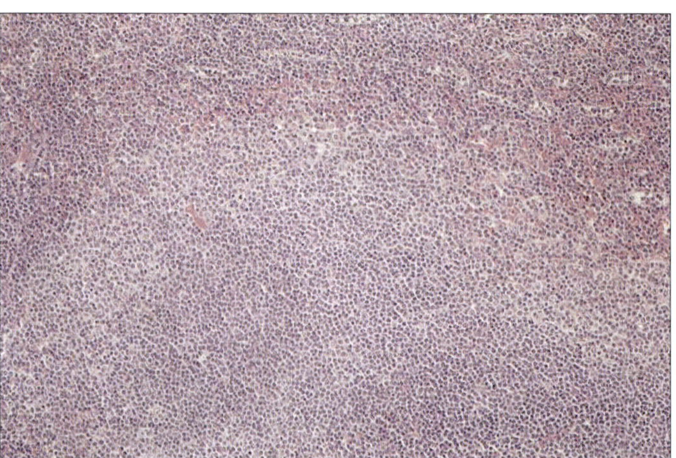

Figure 4.4 Section of spleen from a patient with PLL showing prominent white pulp infiltration. H&E, x 10 objective.

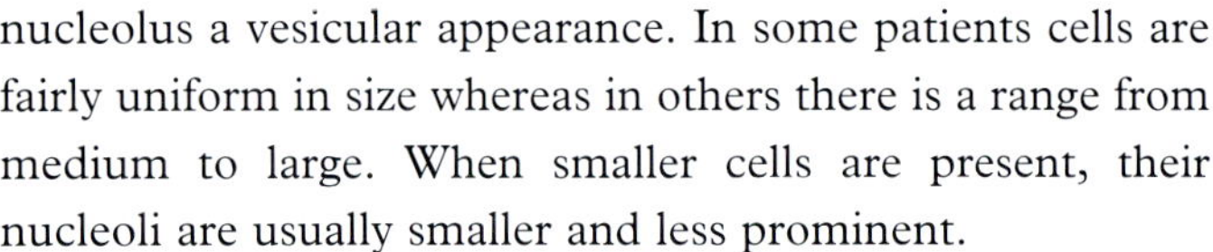

nucleolus a vesicular appearance. In some patients cells are fairly uniform in size whereas in others there is a range from medium to large. When smaller cells are present, their nucleoli are usually smaller and less prominent.

The trephine biopsy shows an interstitial/nodular or diffuse pattern of infiltration. Lymph node infiltration is diffuse, sometimes with a vaguely nodular pattern. Splenic infiltration is in both red and white pulp and in the white pulp it may be nodular (Figures **4.4** and **4.5**).

A low concentration paraprotein, most often IgM, may be present.

Immunophenotype

The immunophenotype (Figure **4.6**) is often not distinguishable from that of non-Hodgkin's lymphoma (NHL) but in some patients it is intermediate between that typical of CLL and that of NHL. There is usually strong expression of IgM, with or without IgD, and strong expression of pan-B markers CD19, CD20, CD22 and CD79b. FMC7 and CD11c are usually expressed. CD10, CD23 and CD25 are not usually expressed. CD5 expression has been reported in about one-third of patients; some of these cases may represent misdiagnosed mantle cell lymphoma (see below) while others are *bona fide* PLL. On immunohistochemistry there is expression of CD20 and CD79a. Cyclin D1 expression has been reported but requires re-evaluation, because of the possibility that such cases were actually mantle cell lymphoma. B-PLL is heterogeneous with regard to CD38 and ZAP70 expression and IG_VH mutational status; CD38 expression and IG_VH mutations are of no prognostic significance whereas ZAP70 correlates with a better prognosis (in contrast to CLL) [4].

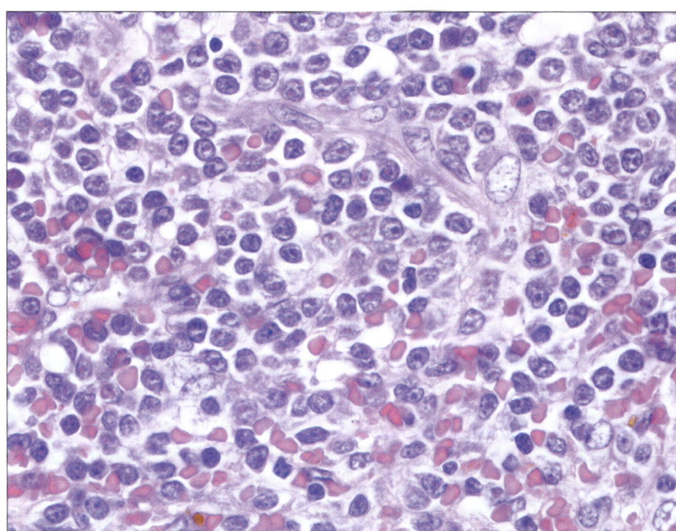

Figure 4.5 Section of spleen from a patient with PLL showing large cells with large nuclei containing prominent eosinophilic nucleoli. H&E, x 100 objective.

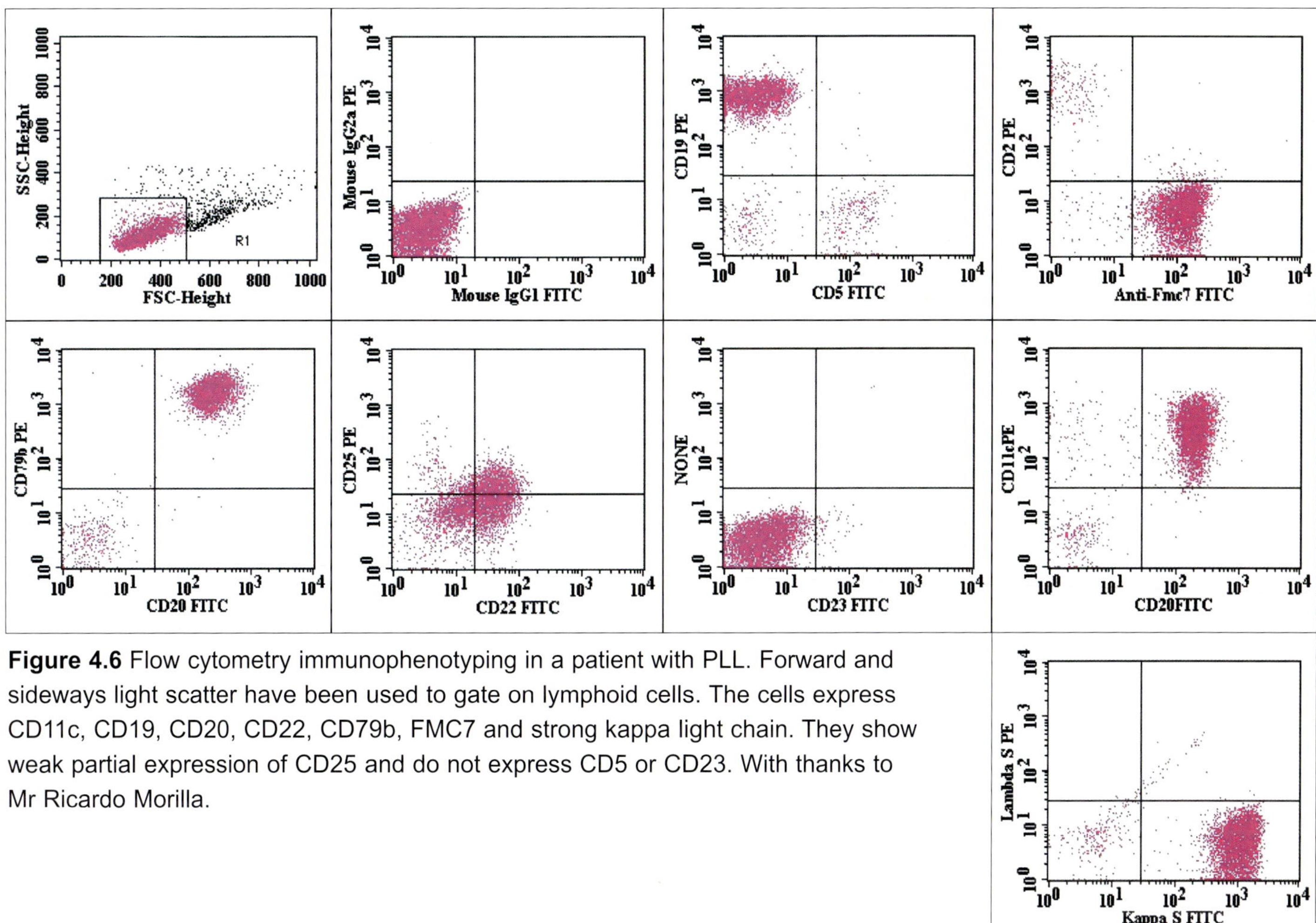

Figure 4.6 Flow cytometry immunophenotyping in a patient with PLL. Forward and sideways light scatter have been used to gate on lymphoid cells. The cells express CD11c, CD19, CD20, CD22, CD79b, FMC7 and strong kappa light chain. They show weak partial expression of CD25 and do not express CD5 or CD23. With thanks to Mr Ricardo Morilla.

Cytogenetic and molecular genetic abnormalities

There is no specific cytogenetic or molecular genetic abnormality. About 20% of cases have been found to have t(11;14) but it is likely that this represents misdiagnosis of mantle cell lymphoma [5]. Deletions of 6q, 11q23 and 13q14, trisomy 3 and mutation of *TP53* are very frequent [6, 7].

Diagnosis and differential diagnosis

The differential diagnosis includes NHL, the mixed cell type of CLL (CLL/PL) and hairy cell leukaemia variant. It is important to recognize cases of mantle cell lymphoma with prolymphocytoid morphology in the peripheral blood [5]. The presence of t(11;14) and expression of CD5 and cyclin D1 permit the distinction.

Prognosis

The prognosis is worse than that of CLL, with the median survival being around 3 years. A high white cell count and anaemia are indicative of a worse prognosis.

Treatment

There is sometimes a response to combination chemotherapy or nucleoside analogues but treatment response is generally poor.

References

1. Galton DAG, Goldman JM, Wiltshaw E, Catovsky D, Henry K and Goldenberg GJ (1974). Prolymphocytic leukaemia. *Br J Haematol*, **27**, 7–23.
2. Shvidel L, Shtalrid M, Bassous L, Klepfish A, Vorst E and Berrebi A (1999). B-cell prolymphocytic leukemia: a survey of 35 patients emphasizing heterogeneity, prognostic factors and evidence for a group with an indolent course. *Leuk Lymphoma*, **33**, 169–179.
3. Melo JV, Catovsky D and Galton DAG (1986). The relationship between chronic lymphocytic leukaemia and prolymphocytic leukaemia. I. Clinical and laboratory features of 300 patients and characterisation of an intermediate group. *Br J Haematol*, **63**, 377–387.
4. Del Guidice I, Davis Z, Matutes E, Osuji N, Parry-Jones N, Morilla A *et al.* (2006). B-cell IgVH genes mutation and usage, ZAP-70 and CD38 expression provide new insights on prolymphocytic leukaemia (B-PLL). *Leukemia*, **20**, 1231–1237.
5. Ruchlemer R, Parry-Jones N, Brito-Babapulle V, Attolico I, Wotherspoon AC, Matutes E and Catovsky D (2004). B-prolymphocytic leukaemia with t(11;14) revisited: a splenomegalic form of mantle cell lymphoma evolving with leukaemia. *Br J Haematol*, **125**, 330–336.
6. Lens D, Matutes E, Catovsky D and Coignet LJA (2000). Frequent deletions at 11q23 and 13q14 in B cell prolymphocytic leukemia (B-PLL). *Leukemia*, **14**, 427–430.
7. Lens D, de Schouwer PJ, Hamoudi RA, Abdul-Rauf M, Farahat N, Matutes E, Crook T, Dyer MJ and Catovsky D (1997). p53 abnormalities in B-cell prolymphocytic leukemia. *Blood*, **89**, 2015–2023.

Chapter 5

Follicular lymphoma

Follicular lymphoma is also referred to as follicle centre cell lymphoma and was previously known as poorly differentiated lymphocytic lymphoma and centroblastic/centrocytic lymphoma. It is a disease of adult life, occurring in young, middle aged and elderly adults. It is rare in children and adolescents. In contrast to most other lymphoproliferative disorders, there is a somewhat higher incidence in women. It is a low-grade malignancy. Although many patients (around 80%) present with widespread disease, median survival is of the order of 9 to 10 years. Follicular lymphoma arises from a germinal centre B cell showing ongoing somatic hypermutation of IG_VH.

Clinical features

Patients usually present with lymphadenopathy [1]. Sometimes the spleen is also enlarged and Waldeyer's ring may be involved. Occasionally the diagnosis is incidental in an asymptomatic patient. Even widespread disease is often relatively asymptomatic but some patients with advanced disease have B symptoms (fever, weight loss and night sweats). Patients with advanced disease may have pleural or pericardial effusions or ascites. Spontaneous remissions, with subsequent relapse, are sometimes observed. Rarely, a spontaneous remission occurs and on prolonged follow-up there is no relapse. Transformation to diffuse high-grade B-cell lymphoma can occur. Follicular lymphoma of the skin differs somewhat from other follicular lymphomas in its pathological features.

Haematological and pathological features

The peripheral blood may be normal or there may be a greater or lesser number of circulating lymphoma cells [2]. Cytological characteristics differ between patients (Figures **5.1–5.3**). Some patients, particularly those with large numbers of circulating lymphoma cells, have very small cells, smaller than those of chronic lymphocytic leukaemia, with scanty cytoplasm; the nuclei show evenly condensed (rather than clumped) chromatin and deep, very narrow clefts. In other patients the cells are larger and more pleomorphic with less condensed cytoplasm and often a visible nucleolus; some cells have nuclear clefts, which are characteristically deep and narrow with parallel edges. Cells are less fragile than those of chronic lymphocytic leukaemia so that smear cells are less often a feature. Anaemia and thrombocytopenia are uncommon at presentation, but may be seen in patients with advanced disease.

The bone marrow is infiltrated in around half of patients. A trephine biopsy characteristically shows paratrabecular infiltration with a variable degree of interstitial infiltration (Figures **5.4** and **5.5**) and, in patients with advanced disease, a 'packed marrow' pattern. A follicular pattern detectable on an H&E stain is decidedly unusual in the bone marrow (Figure **5.6**) but when present the follicle centres are BCL2 positive. Often the bone marrow shows only small cells (centrocytes) when lymph node biopsy shows both small and large (centrocytes and centroblasts). Reticulin deposition is increased in infiltrated areas and serves to highlight them. A trephine biopsy is more sensitive than a bone marrow aspirate for the detection of infiltration. Sometimes the aspirate is normal both on light microscopy and on flow cytometry immunophenotyping despite trephine biopsy sections showing paratrabecular infiltration.

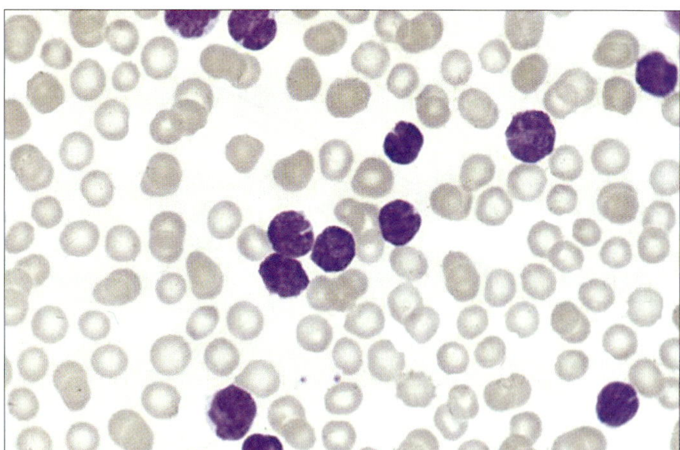

Figure 5.1 Peripheral blood film in follicular lymphoma showing mature lymphocytes with cleft nuclei and condensed chromatin. Romanowsky, x 60 objective.

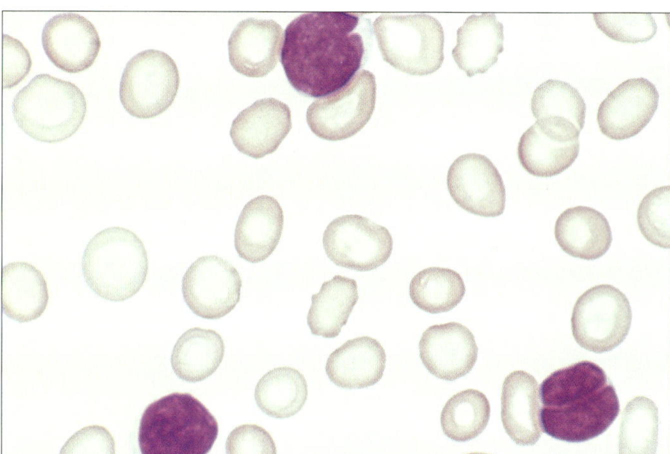

Figure 5.2 Peripheral blood film in follicular lymphoma showing showing mature lymphocytes with very scanty cytoplasm and in two of the three cells, cleft or notched nuclei; chromatin is fairly evenly condensed. Romanowsky, x 100 objective.

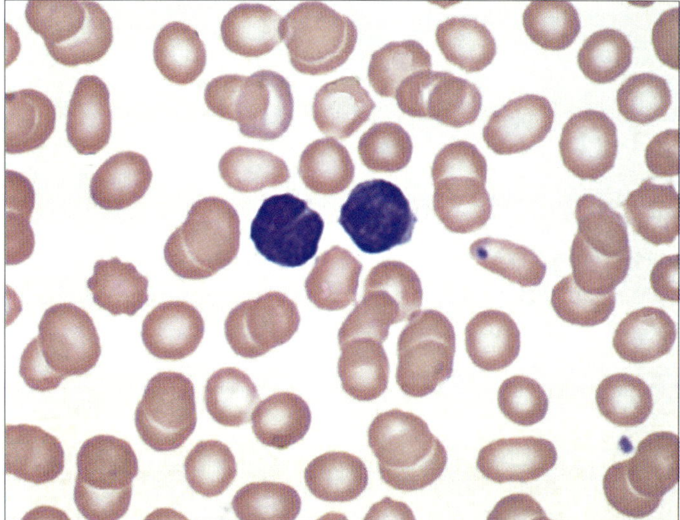

Figure 5.3 Peripheral blood film in follicular lymphoma showing two lymphoma cells, one of which has a nuclear cleft. Romanowsky, x 100 objective.

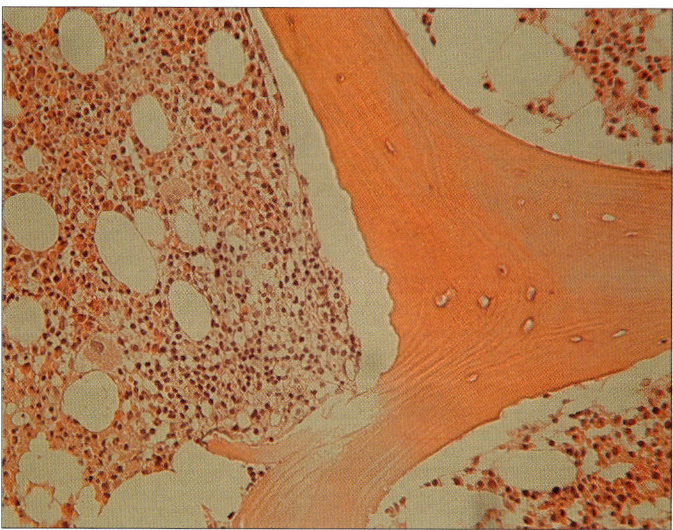

Figure 5.4 Trephine biopsy section from a patient with follicular lymphoma showing paratrabecular infiltration. H&E, x 4 objective. With thanks to Dr Alexandra Rice.

Immunohistochemistry (see below) is useful for showing the extent of disease and for detecting small inconspicuous infiltrates.

Lymph node biopsy shows a follicular pattern with the dominant cell usually being a small angular cell, analogous to a centrocyte. Follicles have lost their normal zoning and the mantle zone and marginal zone are inconspicuous or absent. Macrophages are inconspicuous. The proportion of large cells, centroblasts, differs between individuals and in the WHO classification this has been used to grade disease as grade 1, grade 2, grade 3a or grade 3b [3] (Figures **5.7–5.10**). There may be some areas of an involved lymph node showing diffuse infiltration and sometimes histology shows only minimal follicularity. Grades 1–3a tend to behave as low-grade lymphomas whereas the behaviour of grade 3b lymphoma may be more aggressive, similar to that of diffuse large B-cell (centroblastic) lymphoma.

High-grade transformation is characterized by large cells,

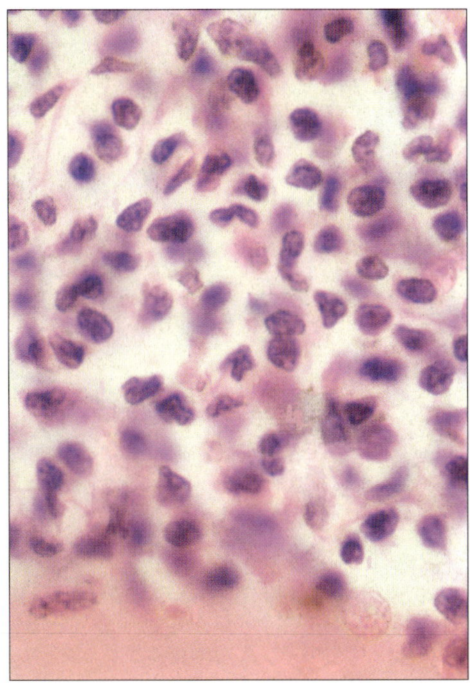

Figure 5.5 Trephine biopsy section from a patient with follicular lymphoma showing infiltration by small angular cells. H&E, x 100 objective.

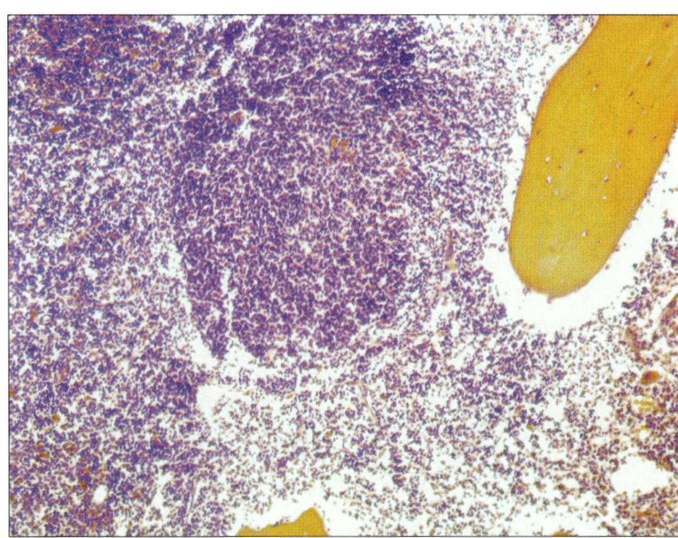

Figure 5.6 Trephine biopsy section from a patient with follicular lymphoma showing a 'packed marrow' pattern with follicle formation. H&E, x 40 objective.

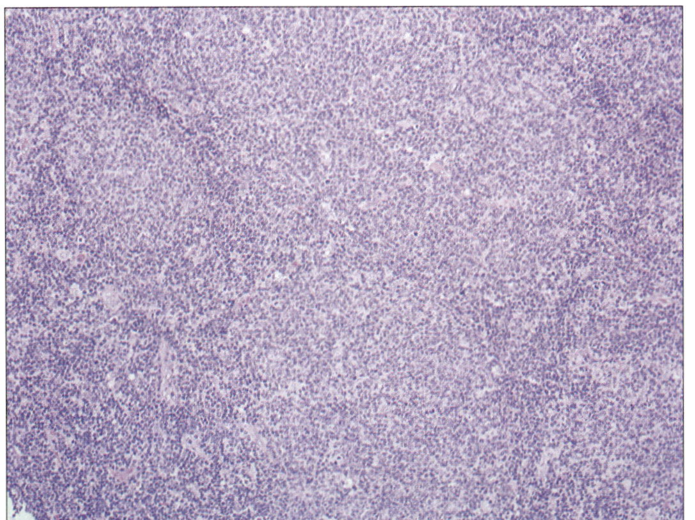

Figure 5.7 Section of lymph node biopsy from a patient with grade 1 follicular lymphoma. H&E, x 20 objective.

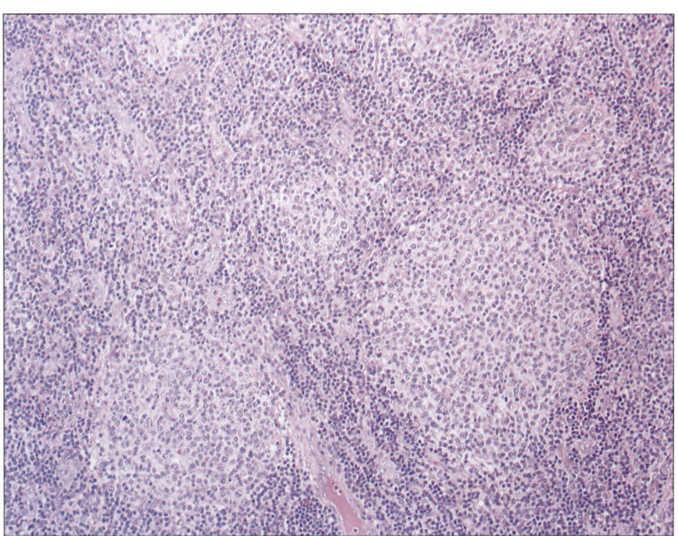

Figure 5.8 Section of lymph node biopsy from a patient with grade 2 follicular lymphoma. H&E, x 20 objective.

often with cleft or irregular nuclei and prominent nucleoli (Figures **5.11** and **5.12**).

Cutaneous follicular lymphoma (Figure **5.13**) appears to be a somewhat different disease from node-based follicular lymphoma. In this condition, follicle centre cells do not usually express BCL2 and the cytogenetic abnormalities typical of node-based lymphoma are not present.

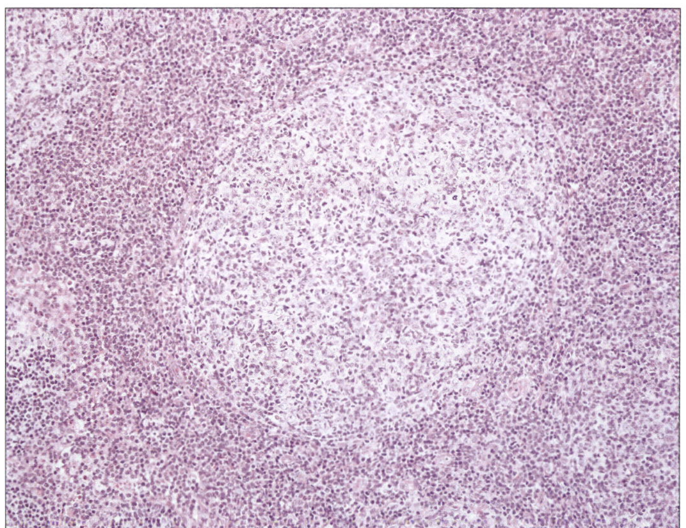

Figure 5.9 Section of lymph node biopsy from a patient with grade 3a follicular lymphoma. H&E, x 20 objective.

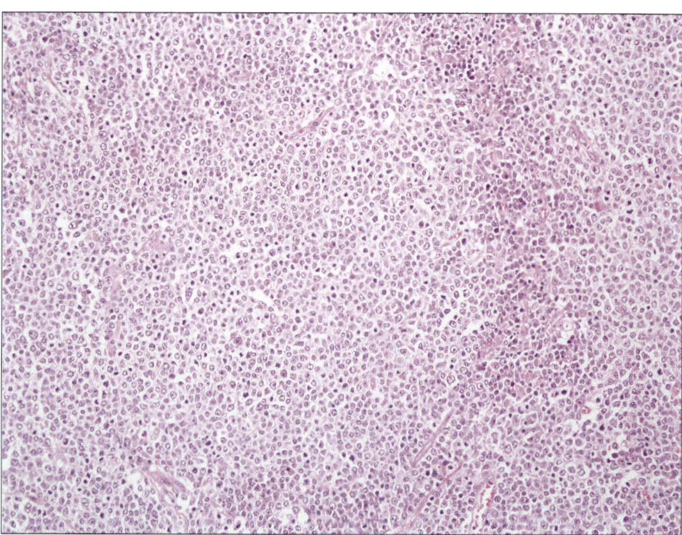

Figure 5.10 Section of lymph node biopsy from a patient with grade 3b follicular lymphoma. H&E, x 20 objective.

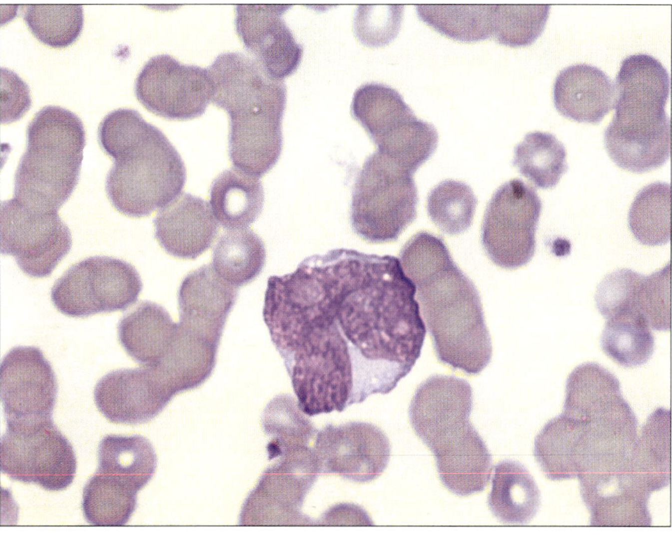

Figure 5.11 Peripheral blood film from a patient with high-grade transformation of follicular lymphoma showing a large lymphoma cell with a deeply cleft nucleus with giant nucleoli. Romanowsky, x 100 objective.

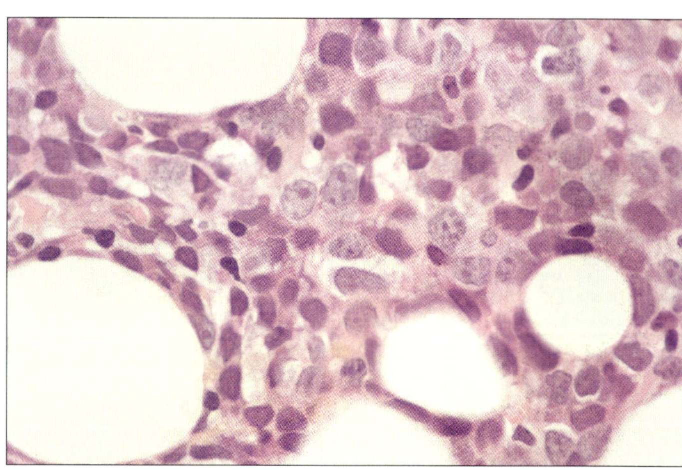

Figure 5.12 Trephine biopsy section from a patient with high-grade transformation of follicular lymphoma showing interstitial infiltration by large nucleolated cells. H&E, x 100 objective.

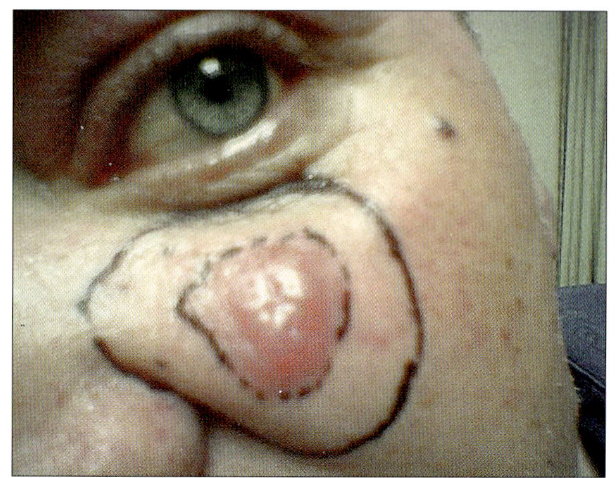

Figure 5.13 Clinical photograph of a patient with a cutaneous follicular lymphoma. With thanks to Dr S. Cleator and the patient.

Immunophenotype

The immunophenotype is that of non-Hodgkin's lymphoma with moderately strong monotypic expression of surface membrane immunoglobulin (usually IgM plus IgD) and expression of pan-B markers such as CD19, CD20, CD22, CD24, CD79a, CD79b and FMC7 (Figure **5.14**). CD5, CD11c, CD23, CD25 and CD103 are not usually expressed. However, in up to one-quarter of patients expression of CD5 is detected. CD10 is often expressed, expression being weaker than in acute lymphoblastic leukaemia.

On immunohistochemical staining of lymph node sections, the follicle centres express BCL2 (Figure **5.15**), whereas in follicular hyperplasia BCL2 is not expressed (see Figure **1.4**). However, sometimes BCL2 is not expressed,

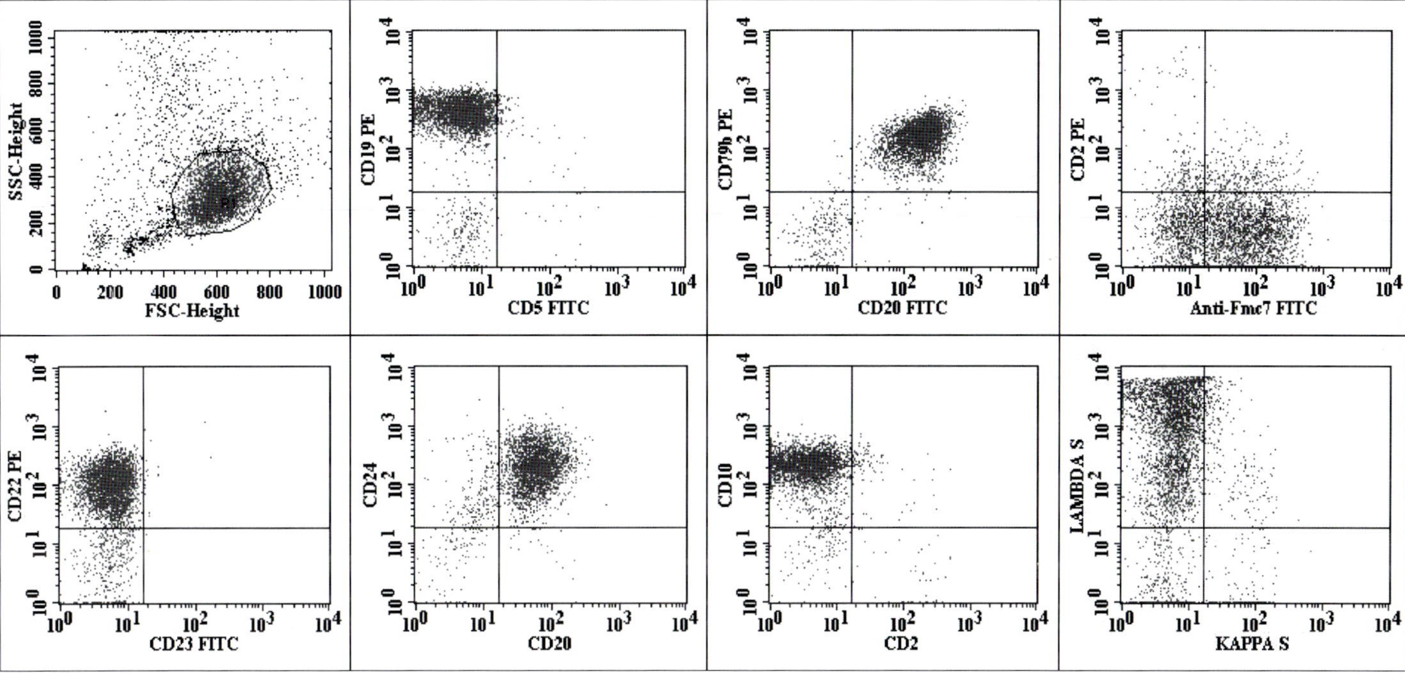

Figure 5.14 Flow cytometry immunophenotyping from a patient with follicular lymphoma. Forward and sideways light scatter have been used to gate on lymphocytes. These express CD10, CD19, CD20, CD22, CD24, CD79b, FMC7 and strong λ light chain. They do not express CD5 or CD23. With thanks to Mr Ricardo Morilla.

Figure 5.15 Section of lymph node biopsy from a patient with follicular lymphoma showing that the follicles are BCL2 positive. Immunoperoxidase, x 20 objective.

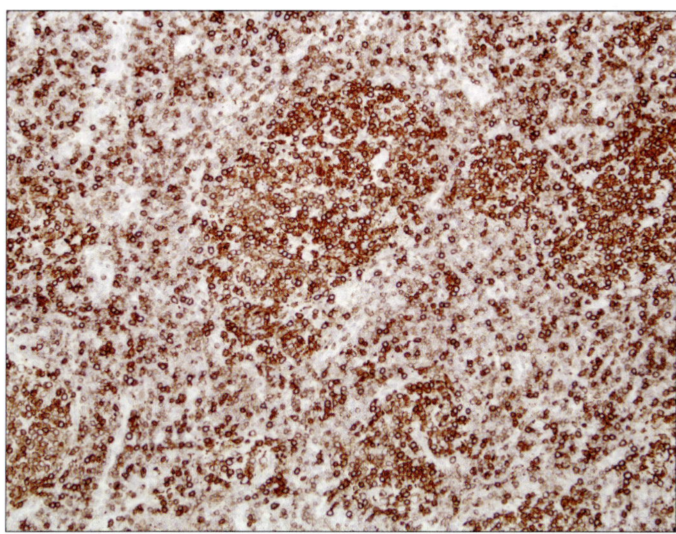

particularly in grade 3 disease. CD10 expression (Figure **5.16**) is often more readily detected by immunohistochemistry than by flow cytometry; CD10-positive neoplastic cells may be found in the interfollicular area as well as within the follicles. BCL6 is expressed (Figure **5.17**). CD43 is usually not expressed. The follicular pattern is highlighted on immunohistochemistry for CD21 or CD23, which shows a network of follicular dendritic cells within the follicles. On trephine biopsy sections, infiltrating cells express CD10, CD20 and CD79a but not CD5 or CD23. BCL2 staining is only useful if interpreted in the context of the architecture [4]. CD3 staining shows that there are some T cells associated with the B-cell infiltrate. Immunohistochemistry is particularly important for assessment of residual disease following immunotherapy. An apparent infiltrate may be found to be just residual T cells.

Cytogenetic and molecular genetic abnormalities

The most characteristic cytogenetic abnormality is t(14;18)(q32;q21) (Figure **5.18**), which leads to dysregulation of *BCL2* at 18q21 by proximity to the immunoglobulin heavy chain gene [5]. In a minority of patients one of the variant translocations, t(2;18)(p12;q21) or t(18;22)(q21;q11), is present; *BCL2* is then dysregulated by proximity to the kappa (κ) or the lambda (λ) gene. One of these three translocations is present in 80–90% of cases of follicular lymphoma. *BCL2* encodes an anti-apoptotic protein, which is believed to contribute to oncogenesis.

In a minority of patients an alternative mechanism of oncogenesis is operating. There is a translocation involving *BCL6* at 3q27, rather than *BCL2*; the most common of these translocations is t(3;14)(q27;q32).

The t(14;18) chromosomal rearrangement can be demonstrated by standard cytogenetic analysis, by fluorescence *in situ* hybridization (FISH) or by both techniques and the molecular rearrangement can also be demonstrated by the polymerase chain reaction (PCR) [6]. FISH analysis with a break-apart *BCL2* probe permits detection of the three rearrangements involving this gene whereas probes for *BCL2* and 14q32 show the most usual t(14;18) rearrangement clearly. *BCL2* expression and t(14;18) are less frequent among large cell follicular lymphoma [7]. There is ongoing IG_VH mutation [8].

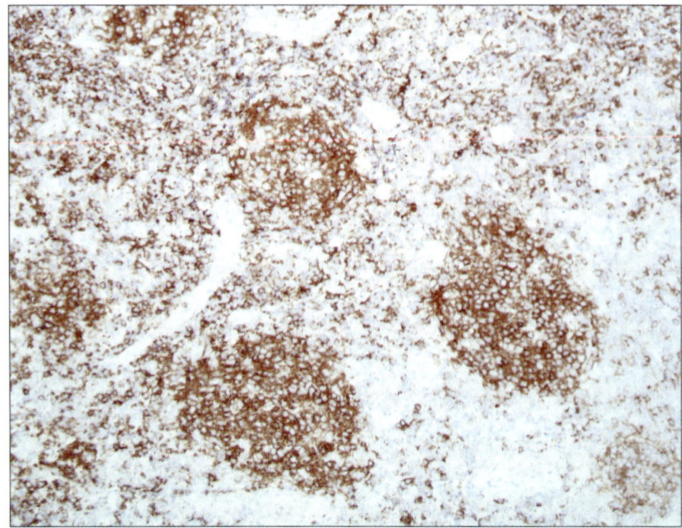

Figure 5.16 Section of lymph node biopsy from a patient with follicular lymphoma showing that the follicles are CD10 positive. There are also CD10-positive lymphocytes in the interfollicular zone whereas normally these are confined to the follicle centre. Immunoperoxidase, x 20 objective.

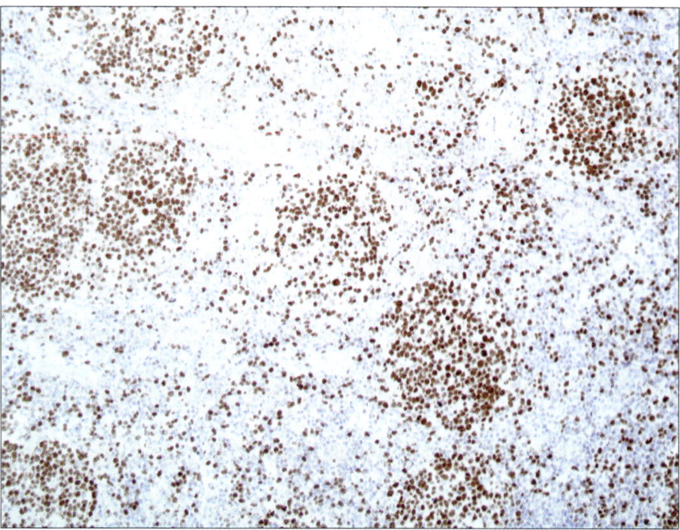

Figure 5.17 Section of lymph node biopsy from a patient with follicular lymphoma showing that the follicles are BCL6 positive. BCL6 is a marker of follicle centre cells. Immunoperoxidase, x 20 objective.

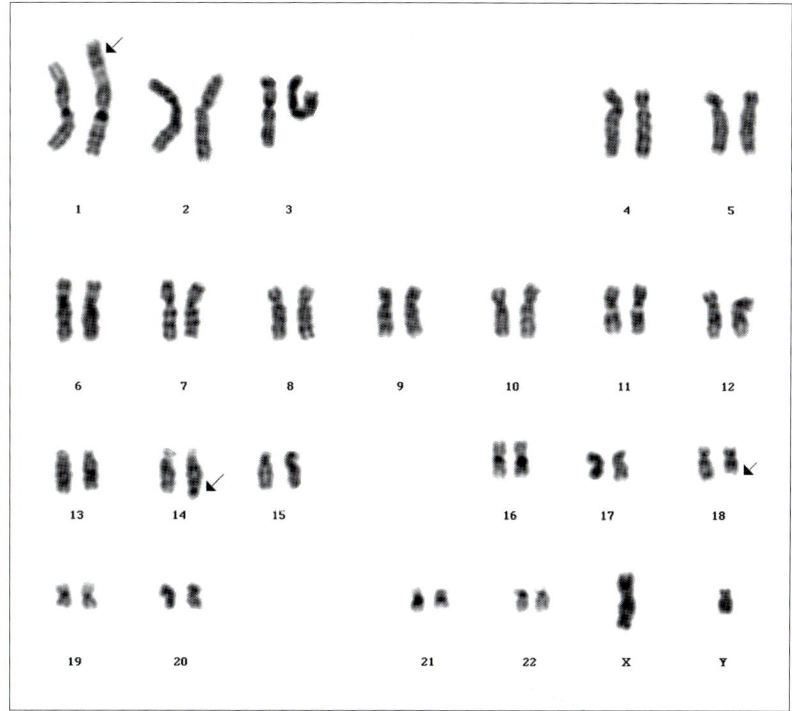

Figure 5.18 Karyogram from a patient with follicular lymphoma showing t(14;18)(q32;q21). There is also additional material added to the short arm of one chromosome 1. The arrows indicate the chromosomes involved in the translocation. With thanks to Dr John Swansbury.

Diagnosis and differential diagnosis

When there is peripheral blood involvement, the differential diagnosis includes chronic lymphocytic leukaemia (CLL), mantle cell lymphoma and other low-grade non-Hodgkin's lymphomas. The immunophenotype is very different from that of CLL but in cases with CD5 expression confusion with atypical CLL or mantle cell lymphoma is possible; lack of expression of cyclin D1 in follicular lymphoma is useful in the latter instance. The differential diagnosis on lymph node biopsy is reactive follicular hyperplasia and nodular lymphocyte-predominant Hodgkin's disease.

Prognosis

Prognosis is related to age of the patient and stage and grade of the disease. A high lactate dehydrogenase (LDH), anaemia and poor performance status are predictive of worse survival. Prognostic markers have been combined in a scoring system, designated Follicular Lymphoma International Prognostic Index (FLIPI) [9]. Microarray analysis may also give prognostic information [10].

Treatment

The minority of patients who present with localized disease are treated with radiotherapy, since this may be curative. In patients with non-localized disease, conventional treatment is not curative and a 'watch and wait' policy is sometimes appropriate. Otherwise treatment is traditionally with non-intensive oral chemotherapy, e.g. with chlorambucil or nucleoside analogues such as fludarabine. Rituximab is likewise effective and a combination of chemotherapy and immunotherapy may be more effective than either alone. Maintenance immunotherapy can improve survival. Radioimmunotherapy with radiolabelled monoclonal antibodies is also possible. Patients with grade 3b disease, and, less often, those with grade 3a disease, may be treated with combination chemotherapy plus immunotherapy. In younger patients allogeneic stem cell transplantation, including stem cell transplantation following non-myeloablative conditioning, requires consideration.

References

1. Armitage JO and Weisenburger DD (1998). New approach to classifying non-Hodgkin's lymphomas: clinical features of the major histologic subtypes. Non-Hodgkin's Lymphoma Classification Project. *J Clin Oncol*, **16**, 2780–2795.
2. Oertel J, Kingree D, Busemann C, Stein H and Dorken B (2002). Morphologic diagnosis of leukaemic B-lymphoproliferative disorders and the role of cyclin D1 expression. *J Cancer Res Clin Oncol*, **128**, 182–188.
3. Ott G, Katzenberger T, Lohr A, Kindelberger S, Rudiger T, Wilhelm M *et al.* (2002). Cytomorphologic, immunohistochemical, and cytogenetic profiles of follicular lymphoma: 2 types of follicular lymphoma grade 3. *Blood*, **99**, 3806–3812.
4. West R, Warnke R and Natkunam Y (2002). The usefulness of immunohistochemistry in the diagnosis of follicular lymphoma in bone marrow biopsy specimens. *Am J Clin Pathol*, **117**, 636–643.
5. de Jong D (2005). Molecular pathogenesis of follicular lymphoma: a cross talk of genetic and immunologic factors. *J Clin Oncol*, **23**, 6358–6363.
6. Horsman DE, Gascoyne RD, Coupland RW, Coldman AJ and Adomat SA (1995). Comparison of cytogenetic analysis, southern blot analysis, and polymerase chain reaction for the detection of t(14;18) in follicular lymphoma. *Am J Clin Pathol*, **103**, 472–478.
7. Weisenburger DD, Gascoyne RD, Bierman PJ, Shenkier T, Horsman D, Lynch JC *et al.* (2000). Clinical significance of the t(14;18) and BCL2 overexpression in follicular large cell lymphoma. *Leuk Lymphoma*, **36**, 513–523.
8. Ottensmeier CH, Thompsett AR, Zhu D, Wilkins BS, Sweetenham JV and Stevenson FK (1998). Analysis of VH genes in follicular and diffuse lymphoma shows ongoing somatic mutation and multiple isotype transcripts in early disease with changes during disease progression. *Blood*, **91**, 4292–4299.
9. Solal-Celigny P, Roy P, Colombat P, White J, Armitage JO, Arranz-Saez R *et al.* (2004). Follicular lymphoma international prognostic index. *Blood*, **104**, 1258–1265.
10. Sigal S, Ninette A and Rechavi G (2005). Microarray studies of prognostic stratification and transformation of follicular lymphomas. *Best Pract Res Clin Haematol*, **18**, 143–156.

Chapter 6

Mantle cell lymphoma

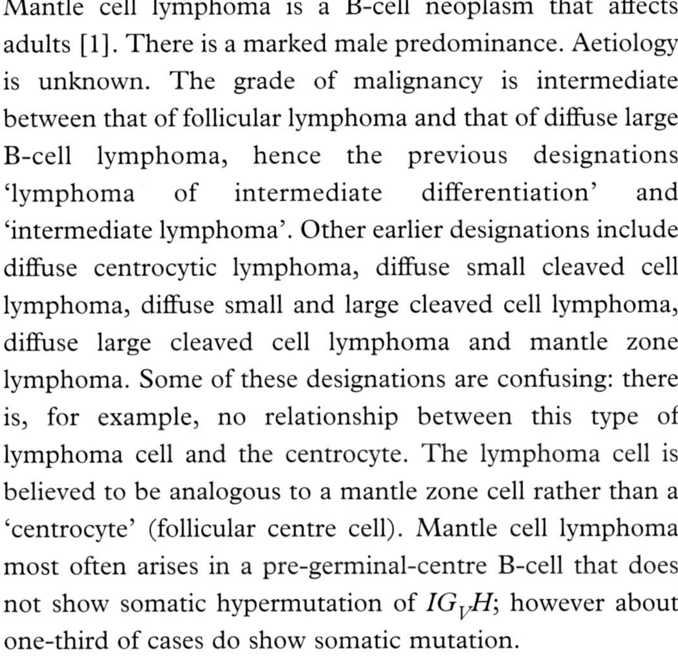

Mantle cell lymphoma is a B-cell neoplasm that affects adults [1]. There is a marked male predominance. Aetiology is unknown. The grade of malignancy is intermediate between that of follicular lymphoma and that of diffuse large B-cell lymphoma, hence the previous designations 'lymphoma of intermediate differentiation' and 'intermediate lymphoma'. Other earlier designations include diffuse centrocytic lymphoma, diffuse small cleaved cell lymphoma, diffuse small and large cleaved cell lymphoma, diffuse large cleaved cell lymphoma and mantle zone lymphoma. Some of these designations are confusing: there is, for example, no relationship between this type of lymphoma cell and the centrocyte. The lymphoma cell is believed to be analogous to a mantle zone cell rather than a 'centrocyte' (follicular centre cell). Mantle cell lymphoma most often arises in a pre-germinal-centre B-cell that does not show somatic hypermutation of IG_VH; however about one-third of cases do show somatic mutation.

Clinical features

Many patients present with advanced disease (stage III or IV) [2]. Lymphadenopathy, hepatomegaly and splenomegaly are common and involvement of bone marrow and peripheral blood is often present. Gastrointestinal involvement, as multiple lymphomatous polyposis, is detected in about one-third of patients but, if biopsies are carried out routinely, some degree of infiltration is found to be much more common, being detected in most patients. Involvement of Waldeyer's ring, including the tonsil, is present in a significant minority of patients.

Haematological and pathological features

Circulating lymphoma cells are often present, being reported in 20–40% of cases [3]. They tend to be medium sized with some degree of pleomorphism with regard to cell size and the shape of the cell and the nucleus (Figures **6.1–6.3**). Some cleft and irregular nuclei are often present and there may be small nucleoli; the chromatin pattern may be condensed or speckled. Cytoplasm is scanty and weakly basophilic. In a minority of patients the disease is characterized as small cell type or as pleomorphic or blastoid variant. In the small cell type there is a round or slightly indented nucleus with dense chromatin; confusion with chronic lymphocytic leukaemia (CLL) can occur. In the pleomorphic variant, cells are medium sized and large with more cytoplasm, in some cases resembling prolymphocytes and in others being more pleomorphic. Cells of the blastoid variant are more monomorphic with a dispersed chromatin pattern (Figure **6.4**) so that confusion with acute lymphoblastic leukaemia can occur.

A significant minority of patients present with or develop an autoimmune haemolytic anaemia.

Bone marrow infiltration is often present [2, 4]. The pattern of infiltration is variable; it may be interstitial with or without nodules, random focal, paratrabecular or diffuse. Heavy interstitial or diffuse infiltration is more often seen in those with leukaemic manifestations. Paratrabecular infiltration is much less common and, when present, is less striking than in follicular lymphoma. Increased reticulin deposition highlights the infiltrated area.

Lymph node involvement (Figure **6.5**) may manifest as an expanded mantle zone that surrounds residual non-neoplastic follicles, or there may be a nodular pattern or a diffuse infiltrate that effaces the node. The proliferation

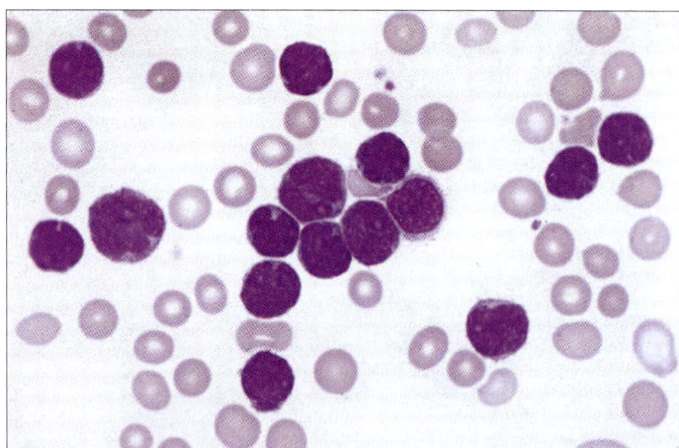

Figure 6.1 Peripheral blood film in mantle cell lymphoma showing pleomorphic cells; some have irregular nuclei and many are nucleolated. Romanowsky, x 60 objective.

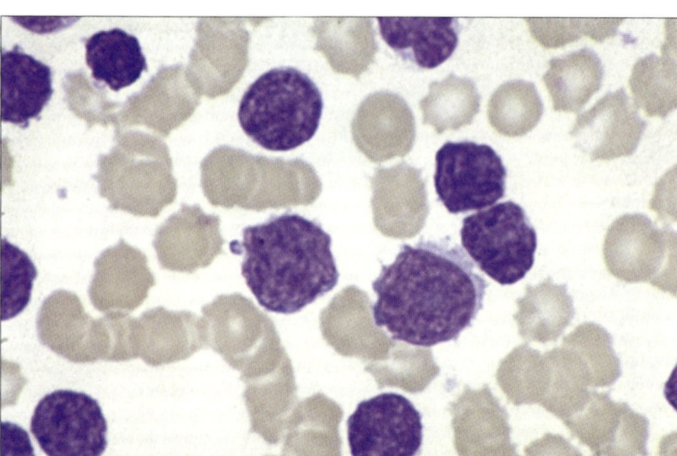

Figure 6.2 Peripheral blood film in mantle cell lymphoma showing pleomorphic cells with variable nuclear shape and variable chromatin condensation.

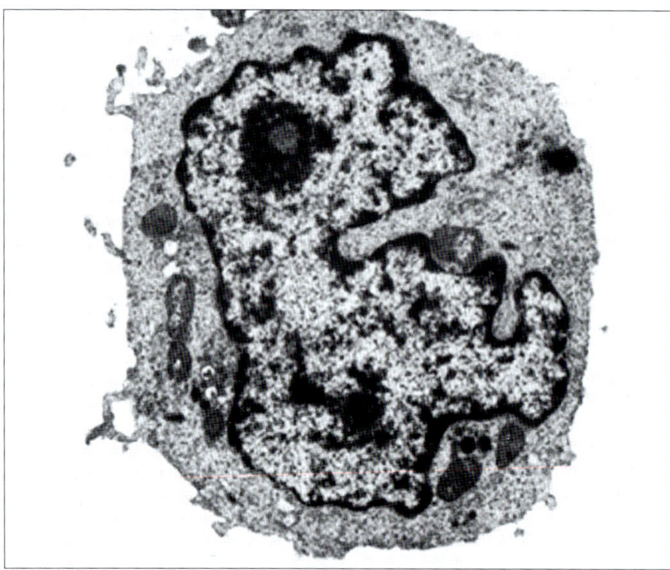

Figure 6.3 Ultrastructure of a lymphoma cell in mantle cell lymphoma showing an irregular nucleus and a prominent nucleolus. Lead nitrate and uranyl acetate stain.

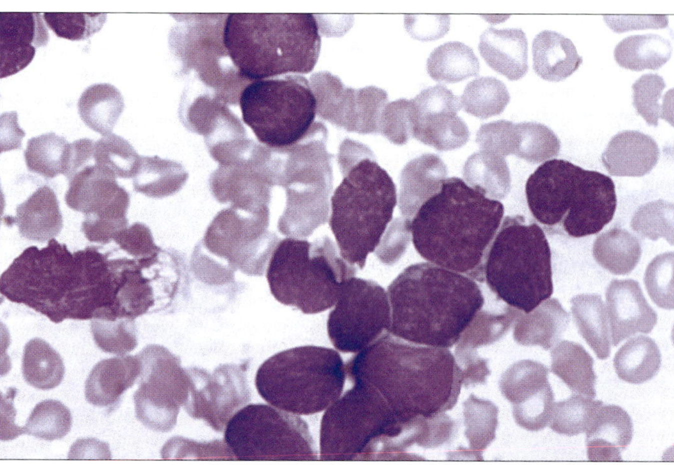

Figure 6.4 Peripheral blood film in blastoid variant of mantle cell lymphoma showing pleomorphic lymphoma cells, some of which have very little chromatin condensation.

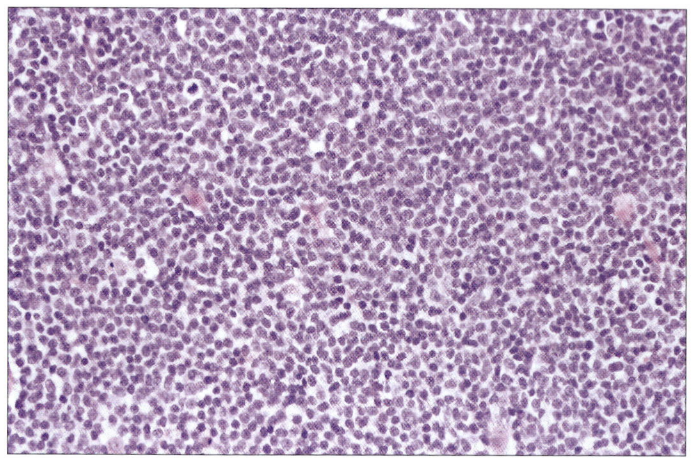

Figure 6.5 Section of lymph node biopsy from a patient with mantle cell lymphoma; the cells are predominantly small but some pleomorphism is apparent. H&E, x 40 objective.

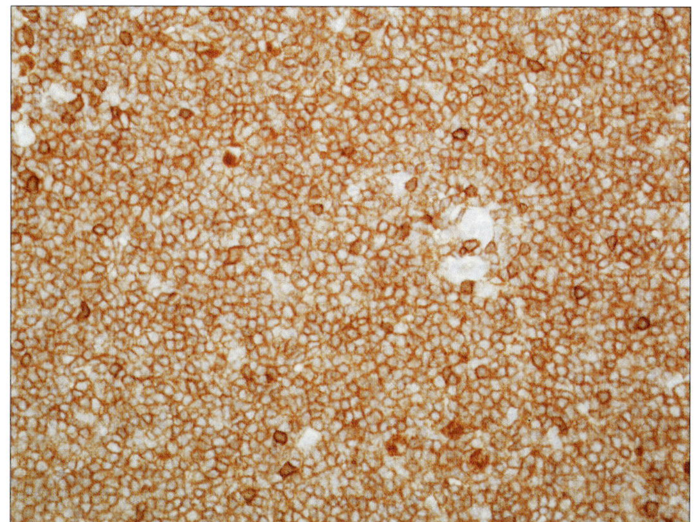

Figure 6.6 Section of lymph node biopsy from a patient with mantle cell lymphoma showing expression of CD5. Immunoperoxidase, x 40 objective.

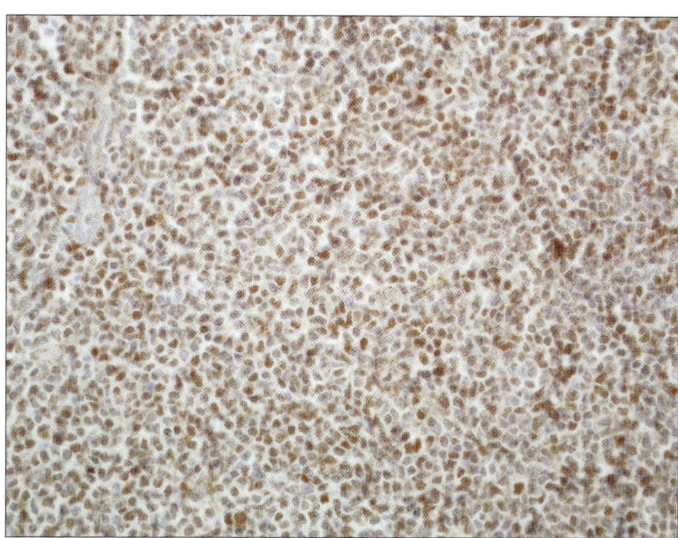

Figure 6.7 Section of lymph node biopsy from a patient with mantle cell lymphoma showing expression of cyclin D1. Immunoperoxidase, x 40 objective.

fraction varies considerably, in one study from 1 to 70%, a higher percentage of positive cells correlating with a worse prognosis [5].

Immunophenotype

The immunophenotype is that of a B-cell non-Hodgkin's lymphoma (NHL) with expression of B-cell-associated antigens (CD20, CD22, CD79a, CD79b and FMC7) and moderate to strong, light-chain restricted, surface membrane immunoglobulin (typically IgM with or without IgD, and more often lambda [λ] than kappa [κ]). CD5 expression (Figure **6.6**) is characteristic but not invariable. CD10, CD11c, CD23 and CD103 are not usually expressed. Immunophenotypic findings observed in 58 patients with disease in leukaemic phase are shown in *Table 6.1* [3]. On histological sections, expression of nuclear cyclin D1 is almost always present (Figure **6.7**) and is very useful in diagnosis. BCL2 is expressed but BCL6 is not. CD43 is usually positive. Staining with Ki67 or MIB1 can be used to evaluate the proliferation fraction.

Table 6.1 Immunophenotypic markers in a personally observed series of 58 patients with mantle cell lymphoma [3]

Marker	*Percentage positive (number tested)*
Kappa	55% (53)
Lambda	45% (53)
CD22 (strong)	70% (47)
CD79b (strong)	70% (34)
CD5	83% (54)*
CD23	16% (51)*
FMC7	91% (53)
CD38	52% (21)

* 15% resembled chronic lymphocytic leukaemia in being CD5+, CD23+. All of these had t(11;14)(q13;q32)

Cytogenetic and molecular genetic abnormalities

The t(11;14)(q13;q32) translocation (Figure **6.8**) is present in most cases and is the hallmark of this disease. The translocation leads to dysregulation of the *BCL1* gene (also known as *cyclin D1*, *CCND1* and *PRAD1*) by proximity to an enhancer of the immunoglobulin heavy chain gene. A variant translocation, t(11;22)(q13;q11), leading to dysregulation of *BCL1* by proximity to the λ light chain gene, is found in a minority of cases. Fluorescence *in situ* hybridization (FISH) analysis (Figure **6.9**) [6] and classical cytogenetic analysis can detect t(11;14)(q13;q32). The relevant molecular rearrangement can also be detected by a reverse transcriptase polymerase chain reaction (RT-PCR) but because of heterogeneity of the breakpoints this is not always positive. FISH is the preferred technique because of its sensitivity and because it will also detect the rearrangement of *BCL1* in patients with the variant translocation. Overexpression of nuclear cyclin D1, detected by immunocytochemistry, is an alternative means of confirming the diagnosis [7]. It should, however, be noted that cyclin D1 expression is not specific for mantle cell lymphoma. In addition, microarray analysis suggests that there are cases of mantle cell lymphoma that lack both t(11;14) and increased cyclin D1 expression but have overexpression of other cyclins [8].

Secondary cytogenetic and molecular genetic abnormalities are very common. These include del 11q23 (*ATM* deletion), +12, del 13q14 and del 17p13 (*TP53* deletion, mutation or both).

Diagnosis and differential diagnosis

The diagnosis is made by observation of typical cytological or histological features or both, aided by demonstration of t(11;14) or cyclin D1 overexpression. The differential diagnosis includes CLL (in cases with relatively small uniform cells), mixed cell type of CLL or atypical CLL, prolymphocytic leukaemia, follicular lymphoma, diffuse large B-cell lymphoma and other types of NHL and, in the blastoid variant, acute lymphoblastic leukaemia.

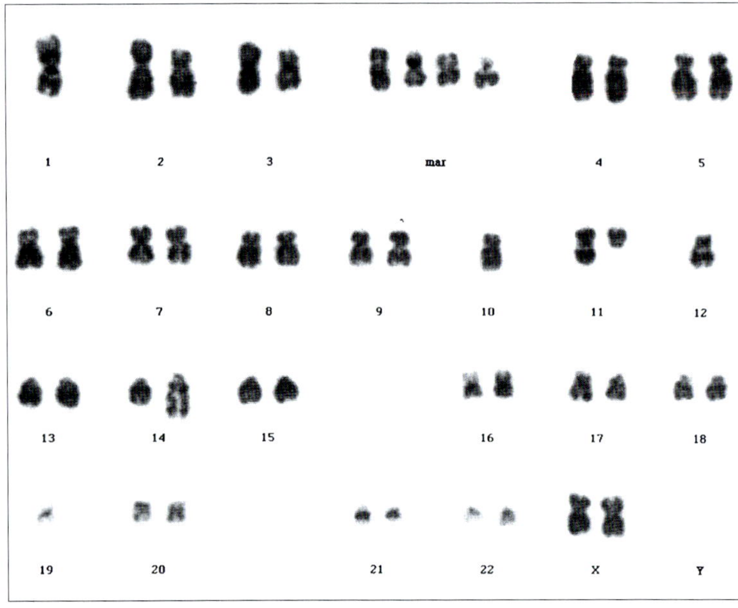

Figure 6.8 Karyogram of a patient with mantle cell lymphoma; the karyotype was 48, XX, t(11;14)(q13;q32), +mar, +mar. With thanks to Dr John Swansbury.

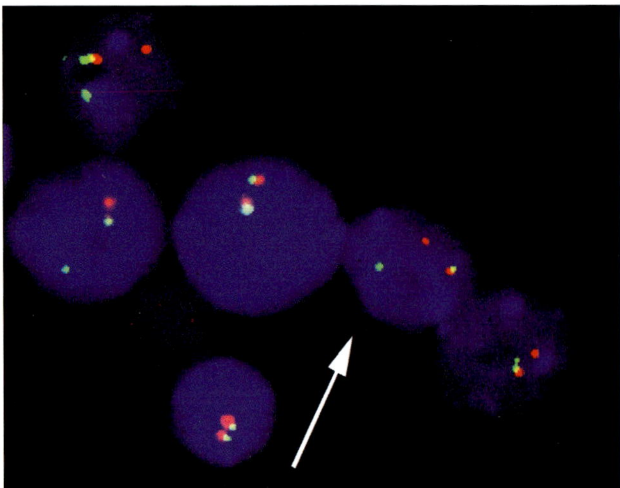

Figure 6.9 FISH analysis in a case of mantle cell lymphoma. Break-apart probes flanking BCL1 have been used. The arrow indicates a cell with a translocation.

Prognosis

Mantle cell lymphoma is usually incurable with current therapy. Median survival is three years or, in some studies, even less [4, 5, 9]. A subset of patients have a longer survival with the five-year survival being 20–25%. Adverse prognostic features include older age, leukaemic phase, anaemia, advanced stage disease, high lactate dehydrogenase (LDH), CD38 expression, a high mitotic rate or proliferation fraction (Ki-67 positivity), blastoid morphology, *TP53* loss or mutation, trisomy 12, chromosomal imbalance, complex karyotype or karyotypic evolution and loss of the tumour suppressor gene *CDKN1A* (p21) [2, 4, 10]. Somatic hypermutation of IG_VH genes correlates with a better prognosis [11]. The Follicular Lymphoma International Prognostic Index is a better indicator of prognosis than the International Prognostic Index, initially devised for large cell lymphoma [9].

Treatment

There is no consensus as to optimal treatment. Therapeutic options include chlorambucil, fludarabine-containing or cladribine-containing regimes (e.g. fludarabine plus cyclophosphamide), other combination chemotherapy and rituximab. There is no clear evidence that regimes containing anthracyclines are more effective than those without. It is possible that rituximab improves overall survival. Splenectomy sometimes has a role in patients with bulky splenomegaly and minor nodal disease.

References

1. Swerdlow SH, Berger F, Isaacson PG, Müller-Hermelink HK, Nathwani BN, Piris MA and Harris NL (2001). Mantle cell lymphoma. *In* Jaffe ES, Harris NL, Stein H and Vardiman JW (Eds). *World Health Organization Classification of Tumours: Pathology and Genetics of Tumours of Haematopoietic and Lymphoid Tissues*, IARC Press, Lyon, pp. 168–170.
2. Bosch F, Lopez-Guillermo A, Campo E, Ribera J, Conde E, Piris MA *et al.* (1998). Mantle cell lymphoma: presenting features, response to therapy, and prognostic factors. *Cancer*, **82**, 567–575.
3. Matutes E, Parry-Jones N, Brito-Babapulle V, Wotherspoon A, Morilla R, Atkinson S *et al.* (2004). The leukemic presentation of mantle-cell lymphoma: disease features and prognostic factors in 58 patients. *Leuk Lymphoma*, **45**, 2007–2015.
4. Pittaluga S, Verhoef G, Criel A, Maes A, Nuyts J, Boogaerts M and de Wolf Peeters C (1996). Prognostic significance of bone marrow trephine and peripheral blood smears in 55 patients with mantle cell lymphoma. *Leuk Lymphoma*, **21**, 115–125.
5. Tiemann M, Schrader C, Klapper W, Dreyling MH, Campo E, Norton A *et al.*; European MCL Network (2005). Histopathology, cell proliferation indices and clinical outcome in 304 patients with mantle cell lymphoma (MCL): a clinicopathological study from the European MCL Network. *Br J Haematol*, **131**, 29–38.
6. Matutes E, Carrara P, Coignet L, Brito-Babapulle V, Villamor N, Wotherspoon A, Catovsky D (1999). FISH analysis for BCL-1 rearrangements and trisomy 12 helps the diagnosis of atypical B cell leukaemias. *Leukemia*, **13**, 1721–1726.
7. Yatabe Y, Suzuki R, Tobinai K, Matsuno Y, Ichinohasama R, Okamoto M *et al.* (2000). Significance of cyclin D1 overexpression for the diagnosis of mantle cell lymphoma: a clinicopathologic comparison of cyclin D1-positive MCL and cyclin D1-negative MCL-like B-cell lymphoma. *Blood*, **95**, 2253–2261.
8. Fu K, Weisenburger DD, Greiner TC, Dave S, Wright G, Rosenwald A *et al.* (2005). Cyclin D1-negative mantle cell lymphoma: a clinicopathologic study based on gene expression profiling. *Blood*, **106**, 4315–4321.
9. Moller MB, Pedersen NT and Christensen BE (2005). Mantle cell lymphoma: prognostic capacity of the Follicular Lymphoma International Prognostic Index. *Br J Haematol*, **133**, 43–49.
10. Bea S, Ribas M, Hernandez JM, Bosch F, Pinyol M, Hernandez L *et al.* (1999). Increased number of chromosomal imbalances and high-level DNA amplifications in mantle cell lymphoma are associated with blastoid variants. *Blood*, **93**, 4365–4374.
11. Orchard J, Garand R, Davis Z, Babbage G, Sahota S, Matutes E *et al.* (2003). A subset of t(11;14) lymphoma with mantle cell features displays mutated IgV_H genes and includes patients with good prognosis, nonnodal disease. *Blood*, **101**, 4975–4981.

Chapter 7

Lymphoplasmacytic lymphoma

Lymphoplasmacytic lymphoma is an uncommon subtype of non-Hodgkin's lymphoma (NHL) occurring mainly in older people. It results from a neoplastic proliferation of post-germinal centre B cells with some degree of maturation to plasma cells [1]. The term encompasses Waldenström's macroglobulinaemia. Various diagnostic criteria have been proposed [2–4].

Clinical features

The clinical presentation is very variable with some clinical features being typical of lymphoma (hepatomegaly, splenomegaly and lymphadenopathy) and others being the result of the paraprotein that is often present [5]. Patients with a high concentration of an IgM paraprotein may have the clinical presentation of Waldenström's macroglobulinaemia, specifically increased plasma volume and hyperviscosity leading to retinal abnormalities, haemorrhage, cardiac failure and cerebral symptoms. Other patients have clinical features resulting from a paraprotein that is a cold agglutinin (chronic cold haemagglutinin disease) or a cryoglobulin (essential or type I cryoglobulinaemia) or has antibody activity leading to peripheral neuropathy. Autoimmune haemolytic anaemia can occur. Transformation to high-grade lymphoma sometimes occurs.

Haematological and pathological features

There may be anaemia and the blood film often shows increased rouleaux formation; sometimes there are red cell agglutinates or cryoglobulin deposits. The lymphocyte count may be normal or there may be mild lymphocytosis (Figure **7.1**). Lymphocytes are small and mature and may

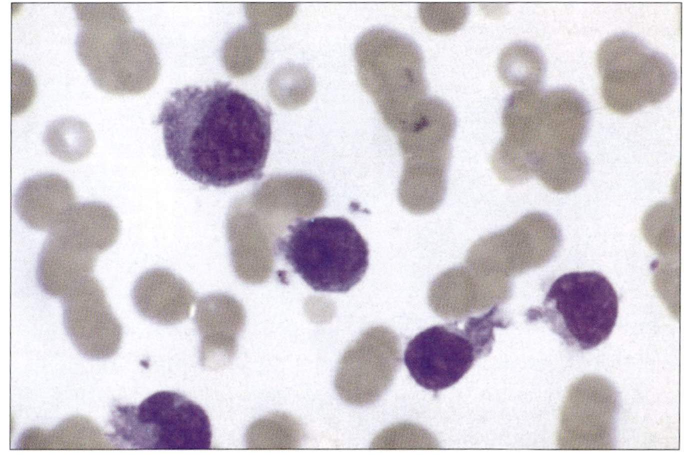

Figure 7.1 Peripheral blood film from a patient with lymphoplasmacytic lymphoma showing rouleaux and one cell with an eccentric nucleus and an ill-defined Golgi zone. Romanowsky, x 100 objective.

show plasmacytoid features – abundant basophilic cytoplasm with a small Golgi zone. Larger cells may be present if transformation occurs (Figure 7.2).

Bone marrow infiltration is characteristically by small lymphocytes, plasmacytoid lymphocytes and plasma cells. Crystals or immunoglobulin inclusions are sometimes present within lymphocytes, the term Russell body being used to indicate a rounded cytoplasmic inclusion and Dutcher body to indicate an apparently intra-nuclear inclusion. Mast cells are often increased. Trephine biopsy shows an interstitial or nodular infiltrate. Lymph node infiltration is diffuse.

A paraprotein is usually present, most often IgM but sometimes IgG or IgA. Bence–Jones protein may be detected in the urine.

Immunophenotype

The immunophenotype is that of a mature B cell with expression of light chain-restricted surface membrane immunoglobulin (most often IgM without IgD but sometimes IgG or IgA) and pan-B markers such as CD19, CD20, CD22 and CD79b. In addition to surface membrane immunoglobulin, some cells have cytoplasmic immunoglobulin (Figure 7.3). FMC7 is usually expressed and there may be expression of CD38. CD25 is often expressed [6]. CD5, CD10, CD11c, CD23 and CD103 are not usually expressed [6]. On immunocytochemistry, expression of CD20 and CD79a is detected and there is monotypic expression of cytoplasmic immunoglobulin in some of the cells.

Cytogenetic and molecular genetic abnormalities

There is no specific cytogenetic abnormality. The translocation t(9;14)(p13;q32), which results in dysregulation of the *PAX5* gene by proximity to the immunoglobulin heavy chain gene, has been reported [7] but has been found to be uncommon [8]. Non-specific abnormalities such as 6q- have been reported [9].

Diagnosis and differential diagnosis

The differential diagnosis includes chronic lymphocytic leukaemia (CLL) and B-NHL, particularly other NHL with plasmacytic differentiation (e.g. mucosa-associated lymphoid tissue [MALT]-type lymphoma or splenic marginal zone lymphoma). Multiple myeloma also needs to be included in the differential diagnosis since some cases of lymphoplasmacytic lymphoma have numerous plasma cells and some cases of multiple myeloma have lymphoplasmacytic rather than plasmacytic morphology.

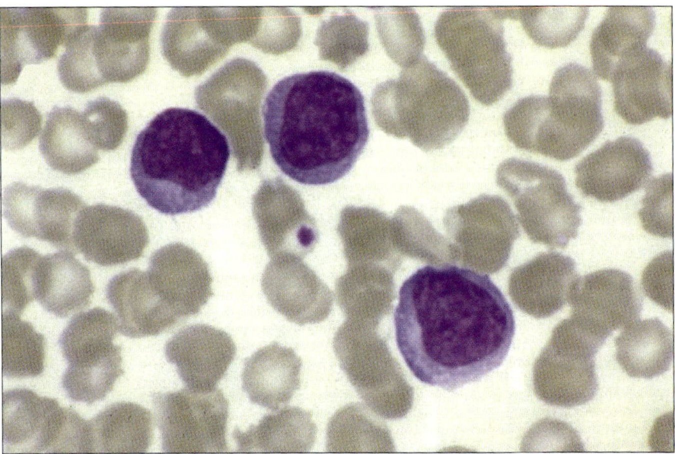

Figure 7.2 Peripheral blood film from a patient with large cell transformation of lymphoplasmacytic lymphoma, showing cells with a high nucleocytoplasmic ratio with a Golgi zone being apparent in two of the three cells. Romanowsky, x 100 objective.

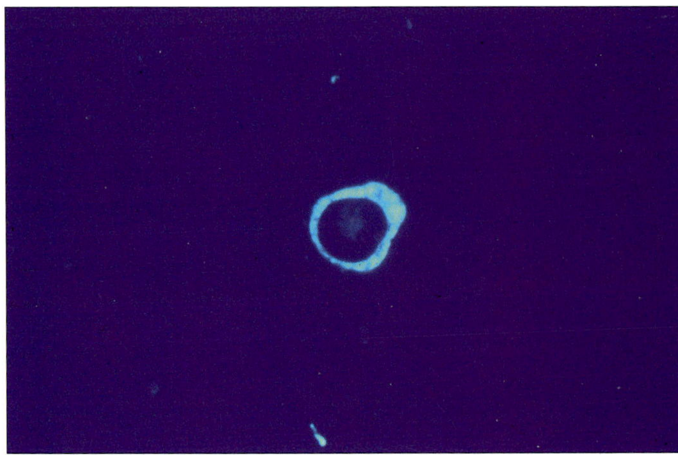

Figure 7.3 Cytoplasmic immunoglobulin demonstrated by immunofluorescence. Immunofluorescence, x 100 objective.

The differential diagnosis also includes other causes of cryoglobulinaemia, e.g. chronic hepatitis C infection, which leads to type II cryoglobulinaemia.

Prognosis

This lymphoma is usually indolent. The effects of a paraprotein may dominate those directly resulting from lymphoproliferation. Anaemia, increased β_2-microglobulin, hyperviscosity and significantly elevated serum immunoglobulin M have been found to be prognostically adverse [5, 10].

Treatment

Not all patients require treatment. Responses occur to chlorambucil, cyclophosphamide, nucleoside analogues and rituximab [10, 11]. Plasmapheresis can be useful to ameliorate the effects of a paraprotein.

References

1. Sahota SS, Forconi F, Ottensmeier CH, Provan D, Oscier DG, Hamblin TJ and Stevenson FK (2002). Typical Waldenström macroglobulinaemia is derived from a B cell arrested after cessation of somatic mutation but prior to isotype switch events. *Blood*, **100**, 1505–1507.
2. Berger F, Isaacson PG, Piris MA, Harris NL, Müller-Hermelink HK, Nathwani BN and Swerdlow SH (2001). Lymphoplasmacytic lymphoma/Waldenström macroglobulinaemia. *In* Jaffe ES, Harris NL, Stein H and Vardiman JW (Eds). *World Health Organization Classification of Tumours: Pathology and Genetics of Tumours of Haematopoietic and Lymphoid Tissues*, IARC Press, Lyon, pp. 132–134.
3. Owen RG, Treon SP, Al-Katib A, Fonseca R, Greipp PR, McMaster ML *et al.* (2003). Clinicopathological definition of Waldenström's macroglobulinemia: consensus panel recommendations from the Second International Workshop on Waldenström's Macroglobulinemia. *Semin Oncol*, **30**, 110–115.
4. Owen RG (2003). Developing diagnostic criteria in Waldenström's macroglobulinemia. *Semin Oncol*, **30**, 196–200.
5. Garcia-Sanz R, Montoto S, Torrequebrada A, de Coca AG, Petit J, Sureda A *et al.*; Spanish Group for the Study of Waldenström Macroglobulinaemia and PETHEMA (Programme for the Study and Treatment of Haematological Malignancies) (2001). Waldenström's macroglobulinaemia: presenting features and outcome in a series with 217 cases. *Br J Haematol*, **115**, 575–582.
6. San Miguel JF, Vidriales MB, Ocio E, Mateo G, Sanchez-Guijo F, Sanchez ML *et al.* (2003). Immunophenotypic analysis in Waldenström's macroglobulinemia. *Semin Oncol*, **30**, 187–195.
7. Iida S, Rao PH, Ueda R, Chaganti RS and Dalla-Favera R (1999). Chromosomal rearrangement of the PAX-5 locus in lymphoplasmacytic lymphoma with t(9;14)(p13;q32). *Leuk Lymphoma*, **34**, 25–33.
8. George TI, Wrede JE, Bangs CD, Cherry AM, Warnke RA and Arber DA (2005). Low-grade B-Cell lymphomas with plasmacytic differentiation lack *PAX5* gene rearrangements. *J Mol Diagn*, **7**, 346–351.
9. Schop RFJ, Kuehl WM, Van Wier SA, Ahmann GJ, Price-Troska T, Bailey RJ *et al.* (2002). Waldenström's macroglobulinaemia neoplastic cells lack immunoglobulin heavy chain locus translocations but have frequent 6q deletions. *Blood*, **100**, 2996–3001.
10. Dhodapkar MV, Jacobson JL, Gertz MA, Rivkin SE, Roodman GD, Tuscano JM *et al.* (2001). Prognostic factors and response to fludarabine therapy in patients with Waldenström's macroglobulinemia: results of United States intergroup trial (Southwest Oncology Group S9003). *Blood*, **98**, 41–48.
11. Kyle RA, Treon SP, Alexanian R, Barlogie B, Bjorkholm M, Dhodapkar M *et al.* (2003). Prognostic markers and criteria to initiate therapy in Waldenström's macroglobulinaemia: consensus panel recommendations from the Second International Workshop on Waldenström's macroglobulinaemia. *Semin Oncol*, **30**, 116–120.

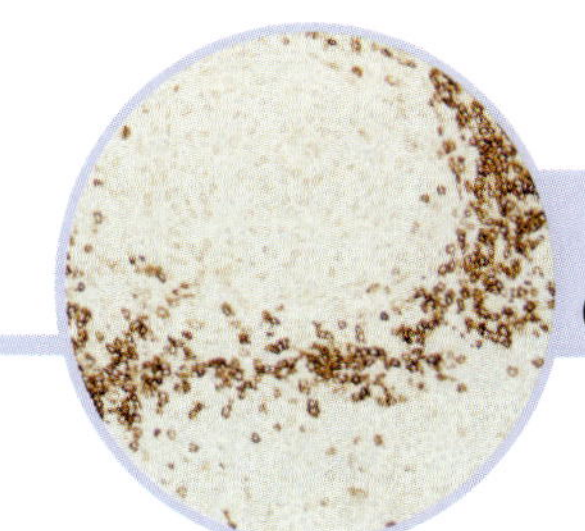

Chapter 8

Nodal marginal zone lymphoma

Nodal marginal zone lymphoma designates a group of lymphomas, possibly heterogeneous, that appear to originate in the marginal zone that surrounds the mantle zone of lymph node follicles [1–3]. This lymphoma was previously known as monocytoid B-cell lymphoma. The clinical presentation is with lymphadenopathy. Some cases may be closely related to extranodal marginal zone lymphoma and others to splenic marginal zone lymphoma. An association with hepatitis C has been observed in a minority of patients [4].

Clinical features

By definition, disease is mainly nodal but otherwise disease characteristics are not well defined. The disease tends to be indolent and most patients present with advanced stage disease.

Haematological and pathological features

Bone marrow and peripheral blood involvement are rare. The lymphoma cells are small to medium sized with a variable amount of cytoplasm, sometimes scanty and sometimes pale and abundant (monocytoid B cell). The nucleus is irregular.

Lymphoma cells occupy the interfollicular region of lymph nodes or the marginal zone of residual follicles or both (Figures **8.1** and **8.2**). Monocytoid B cells may be prominent but in other patients cells more closely resemble small lymphocytes. Follicular colonization can occur. Bone marrow infiltration may be random focal, paratrabecular or nodular. Neoplastic cells may be small or medium sized and sometimes have irregular nuclei and abundant pale cytoplasm.

Some patients have a serum paraprotein.

Immunophenotype

Lymphoma cells express weak monoclonal immunoglobulin and B-cell-associated antigens such as CD20, CD22, CD79a and CD79b. They do not usually express CD5, CD10, CD23, CD43, cyclin D1 or BCL6. CD11c is sometimes expressed.

Cytogenetic and molecular genetic abnormalities

Genetic abnormalities are not well characterized.

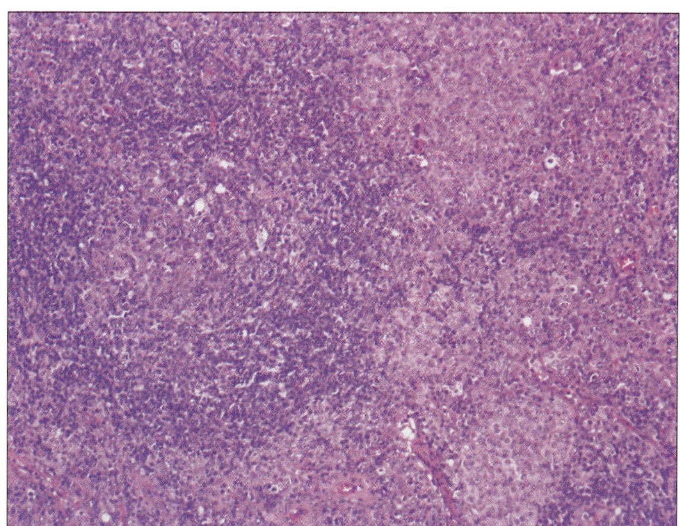

Figure 8.1 Section of lymph node biopsy from a patient with nodal marginal zone lymphoma, showing marginal zone infiltration. H&E, x 20 objective.

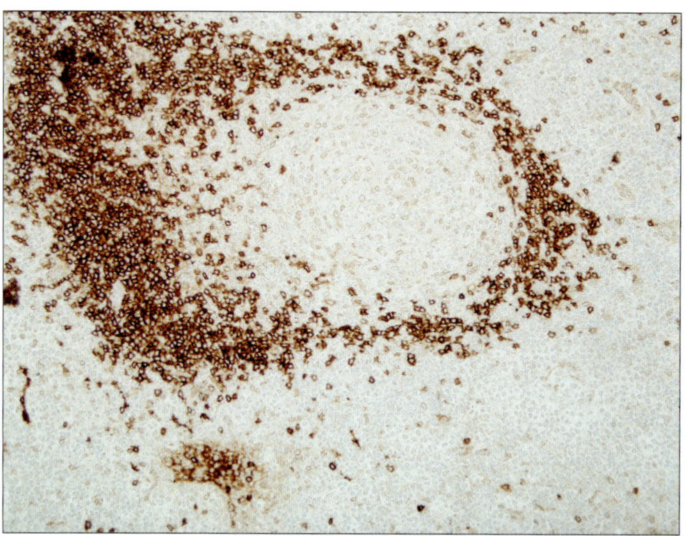

Figure 8.2 Section of lymph node biopsy from a patient with nodal marginal zone lymphoma, showing marginal zone infiltration, which is accentuated by immunohistochemistry for immunoglobulin D. Immunoperoxidase, x 20 objective.

Diagnosis and differential diagnosis

The differential diagnosis includes (i) marginal zone/monocytoid B-cell hyperplasia, (ii) secondary nodal involvement by extranodal and splenic marginal zone lymphoma and (iii) other low-grade B-cell non-Hodgkin's lymphoma, particularly lymphoplasmacytic lymphoma.

Prognosis

This lymphoma is indolent but not curable.

Treatment

Treatment is as for other low-grade lymphomas with there being no consensus as to the optimal agent [5].

References

1. Dogan A (2005). Modern histological classification of low grade B-cell lymphomas. *Best Prac Research Clin Haematol*, **18**, 11–26.
2. Conconi A, Bertoni F, Pedrinis E, Motta T, Roggero E, Luminari S *et al.* (2001). Nodal marginal zone B-cell lymphomas may arise from different subsets of marginal zone B lymphocytes. *Blood*, **98**, 781–786.
3. Arcaini L, Paulli M, Boveri E, Magrini U and Lazzarino M (2003). Marginal zone-related neoplasms of splenic and nodal origin. *Haematologica*, **88**, 80–93.
4. Arcaini L, Paulli M, Boveri E, Vallisa D, Bernuzzi P, Orlando E *et al.* (2004). Splenic and nodal marginal zone lymphomas are indolent disorders at high hepatitis C virus seroprevalence with distinct presenting features but similar morphologic and phenotypic profiles. *Cancer*, **100**, 107–115.
5. Bertoni F and Zucca E (2005). State-of-the-art therapeutics: marginal-zone lymphoma. *J Clin Oncol*, **23**, 6415–6420.

Chapter 9

Extranodal marginal zone lymphoma of MALT type

Extranodal marginal zone lymphoma of mucosa-associated lymphoid tissue (MALT) designates a group of closely related lymphomas that probably arise in marginal zone/memory B cells [1–6]. Similar lymphomas arise in non-mucosal sites, particularly when there is a lymphoid infiltrate as a result of an autoimmune disease (e.g. Sjögren's syndrome or Hashimoto's thyroiditis). Antigenic stimulation appears to be important in the aetiology of MALT lymphomas and ongoing antigenic stimulation may continue to drive the lymphoma, which may not be fully autonomous. Responsible antigens may be autoantigens or foreign antigens resulting from infection, e.g. *Helicobacter pylori* infection in gastric MALT lymphoma, *Borrelia burgdorferi* infection in cutaneous MALT lymphoma and *Chlamydia psittaci* in ocular adnexal MALT lymphoma. In some but not all countries an association with hepatitis C infection is found. Immunoproliferative small intestinal disease (IPSID), often with synthesis of α immunoglobulin heavy chains, is the result of small intestinal MALT lymphoma.

Clinical features

Clinical presentation is dependent on the organ that is involved. Typically, presentation is with gastrointestinal symptoms.

Haematological and pathological features

Infiltration is in the marginal zone of reactive follicles associated with mucous membranes, outside a preserved mantle zone. Follicular colonization sometimes occurs. The infiltrate is often closely related to a mucous membrane, which may be invaded (lymphoepithelial lesions) (Figures **9.1**–**9.3**). Lymphoma cells are pleomorphic, sometimes described as centrocyte-like and sometimes as monocytoid; they are small or medium sized and the latter have abundant pale cytoplasm. Plasmacytic differentiation is common.

The peripheral blood and bone marrow are often normal, although bone marrow infiltration is sometimes observed and rarely there are circulating lymphoma cells. Bone marrow infiltration can be nodular or paratrabecular.

Detailed investigation shows that disease is disseminated at presentation in a third of patients [7].

Immunophenotype

Neoplastic cells express weak monotypic immunoglobulin, most often IgM but in the case of IPSID, α chain only. There is expression of B-cell-associated antigens such as CD20, CD22, CD79a and CD79b. Lymphoma cells do not usually express CD5, CD23, FMC7 or cyclin D1. CD11c is sometimes expressed. BCL2 is expressed and BCL6 is not.

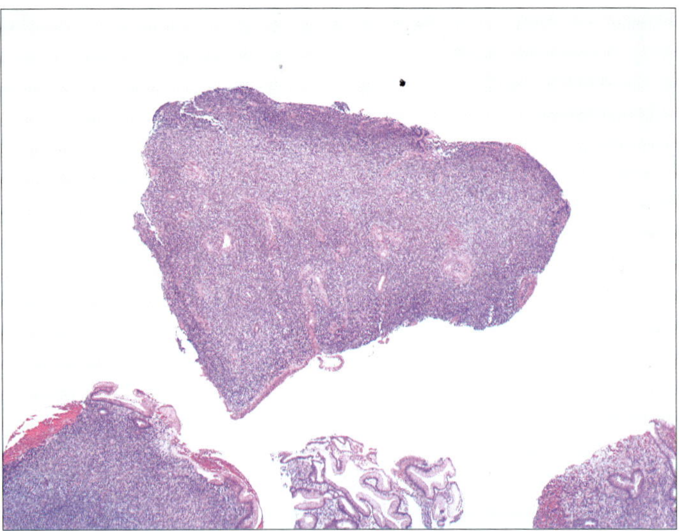

Figure 9.1 Gastric biopsy from a patient with extranodal marginal zone lymphoma of MALT type. H&E, x 4 objective.

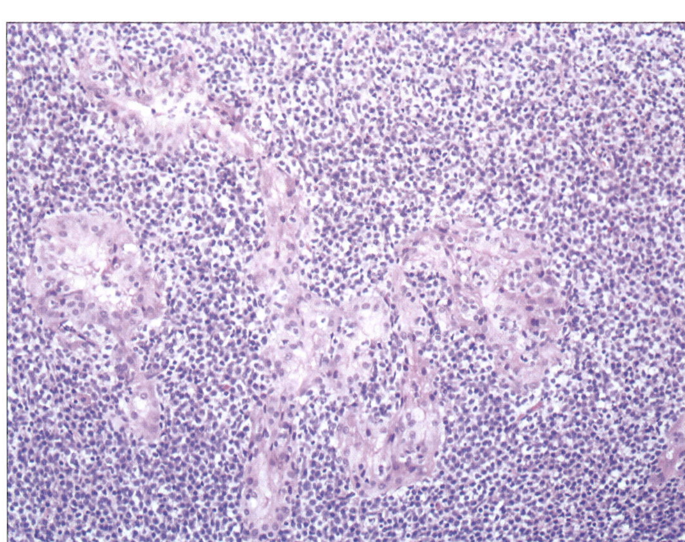

Figure 9.2 Gastric biopsy from a patient with extranodal marginal zone lymphoma of MALT type, showing lymphoepithelial lesions. H&E, x 20 objective.

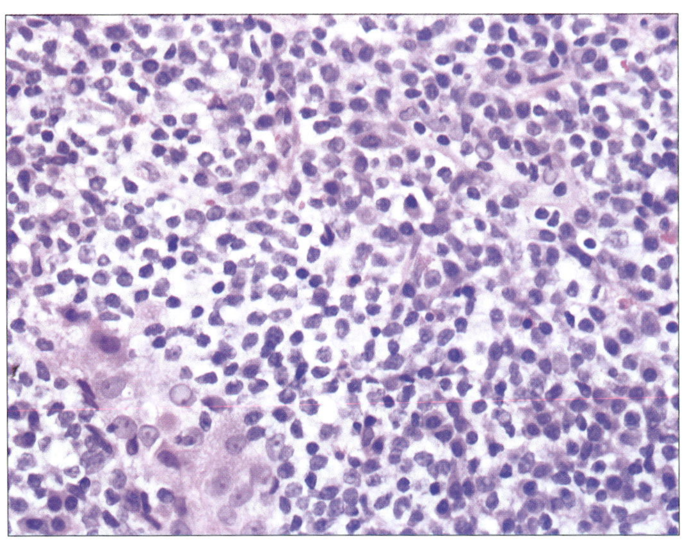

Figure 9.3 Gastric biopsy from a patient with extranodal marginal zone lymphoma of MALT type, showing lymphoepithelial lesions. H&E, x 60 objective.

Cytogenetic and molecular genetic abnormalities

Trisomy 3 is the most frequently observed abnormality [8]. Also quite common is t(11;18)(q21;q21), leading to formation of an *API2-MLT* fusion gene [9]. The presence of t(11;18) is associated with a worse prognosis. Translocations that dysregulate *BCL10* by proximity to an immunoglobulin gene locus, t(1;14)(p22;q32) and t(1;2)(p22;p12), are found in less than 5% of MALT lymphomas and a t(14;18)(q32;q21) leading to dysregulation of *MLT* by proximity to *IGH* in a small percentage [6, 10–13].

Diagnosis and differential diagnosis

The differential diagnosis includes both the autoimmune and infective lesions that may be a precursor of MALT lymphoma (e.g. *Helicobacter pylori*-related gastritis, autoimmune thyroiditis and autoimmune sialadenitis) and other low-grade lymphomas.

Prognosis

The prognosis is generally good although evolution to high-grade lymphoma can occur. Prognosis is no worse in those with disseminated disease at presentation [7]. The lymphoma may respond to elimination of causative bacteria, e.g. *Helicobacter pylori* or intestinal organisms in IPSID. In other patients, chemotherapy suitable for low-grade lymphoma is needed. Patients with gastric MALT lymphoma with t(11;18) or t(1;14)(p22;q32) do not respond to elimination of Helicobacter [11, 14].

Treatment

Gastric MALT lymphoma in patients with *Helicobacter pylori* infection may regress completely following elimination of the organism by treatment with proton pump inhibitors and antibiotics [15]. IPSID can show a similar response to antibiotics. Refractory cases of gastric MALT lymphoma and cases unrelated to Helicobacter can be treated with single agent chemotherapy (chlorambucil), radiotherapy, surgery or rituximab; a similar range of treatment is used for MALT lymphomas at other sites.

References

1. Wotherspoon AC, Ortiz-Hidalgo C, Falcon MR and Isaacson PG (1991). *Helicobacter pylori*-associated gastritis and primary B-cell gastric lymphoma. *Lancet*, **338**, 1175–1176.
2. Isaacson PG (1994). Gastrointestinal lymphoma. *Hum Pathol*, **25**, 1020–1029.
3. Wotherspoon AC, Dogan A and Du M-Q (2002). MALT lymphoma. *Curr Opin Haematol*, **9**, 50–55.
4. Arcaini L, Paulli M, Boveri E, Magrini U and Lazzarino M (2003). Marginal zone-related neoplasms of splenic and nodal origin. *Haematologica*, **88**, 80–93.
5. Zucca E, Conconi A, Pedrinis E, Cortelazzo S, Motta T, Gospodarowicz MK *et al.* (2003). Nongastric marginal zone B-cell lymphoma of mucosa-associated lymphoid tissue. *Blood*, **101**, 2489–2495.
6. Isaacson PG (2005). Update in MALT lymphomas. *Best Prac Res Clin Haematol*, **18**, 57–68.
7. Thieblemont C, Berger F, Dumontet C, Moullet I, Bouafia F, Felman P *et al.* (2000). Mucosa-associated lymphoid tissue lymphoma is a disseminated disease in one third of 158 patients analyzed. *Blood*, **95**, 802–806.
8. Wotherspoon AC, Finn TM and Isaacson PG (1995). Trisomy 3 in low grade B-cell lymphomas of mucosa-associated lymphoid tissue. *Blood*, **85**, 2000–2004.
9. Auer IA, Gascoyne RD, Conners JM, Cotter FE, Greiner TC, Sanger WG and Horsman DE (1997). t(11;18)(q21;q21) is the most common translocation in MALT lymphomas. *Ann Oncol*, **8**, 979–985.
10. Willis TG, Jadayel DM, Du MQ, Peng H, Perry AR, Abdul Rauf M *et al.* (1999). *Bcl10* is involved in t(1;14)(p22;q32) in MALT B cell lymphoma and mutated in multiple tumor types. *Cell*, **96**, 35–45.
11. Du M-Q, Peng H, Liu H, Hamoudi RA, Diss TC, Willis TG *et al.* (2000). *BCL10* gene mutation in lymphoma. *Blood*, **95**, 3885–3890.
12. Streubel B, Lamprecht A, Dierlamm J, Cerroni L, Stolte M, Ott G *et al.* (2003). T(14;18)(q32;q21) involving IGH and MALT1 is a frequent chromosomal aberration in MALT lymphoma. *Blood*, **101**, 2335–2339.
13. Farinha P and Gascoyne RD (2005). Molecular pathogenesis of mucosa-associated lymphoid tissue lymphoma. *J Clin Oncol*, **23**, 6370–6378.
14. Liu H, Ye H, Ruskone-Fourmestraux A, De Jong D, Pileri S, Thiede C *et al.* (2002). t(11;18) is a marker for all stage gastric MALT lymphomas that will not respond to *H. pylori* eradication. *Gastroenterology*, **122**, 1286–1294.
15. Bertoni F and Zucca E (2005). State-of-the-art therapeutics: marginal-zone lymphoma. *J Clin Oncol*, **23**, 6415–6420.

Chapter 10

Splenic marginal zone lymphoma, including splenic lymphoma with villous lymphocytes

Splenic marginal zone lymphoma is a lymphoma that infiltrates the marginal and mantle zones of splenic follicles [1–3]; whether the disease actually arises in splenic marginal zone memory B cells is uncertain [4]. Analysis of immunoglobulin genes suggests that about one-third of cases arise in a pre-germinal-centre naïve B cell and the other two-thirds in a post-germinal-centre memory B cell. On-going immunoglobulin gene mutations occur [5].

Splenic lymphoma with villous lymphocytes is a morphological subset of splenic marginal zone lymphoma characterized by circulating lymphoma cells with fine cytoplasmic projections.

Clinical features

There is usually significant splenomegaly with minimal lymphadenopathy. In some patients the disease is associated with hepatitis C infection, this association being observed particularly around the Mediterranean area [6]. Transformation to diffuse large B-cell lymphoma occurs in about 10% of cases.

Haematological and pathological features

The peripheral blood may be normal or there may be a moderate lymphocytosis with the lymphoma cells either being small lymphocytes with no distinguishing features or 'villous' lymphocytes; the latter have fine cytoplasmic projections, sometimes at one or both poles of the cell (Figures **10.1** and **10.2**). Chromatin is condensed and sometimes there are small nucleoli. There may also be circulating plasmacytoid lymphocytes. Pancytopenia may be present as a result of splenomegaly and hypersplenism.

Bone marrow infiltration, when present, may be interstitial, nodular or paratrabecular; a strikingly paratrabecular pattern of infiltration is less common than in follicular lymphoma. Occasionally, neoplastic cells surround a reactive germinal centre. Intra-sinusoidal infiltration, marked or subtle, is common. The presence of isolated intra-sinusoidal infiltration is particularly suggestive of this type of lymphoma.

Lymph node infiltration, e.g. in splenic hilar lymph nodes, is also around germinal centres.

Splenic infiltration is around pre-existing white pulp follicles (Figures **10.3**–**10.9**), which are atrophic (Figure **10.10**), and involves the marginal zone as well as the mantle zone [7]. There is a distinct zoning of the infiltration with an outer paler zone being composed of larger cells with a high proliferative rate and an inner zone composed of smaller darker cells with a lower proliferative rate. The red pulp is also infiltrated.

A paraprotein is often present (about one-third of patients) but the concentration is low. It may be IgM or IgG.

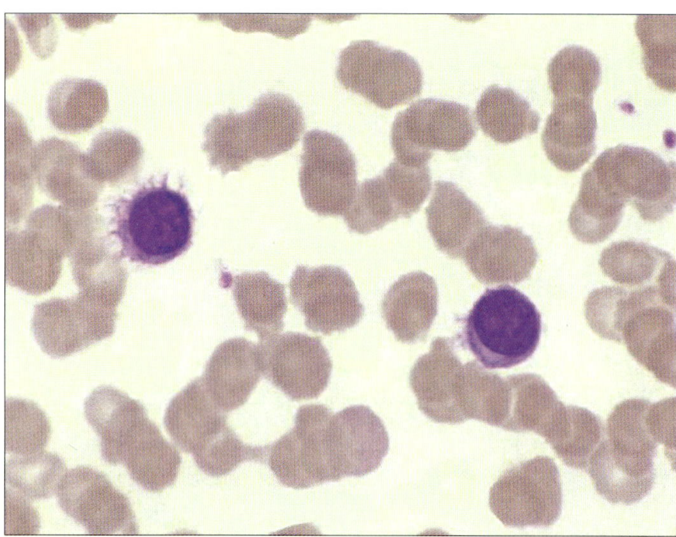

Figure 10.1 Peripheral blood film of a patient with splenic marginal zone lymphoma (splenic lymphoma with villous lymphocytes) showing rouleaux and two villous lymphocytes; one of the lymphocytes has a detectable Golgi zone. Romanowsky, x 100 objective.

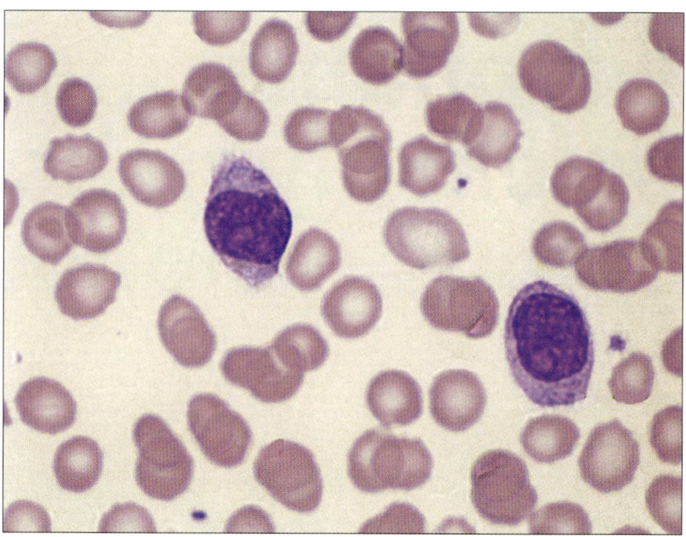

Figure 10.2 Peripheral blood film of a patient with splenic marginal zone lymphoma (splenic lymphoma with villous lymphocytes) showing two nucleolated lymphocytes, one of which has villi at both poles of the cell. Romanowsky, x 100 objective.

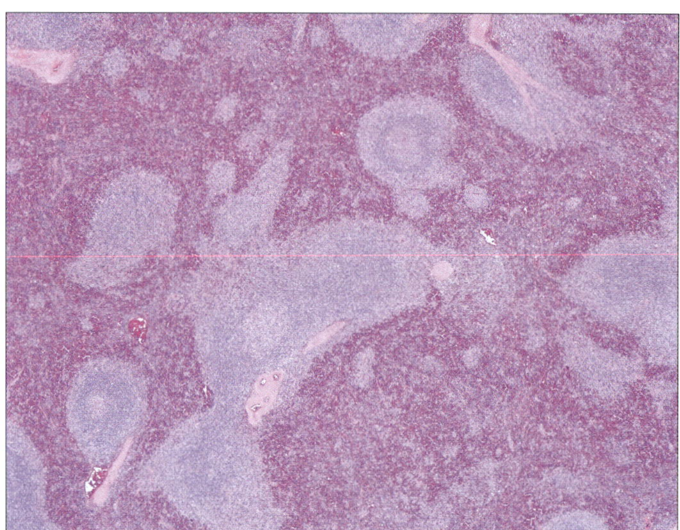

Figure 10.3 Section of spleen from a patient with splenic marginal zone lymphoma showing infiltration of the marginal zone of follicles. H&E, x 4 objective.

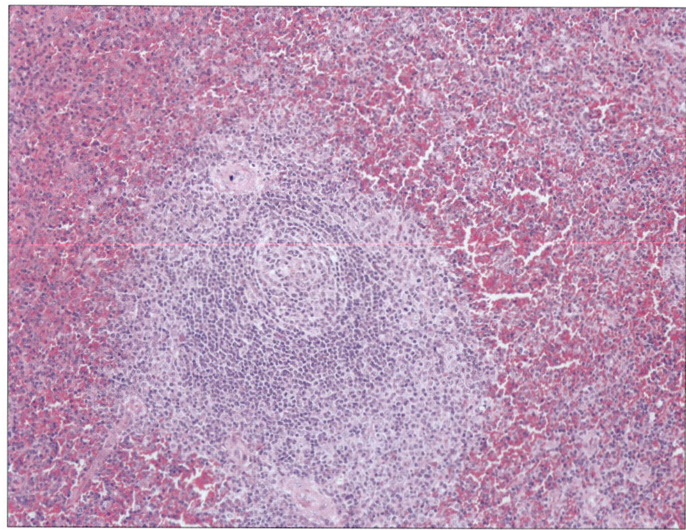

Figure 10.4 Section of spleen from a patient with splenic marginal zone lymphoma showing infiltration of the marginal zone of follicles. H&E, x 20 objective.

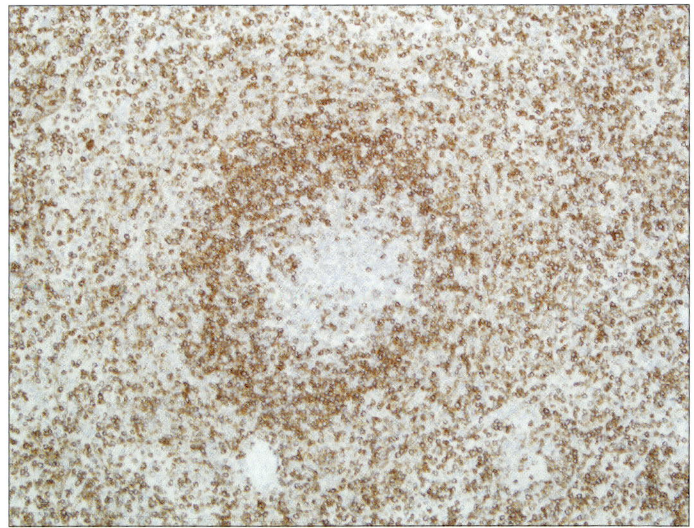

Figure 10.5 Section of spleen from a patient with splenic marginal zone lymphoma showing infiltration of the marginal zone of a residual normal follicle, which is BCL2 negative. Immunoperoxidase, x 20 objective.

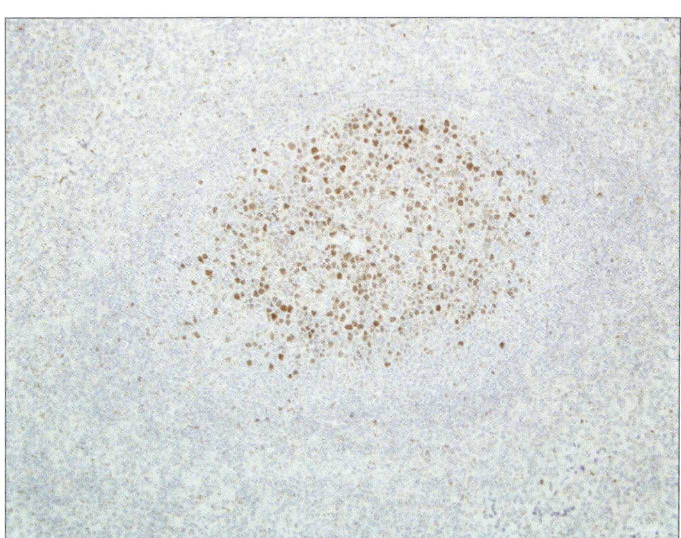

Figure 10.6 Section of spleen from a patient with splenic marginal zone lymphoma showing infiltration of the marginal zone of a residual normal follicle, which is BCL6 positive. Immunoperoxidase, x 20 objective.

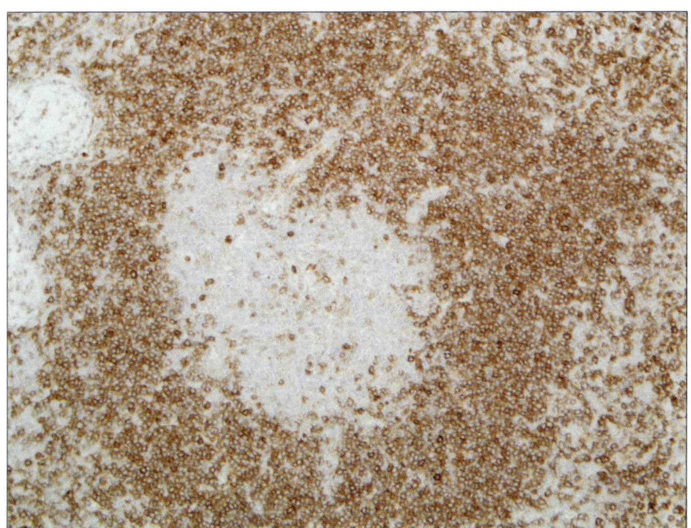

Figure 10.7 Section of spleen from a patient with splenic marginal zone lymphoma showing infiltration of the marginal zone of a residual normal follicle; the lymphoma cells are positive for immunoglobulin D. Immunoperoxidase, x 20 objective.

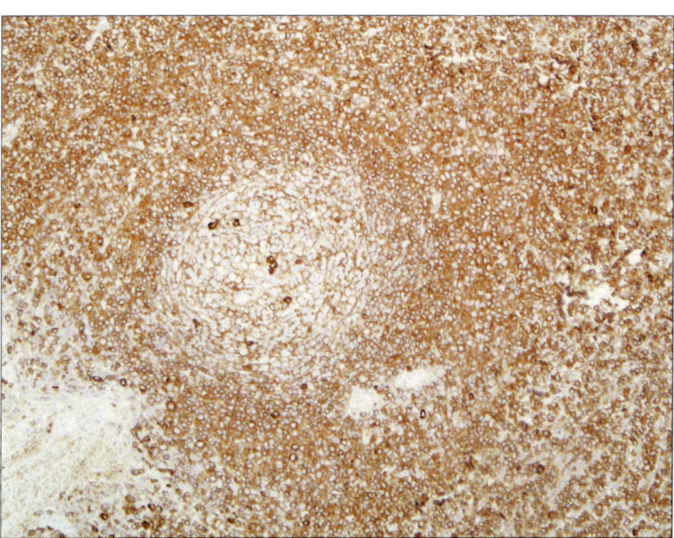

Figure 10.8 Section of spleen from a patient with splenic marginal zone lymphoma showing infiltration of the marginal zone of a residual normal follicle; the lymphoma cells are positive for κ light chain. Immunoperoxidase, x 20 objective.

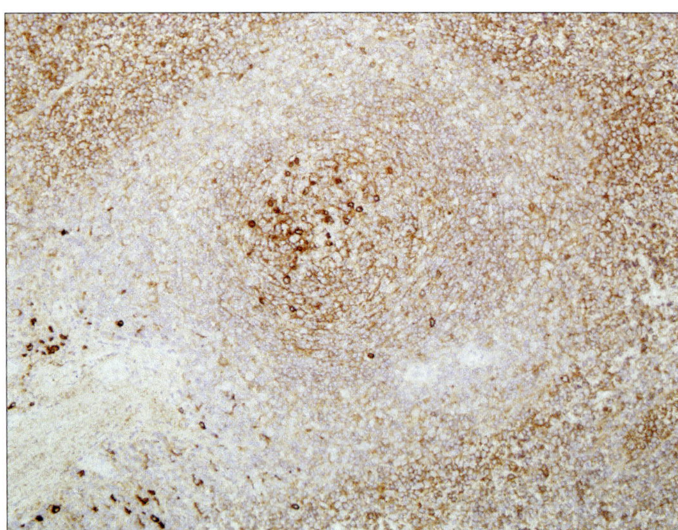

Figure 10.9 Section of spleen from a patient with splenic marginal zone lymphoma showing infiltration of the marginal zone of a residual normal follicle; the lymphoma cells are negative for λ light chain. Immunoperoxidase, x 20 objective.

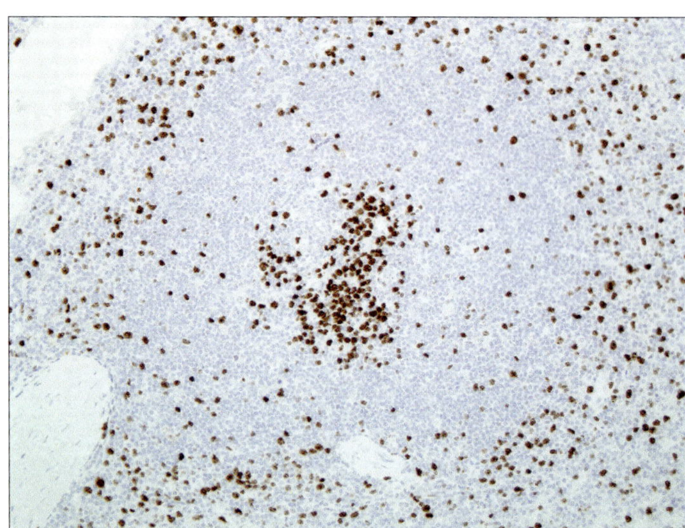

Figure 10.10 Section of spleen from a patient with splenic marginal zone lymphoma showing infiltration of the marginal zone of a residual follicle; there are proliferating cells in the follicle centre, highlighted with the MIB1 monoclonal antibody. Immunoperoxidase, x 20 objective.

Immunophenotype

Lymphoma cells usually express monotypic IgM and IgD plus pan-B markers such as CD19, CD20, CD79b and CD79a [8] (Figure **10.11**). They express FMC7 and BCL2 but do not usually express CD5, CD10, CD23, CD43, CD103, CD123 or cyclin D1. BCL6 expression is heterogeneous. CD11c is often expressed (about one-half of cases) and CD25 sometimes (about one-third of cases).

Cytogenetic and molecular genetic abnormalities

The most characteristic genetic abnormality is loss of 7q31–32. Trisomy 3 is seen in up to 17% of patients with splenic lymphoma with villous lymphocytes [9] and in a minority there are abnormalities of *TP53* [10].

Diagnosis and differential diagnosis

The differential diagnosis includes reactive marginal zone hyperplasia, chronic lymphocytic leukaemia, hairy cell leukaemia, hairy cell leukaemia variant and low-grade B-cell non-Hodgkin's lymphoma. If t(11;14) or cyclin D1 expression is detected a diagnosis of mantle cell lymphoma should be suspected.

Prognosis

The disease is indolent with a median survival of more than eight years. Although compatible with long survival, this lymphoma is not curable with current treatment. High-grade transformation occurs in a minority of patients. In splenic lymphoma with villous lymphocytes, anaemia and a lymphocyte count of greater than 16×10^9/l correlate with worse prognosis [11].

Treatment

Splenectomy may be followed by long remissions and is generally preferred to chemotherapy. The disease is responsive to chlorambucil in a minority of patients and is responsive to fludarabine and rituximab in a larger number. Interferon plus ribaravin is indicated in patients with associated hepatitis C infection since remission may occur [12].

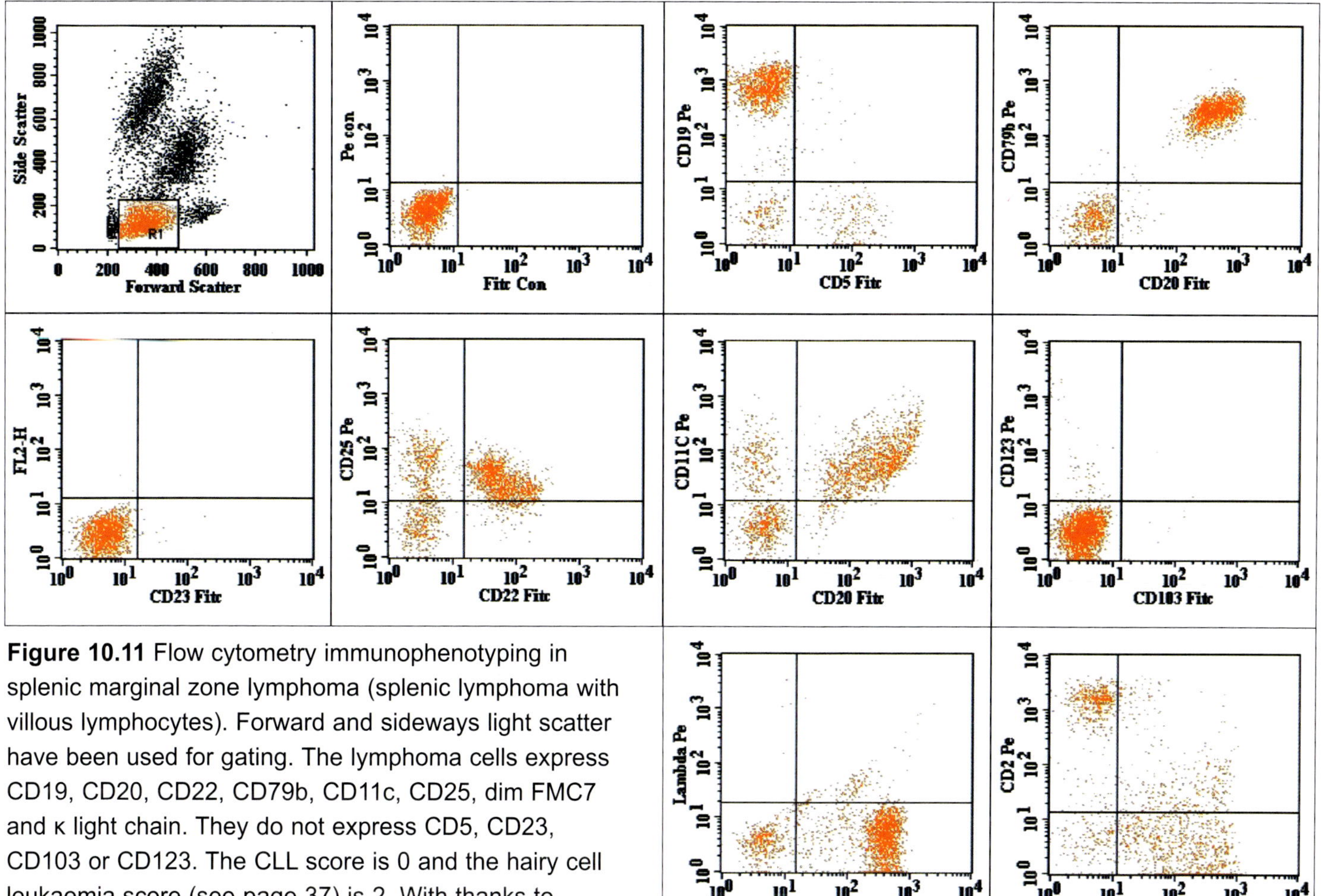

Figure 10.11 Flow cytometry immunophenotyping in splenic marginal zone lymphoma (splenic lymphoma with villous lymphocytes). Forward and sideways light scatter have been used for gating. The lymphoma cells express CD19, CD20, CD22, CD79b, CD11c, CD25, dim FMC7 and κ light chain. They do not express CD5, CD23, CD103 or CD123. The CLL score is 0 and the hairy cell leukaemia score (see page 37) is 2. With thanks to Mr Ricardo Morilla.

References

1. Catovsky D and Matutes E (1999). Splenic lymphoma with circulating villous lymphocytes/splenic marginal-zone lymphoma. *Semin Hematol*, **36**, 148–154.
2. Isaacson PG, Piris MA, Catovsky D, Swerdlow S, Montserrat E, Berger F *et al.* (2001). Splenic marginal zone lymphoma. *In* Jaffe ES, Harris NL, Stein H and Vardiman JW (Eds). *World Health Organization Classification of Tumours: Pathology and Genetics of Tumours of Haematopoietic and Lymphoid Tissues*, IARC Press, Lyon, pp. 135–137.
3. Franco V, Florena AM and Iannitto E (2003). Splenic marginal zone lymphoma. *Blood*, **101**, 2464–2472.
4. Dogan A (2005). Modern histological classification of low grade B-cell lymphomas. *Best Prac Research Clin Haematol*, **18**, 11–26.
5. Tierens A, Delabie J, Malecka A, Wang J, Gruszka-Westwood A, Catovsky D and Matutes E (2003). Splenic marginal zone lymphoma with villous lymphocytes shows on-going immunoglobulin gene mutations. *Am J Pathol*, **162**, 681–689.
6. Talamini R, Montella M, Crovatto M, Dal Maso L, Crispo A, Negri E *et al.* (2004). Non-Hodgkin's lymphoma and hepatitis C virus: a case-control study from northern and southern Italy. *Int J Cancer*, **110**, 380–385.
7. Isaacson PG, Matutes E, Burke M and Catovsky D (1994). The histopathology of splenic lymphoma with villous lymphocytes. *Blood*, **84**, 3828–3834.

8. Matutes E, Morilla R, Owusu-Ankomah K, Houlihan A and Catovsky D (1994). The immunophenotype of splenic lymphoma with villous lymphocytes and its relevance to the differential diagnosis with other B-cell disorders. *Blood*, **83**, 1558–1562.
9. Gruszka-Westwood AM, Matutes E, Coignet LJ, Wotherspoon A and Catovsky D (1999). The incidence of trisomy 3 in splenic lymphoma with villous lymphocytes: a study by FISH. *Br J Haematol*, **104**, 600–604.
10. Gruszka-Westwood AM, Hamoudi RA, Matutes E, Tuset E, Catovsky D (2001). p53 abnormalities in splenic lymphoma with villous lymphocytes. *Blood*, **97**, 3552–3558.
11. Parry-Jones N, Matutes E, Gruszka-Westwood AM, Swansbury GJ, Wotherspoon AC and Catovsky D (2003). Prognostic features of splenic lymphoma with villous lymphocytes: a report on 129 patients. *Br J Haematol*, **120**, 759–764.
12. Hermine O, Lefrere F, Bronowicki J, Mariette X, Jondeau K, Eclache-Saudreau V *et al.* (2002). Regression of splenic lymphoma with villous lymphocytes after treatment of hepatitis C virus infection. *N Engl J Med*, **347**, 89–94.

Chapter 11

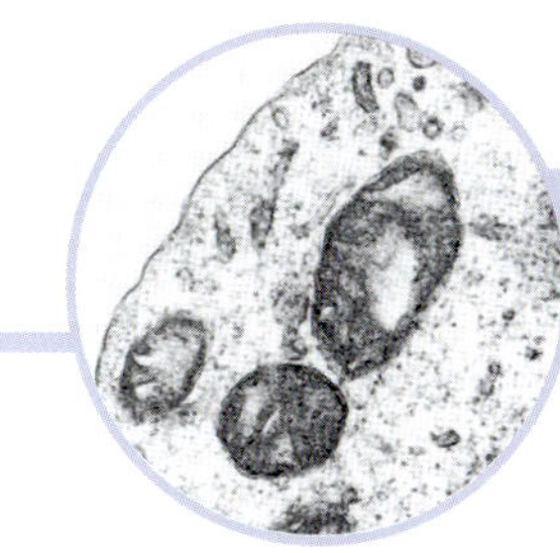

Hairy cell leukaemia

Hairy cell leukaemia is an indolent lymphoproliferative disorder resulting from the proliferation of a neoplastic clone of morphologically and immunophenotypically distinctive mature B lymphocytes [1, 2]. Most patients are middle aged with a marked male predominance. Patients who present with advanced disease often show immune deficiency.

Clinical features

Characteristically there is splenomegaly without palpable lymphadenopathy, although up to one-third of patients have abdominal lymphadenopathy on CT scanning. Prominent abdominal lymphadenopathy may be detected at relapse [3]. Presentation may be with mycobacterial or other opportunistic infection.

Haematological and pathological features

There is cytopenia (sometimes bicytopenia or pancytopenia) with prominent monocytopenia. It is uncommon for the white cell count to be elevated. Monocytopenia is not a feature of other lymphoproliferative disorders and can thus be a useful clue to diagnosis. Hairy cells are medium sized with plentiful weakly basophilic cytoplasm with irregular margins (Figure **11.1**). The nucleus may be round, oval, bean-shaped or dumb-bell-shaped and characteristically has a delicate chromatin pattern without an obvious nucleolus. Hairy cells may be infrequent in the peripheral blood and concentrating them in a buffy coat preparation can be useful. The degree of 'hairiness' of the neoplastic cells varies between films and even between different parts of the one blood film. Cells express tartrate-resistant acid phosphatase (Figure **11.2**). On ultrastructural examination, a ribosomal

Figure 11.1 Peripheral blood film in hairy cell leukaemia showing a hairy cell with a bean-shaped nucleus and plentiful weakly basophilic irregular cytoplasm. Romanowsky, x 100 objective.

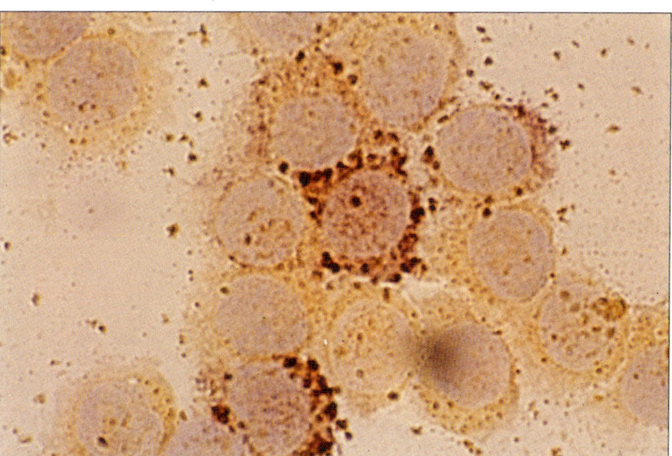

Figure 11.2 Tartrate-resistant acid phosphatase activity in hairy cells.

lamellar complex is characteristic (Figure **11.3**).

The bone marrow is usually hard to aspirate and often aspiration is impossible. If an aspirate is obtained, hairy cells are usually more easily detectable than in the peripheral blood. If bone marrow cannot be aspirated, an imprint should be made from the trephine biopsy specimen. Trephine biopsy sections show bone marrow infiltration to be initially random focal and interstitial but with advanced disease it becomes diffuse (Figure **11.4**). Cytological features on sections are very distinctive. The pale, rather bland, irregularly shaped nucleus is apparent and is surrounded by scanty irregular cytoplasm and then by an artefactual space, which is the result of cytoplasmic shrinkage. The result is that the neoplastic cells appear to be spaced apart (so called 'fried-egg' pattern). Erythrocytes may be present in the interstitium. Reticulin deposition is usually increased.

Lymph node biopsy is rarely performed (except in conjunction with splenectomy); infiltration is mainly paracortical. Splenic infiltration is characteristically in the red pulp with the white pulp being atrophic. There may be lakes of red cells surrounded by hairy cells.

The presence of large neoplastic cells has been observed in the bone marrow and lymph nodes at relapse [3].

Immunophenotype

Hairy cells are late mature B cells expressing strong monotypic surface membrane immunoglobulin. This is most often IgM or IgG with or without IgD and IgA and in some patients multiple heavy chains are expressed (e.g. IgG, IgA and IgM). The cells demonstrate B-cell-associated antigens such as CD19, CD20 (strong expression), CD22, CD79b and FMC7 (Figure **11.5**). They also express a characteristic set of antigens that are much less often expressed in other B-cell lymphoproliferative disorders, specifically CD11c, CD25, CD103, CD123 and the antigen detected by the HC2 monoclonal antibody [4, 5]. A scoring system using four of these antigens can be applied with cases of hairy cell leukaemia typically scoring 3 or 4. Absence of surface CD27 expression also distinguishes hairy cell leukaemia from other B-cell disorders [6]. Hairy cells do not usually express CD5, CD10 or CD23, although approaching one in five patients show expression of CD23 [7]. In tissue sections, expression of CD20, CD79a and CD25 (Figure **11.6**) can be detected. A monoclonal antibody to tartrate-resistant acid phosphatase can be used to highlight hairy cells (Figure **11.7**), as can DBA44 [8]

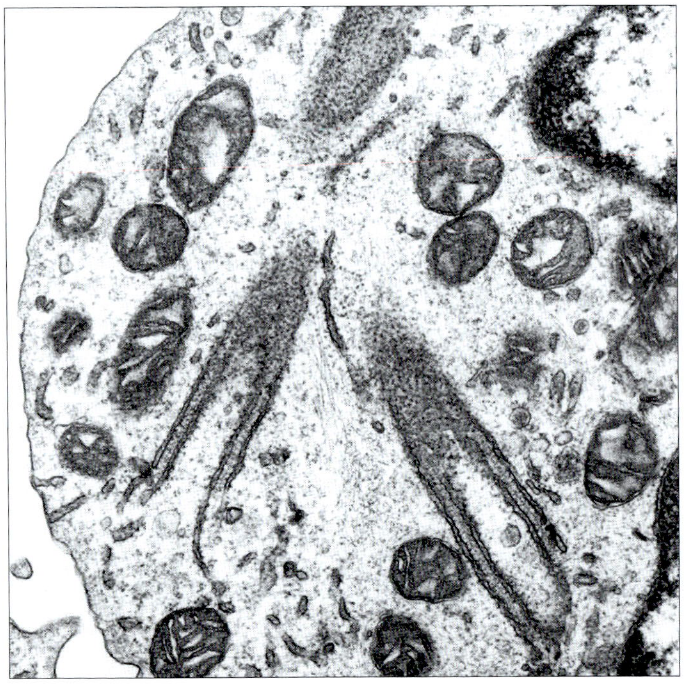

Figure 11.3 Ultrastructural features of a hairy cell, including ribosomal lamellar complexes. Electron microscopy.

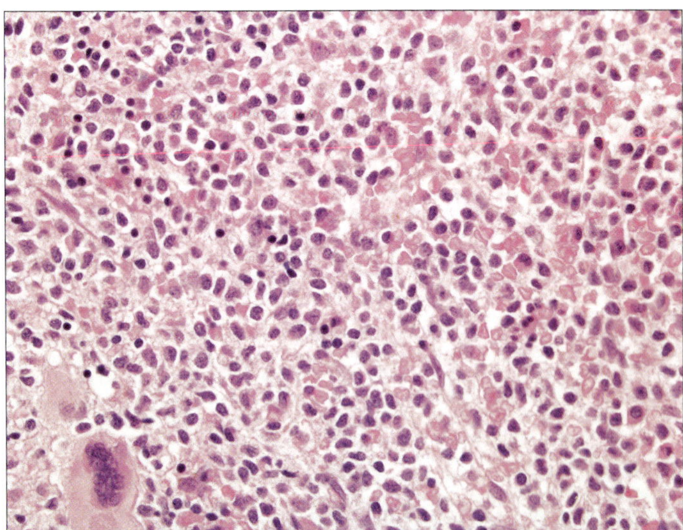

Figure 11.4 Section of a trephine biopsy specimen from a patient with hairy cell leukaemia showing characteristically spaced cells, the nuclei of which show considerable variation in shape. H&E, x 60 objective.

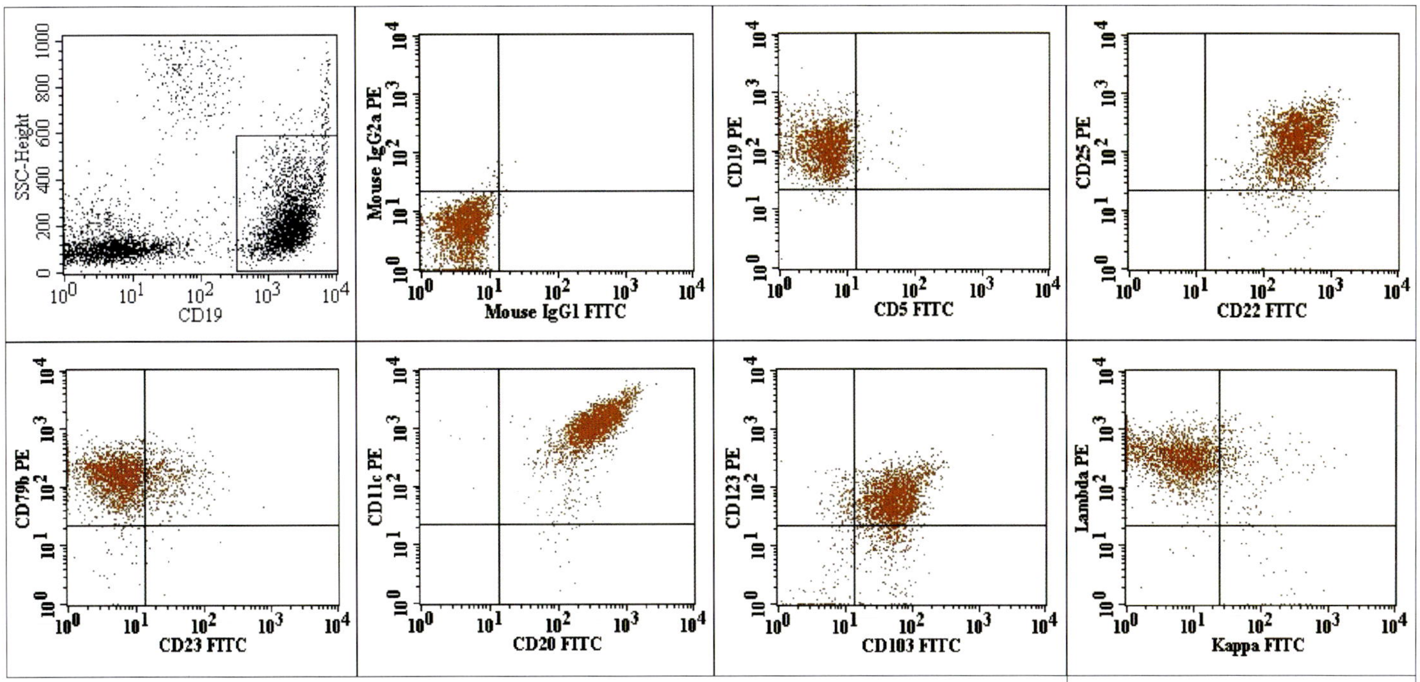

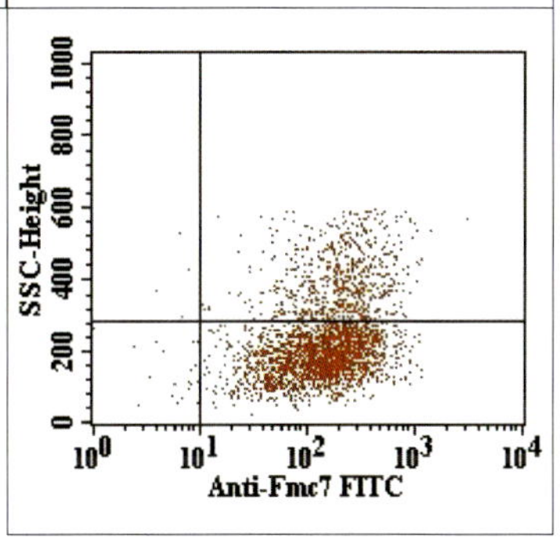

Figure 11.5 Flow cytometry immunophenotyping in hairy cell leukaemia. Sideways light scatter and CD19 expression have been used for gating. In addition to CD19, cells express CD20, CD22, CD79b, FMC7, CD11c, CD25, CD103, CD123 and λ. They do not express CD23. The CLL score is 0 and the hairy cell score is 4. With thanks to Mr Ricardo Morilla.

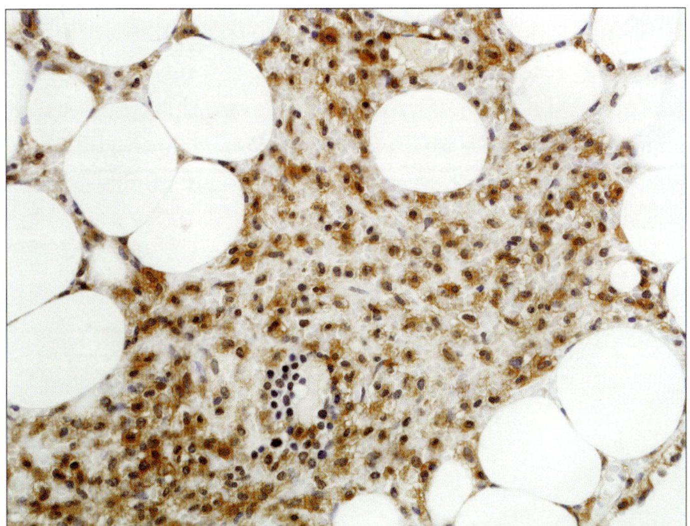

Figure 11.6 Section of a trephine biopsy specimen from a patient with hairy cell leukaemia showing expression of CD25. Immunoperoxidase, x 40 objective.

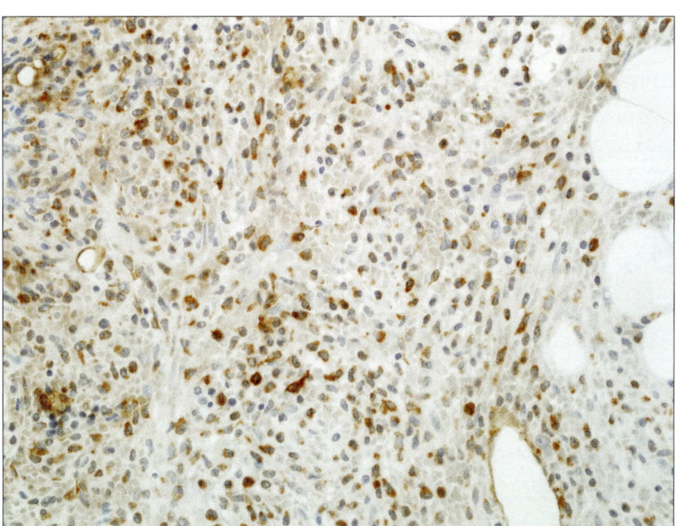

Figure 11.7 Section of a trephine biopsy specimen from a patient with hairy cell leukaemia showing expression of tartrate-resistant acid phosphatase antigen. Immunoperoxidase, x 40 objective.

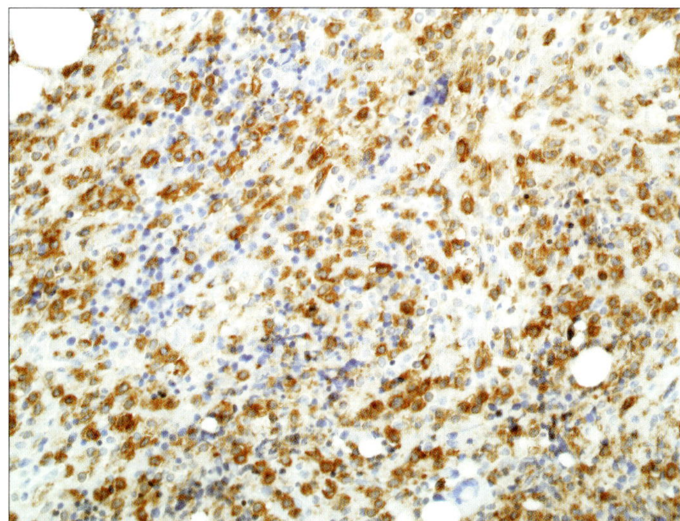

Figure 11.8 Section of a trephine biopsy specimen from a patient with hairy cell leukaemia showing expression of DBA44. Immunoperoxidase, x 40 objective.

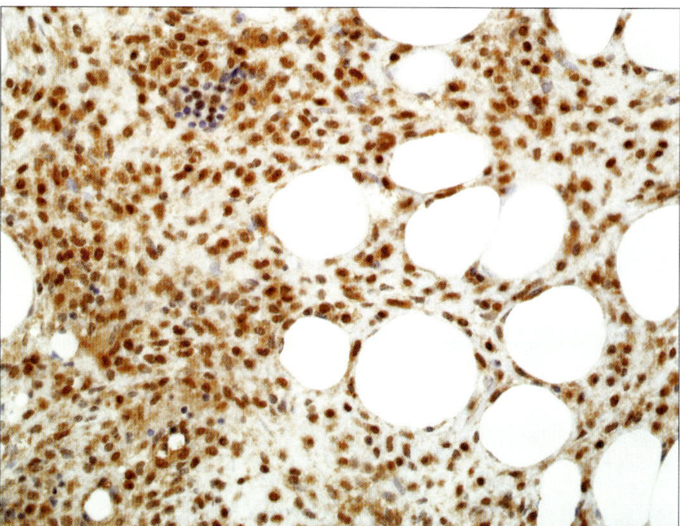

Figure 11.9 Section of a trephine biopsy specimen from a patient with hairy cell leukaemia showing expression of cyclin D1. Immunoperoxidase, x 40 objective.

(Figure **11.8**). Cyclin D1 is often overexpressed, in the absence of t(11;14) [9] (Figure **11.9**). Annexin 1A is expressed in virtually all patients and is negative in other B-cell disorders [10].

Cytogenetic and molecular genetic abnormalities

No specific cytogenetic or molecular genetic abnormality has yet been recognized. When an abnormality is detected it may be in only a low proportion of cells and is thus not the primary abnormality [11]. In contrast to hairy cell leukaemia variant, *TP53* deletions are not a feature [11].

Diagnosis and differential diagnosis

The differential diagnosis includes aplastic anaemia (since the marrow may be hypocellular and difficult to aspirate), myelofibrosis (also characterized by splenomegaly and difficulty in aspiration of bone marrow) and other B-cell lymphoproliferative disorders, particularly hairy cell leukaemia variant and splenic marginal zone lymphoma (splenic lymphoma with villous lymphocytes). A variant of hairy cell leukaemia with unusual features has been reported from Japan [12]. Usually hairy cell leukaemia is sufficiently distinctive for diagnosis to be easy.

Prognosis

The prognosis is good, except in those patients who present with very advanced disease, immune deficiency and opportunistic infection.

Treatment

There is an excellent response to nucleoside analogues, cladribine and pentostatin being most often used (95% response rate and 75% complete response) [13–15]. Interferon is also effective but less so than nucleoside analogues so is now much less used. Splenectomy still has a place in patients with marked cytopenia and a bulky spleen. Rituximab can be effective.

References

1. Foucar K and Catovsky D (2001). Hairy cell leukaemia. *In* Jaffe ES, Harris NL, Stein H and Vardiman JW (Eds). *WHO classification of Haematopoietic and Lymphoid tumours*, IARC Press, Lyon, pp. 138–141.
2. Tallman MS and Polliack A (Eds) (2000). *Hairy Cell Leukemia*, Harwood Academic Publishers, Amsterdam.
3. Mercieca J, Matutes E, Moskovic E, McLennan K, Matthey F, Costello C *et al.* (1992). Massive lymphadenopathy in hairy cell leukaemia: a report of 12 cases. *Br J Haematol*, **82**, 547–554.
4. Matutes E, Morilla R, Owusu-Ankomah K, Houlihan A, Meeus P and Catovsky D (1994). The immunophenotype of hairy cell leukemia (HCL). Proposal for a scoring system to distinguish HCL from B-cell disorders with hairy or villous lymphocytes. *Leuk Lymphoma*, **14**, Suppl. 1, 57–61.
5. Del Giudice I, Matutes E, Morilla R, Morilla A, Owusu-Ankomah K, Rafiq F *et al.* (2004). The diagnostic value of CD123 in B-cell disorders with hairy or villous lymphocytes. *Haematologica*, **89**, 303–308.
6. Forconi F, Raspadori D, Lenoci M and Lauria F (2005). Absence of surface CD27 distinguishes hairy cell leukemia from other leukemic B-cell malignancies. *Haematologica*, **90**, 144–146.
7. Chen YH, Tallman MS, Goolsby C and Peterson L (2006). Immunophenotypic variations in hairy cell leukemia. *Am J Clin Pathol*, **125**, 251–259.
8. Salomon-Nguyen F, Valensi F, Troussard X and Flandrin G (1996). The value of the monoclonal antibody, DBA44, in the diagnosis of B-lymphoid disorders. *Leuk Res*, **20**, 909–913.
9. Bosch F, Campo E, Jares P, Pittaluga S, Munoz J, Nayach I *et al.* (1995). Increased expression of the PRAD-1/CCND1 gene in hairy cell leukaemia. *Br J Haematol*, **91**, 1025–1030.
10. Falini B, Tiacci E, Liso A, Basso K, Sabatini E, Pacini R *et al.* (2004). Simple diagnostic assay for hairy cell leukaemia by immunocytochemical detection of annexin A1 (ANXA1). *Lancet*, **363**, 1869–1870. Erratum in: *Lancet*, 2004, **363**, 2194.
11. Vallianatou K, Brito-Babapulle V, Matutes E, Atkinson S and Catovsky D (1999). p53 gene deletion and trisomy 12 in hairy cell leukemia and its variant. *Leuk Res*, **23**, 1041–1045.
12. Machii T, Tokumine Y, Inoue R and Kitani T (1993). Predominance of a distinct subtype of hairy cell leukemia in Japan. *Leukemia*, **7**, 181–186.
13. Saven A, Burian C, Koziol JA and Piro LD (1998). Long-term follow-up of patients with hairy cell leukemia after cladribine treatment. *Blood*, **92**, 1918–1926.
14. Dearden CE, Matutes E, Hilditch BL, Swansbury GJ and Catovsky D (1999). Long-term follow-up of patients with hairy cell leukaemia after treatment with pentostatin or cladribine. *Br J Haematol*, **106**, 515–519.
15. Robak T (2006). Current treatment options in hairy cell leukemia and hairy cell leukemia variant. *Cancer Treat Rev*, **32**, 365–376.

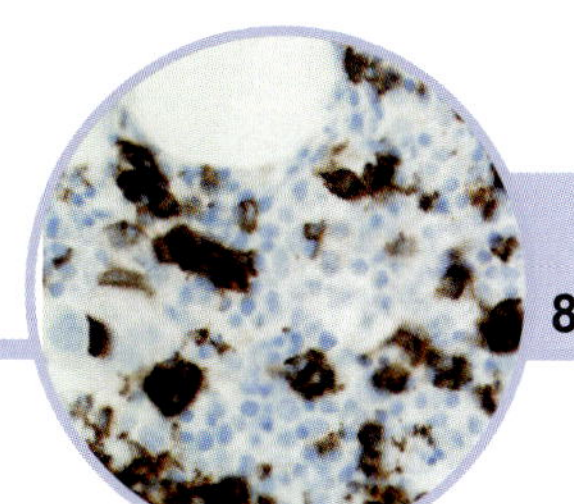

Chapter 12

Hairy cell leukaemia variant

Hairy cell leukaemia variant is a very rare B-lineage lymphoproliferative disorder characterized by a clonal proliferation of B cells that morphologically resemble hairy cells but have a prominent nucleolus, resembling that of a prolymphocyte [1–3]. This disease occurs in the elderly without any male predominance.

Clinical features

Splenomegaly is characteristic while lymphadenopathy is usually minor.

Haematological and pathological features

In contrast to hairy cell leukaemia, the white cell count is moderately elevated (5–300, median around 80 × 10^9/l) [4–7]. There may be mild anaemia and thrombocytopenia. The monocyte count is preserved. The neoplastic cells have moderately plentiful cytoplasm with irregular margins and a round nucleus with a large prominent nucleolus and some chromatin condensation (Figure **12.1**). There may be some binucleated cells. The tartrate-resistant acid phosphatase reaction is usually negative. Bone marrow infiltration is usually interstitial and often intrasinusoidal [8] (Figure **12.2**). Cells may be spaced, as in hairy cell leukaemia, but

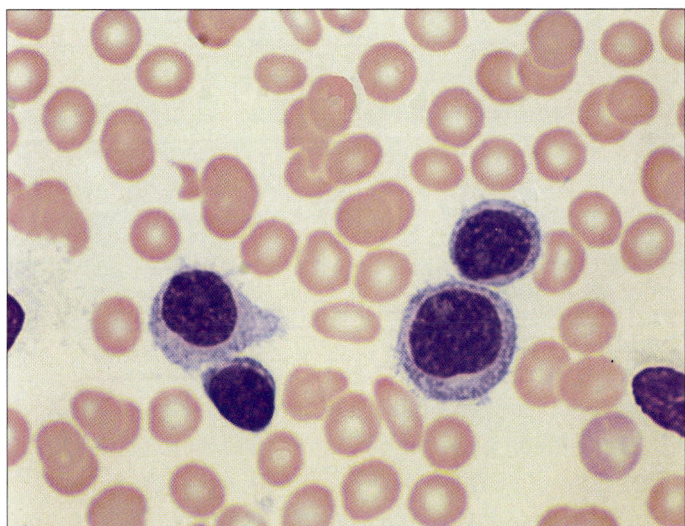

Figure 12.1 Peripheral blood film of a patient with hairy cell leukaemia variant showing characteristic cells. Romanowsky, x 100 objective.

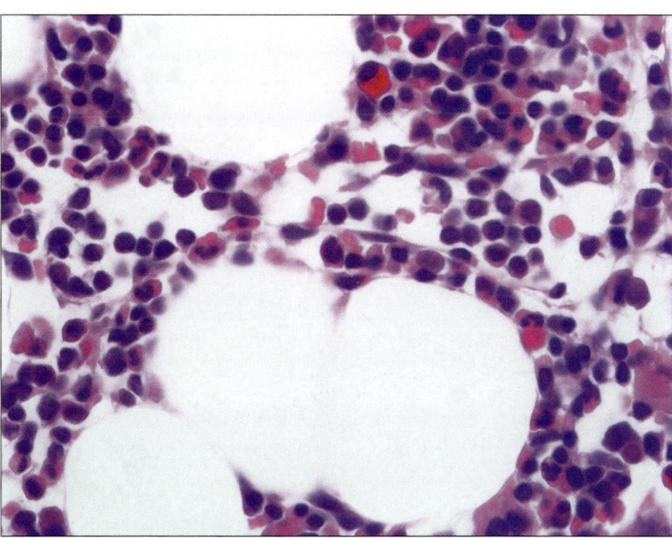

Figure 12.2 Section of a trephine biopsy specimen showing, in the centre of the photograph, intra-sinusoidal infiltration. H&E, x 100 objective.

this feature is not so consistently present. Reticulin deposition is increased but not to the extent that is usual in hairy cell leukaemia so that it is usually possible to aspirate bone marrow. Splenic infiltration is preferentially in the red pulp and may be indistinguishable from that of hairy cell leukaemia.

Immunophenotype

The immunophenotype is useful in distinguishing these cases from hairy cell leukaemia. CD11c is positive in the majority of patients and CD103 is positive in approaching two-thirds but CD25 and CD123 are usually negative [9, 10] (Figure **12.3**). If these four markers are used, cases of hairy cell variant score 0–2 whereas cases of hairy cell leukaemia score 3–4. In contrast to most B-lineage lymphoproliferative disorders, CD79b is more often negative than positive. On immunohistochemistry there is expression of B-lineage markers such as CD20 (Figure **12.4**) and DBA44 (Figure **12.5**).

Cytogenetic and molecular genetic abnormalities

Complex karyotypes and deletion of one *TP53* allele in a proportion of cells are common [8, 11].

Diagnosis and differential diagnosis

The differential diagnosis includes hairy cell leukaemia, splenic marginal zone lymphoma/splenic lymphoma with villous lymphocytes and prolymphocytic leukaemia. Cytology, immunophenotyping, trephine biopsy histology and cytochemistry are all useful in making the distinction.

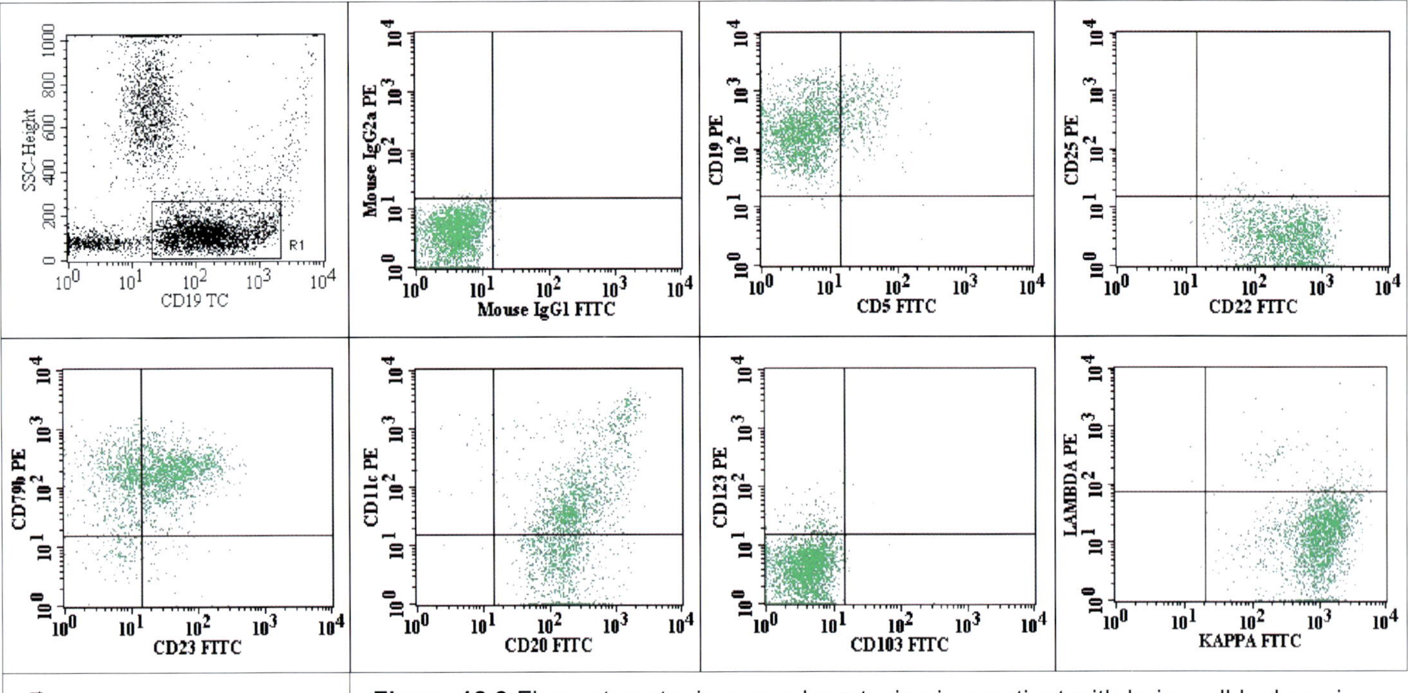

Figure 12.3 Flow cytometry immunophenotyping in a patient with hairy cell leukaemia variant. Sideways scatter and CD19 have been used for gating. In addition to CD19, the leukaemic cells express CD20, CD22 (strong), CD79b, FMC7 and strong κ light chain. There is partial expression of CD11c. The case is unusual in also expressing CD23. There is no expression of CD5, CD25, CD103 or CD123. The CLL score and the hairy cell leukaemia score are both 1. With thanks to Mr Ricardo Morilla.

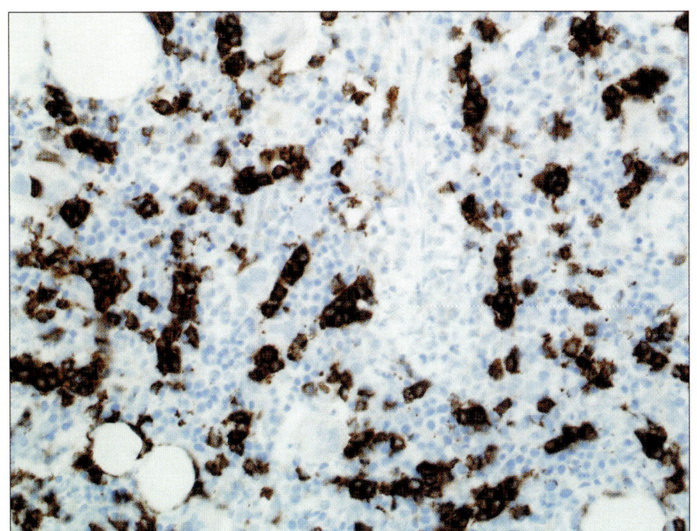

Figure 12.4 Section of a trephine biopsy specimen showing CD20 expression. Immunoperoxidase, x 40 objective.

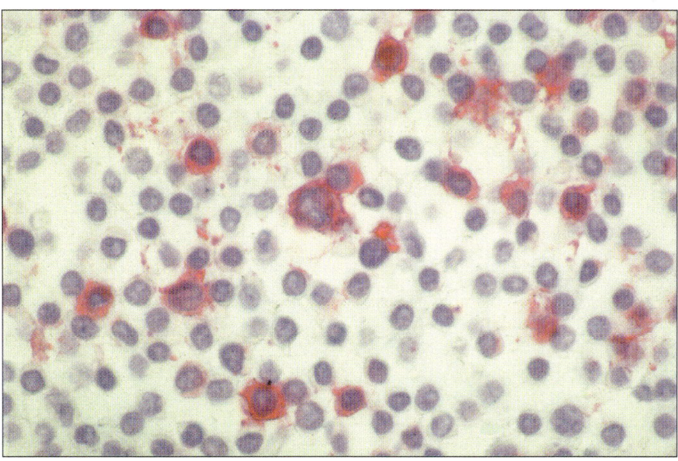

Figure 12.5 Section of a trephine biopsy specimen showing DBA44 expression. Immunoalkaline phosphatase, x 100 objective.

Prognosis

The disease is indolent so that the median survival is around seven years, despite the lack of response to most treatment modalities [6].

Treatment

Nucleoside analogues and interferon, both effective in hairy cell leukaemia, are usually ineffective (partial responses in only around one-half of patients) [6, 12]. Alkylating agents and interferon are usually not useful. Splenectomy can be effective.

References

1. Cawley JC, Burns GF and Hayhoe FGJ (1980). A chronic lymphoproliferative disorder with distinctive features: a distinct variant of hairy cell leukemia. *Leuk Res*, **4**, 547–559.
2. Catovsky D, O'Brien M, Melo JV, Wardle J and Brozovic M (1984). Hairy cell leukemia (HCL) variant: an intermediate disease between HCL and B prolymphocytic leukemia. *Semin Oncol*, **11**, 362–369.
3. Foucar K and Catovsky D (2001). Hairy cell leukaemia. *In* Jaffe ES, Harris NL, Stein H and Vardiman JW (Eds). *WHO classification of Haematopoietic and Lymphoid tumours*, IARC Press, Lyon, pp. 138–141.
4. Zinzani PL, Lauria F, Buzzi M, Raspadori D, Gugliotta L, Bocchia M *et al.* (1990). Hairy cell leukemia variant: a morphologic, immunologic and clinical study of 7 cases. *Haematologica*, **75**, 54–57.
5. Sainati L, Matutes E, Mulligan S, de Oliveira MP, Rani S, Lampert IA and Catovsky D (1990). A variant form of hairy cell leukemia resistant to alpha-interferon: clinical and phenotypic characteristics of 17 patients. *Blood*, **76**, 157–162.
6. Matutes E, Wotherspoon A, Brito-Babapulle V and Catovsky D (2001). The natural history and clinico-pathological features of the variant form of hairy cell leukemia. *Leukemia*, **15**, 184–186.
7. Matutes E, Wotherspoon A and Catovsky D (2003). The variant form of hairy-cell leukaemia. *Best Pract Res Clin Haematol*, **16**, 41–56.
8. Wotherspoon A and Matutes E (2004). Recent advances in understanding small B-cell leukaemias and lymphomas. *Curr Diag Pathol*, **10**, 374–384.

9. Matutes E, Morilla R, Owusu-Ankomah K, Houlihan A, Meeus P and Catovsky D (1994). The immunophenotype of hairy cell leukemia (HCL). Proposal for a scoring system to distinguish HCL from B-cell disorders with hairy or villous lymphocytes. *Leuk Lymphoma*, **14**, 57–61.
10. Del Giudice I, Matutes E, Morilla R, Morilla A, Owusu-Ankomah K, Rafiq F *et al.* (2004). The diagnostic value of CD123 in B-cell disorders with hairy or villous lymphocytes. *Haematologica*, **89**, 303–308.
11. Vallianatou K, Brito-Babapulle V, Matutes E, Atkinson S and Catovsky D (1999). p53 gene deletion and trisomy 12 in hairy cell leukemia and its variant. *Leuk Res*, **23**, 1041–1045.
12. Robak T (2006). Current treatment options in hairy cell leukemia and hairy cell leukemia variant. *Cancer Treat Rev*, **32**, 365–376.

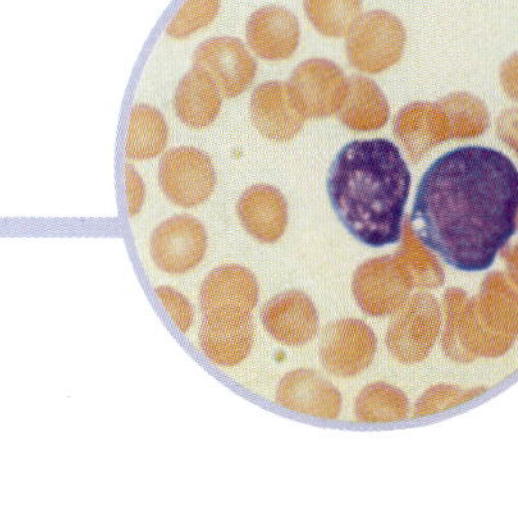

Chapter 13

Burkitt's lymphoma

Burkitt's lymphoma is a highly aggressive lymphoma of mature B cells. In the majority of patients it is an extra-nodal lymphoma but some patients have leukaemic manifestations. Three variants are recognized on the basis of epidemiological and clinicopathological features – endemic, sporadic and human immunodeficiency virus (HIV)-related [1, 2]. Endemic Burkitt's lymphoma occurs in equatorial Africa and in Papua New Guinea where malaria is hyperendemic, is strongly related to Epstein–Barr virus (EBV) infection, occurs in children and usually affects the jaw bones. Sporadic lymphoma occurs in developed countries, is related to EBV in only about 10% of cases, occurs in children and young adults and most often affects the gastrointestinal tract. HIV-related Burkitt's lymphoma is associated with EBV in about one-third of cases and often presents with disseminated disease, e.g. involving lymph nodes and bone marrow. Burkitt's lymphoma is derived from a germinal centre B cell without somatic hypermutation. Recently, gene expression analysis has produced evidence that Burkitt's lymphoma and a sub-set of diffuse large B-cell lymphoma are much more closely related than had previously been realized [3, 4]. In addition to cases of *de novo* Burkitt's lymphoma, there are cases that represent transformation of a pre-existing low-grade lymphoma.

Clinical features

Clinical features vary according to whether the disease is endemic, sporadic or HIV-related, but may include tumours of the mandible or maxilla, orbit, gastrointestinal tract, ovaries, breasts or kidneys. The tumours are remarkable for their high rate of growth, as a result of which patients often present with bulky, locally advanced disease. Central nervous system and bone marrow involvement are common and lymphadenopathy and leukaemia occur in a minority of patients.

Haematological and pathological features

In patients with peripheral blood and bone marrow involvement, the lymphoma cells have the features described by the French–American–British (FAB) group as L3 acute lymphoblastic leukaemia (ALL). It should, however, be noted that this condition is correctly classified as a lymphoma (as in the WHO classification), not as ALL, since the cells are mature B cells. Neoplastic cells are medium sized with strongly basophilic vacuolated cytoplasm (Figures **13.1** and **13.2**). The vacuoles contain lipid and stain with Oil Red O. The same cytological features are apparent in films from fine needle aspirates and in imprints from tissue sections (Figure **13.3**).

In histological sections there is diffuse infiltration by medium sized lymphoid cells with a regular cellular outline; cytoplasmic vacuoles are less apparent than in cytological preparations (Figure **13.4**). The cytoplasm is strongly positive with methyl green pyronine. The high proliferative rate and high rate of cell death are apparent: mitotic figures and apoptotic cells are common and monoclonal antibodies that recognize proliferating cells, such as Ki67 and MIB1, are positive in around 99% of cells (Figure **13.5**). As a result of the high cell turnover, macrophages containing apoptotic cells and cell debris are increased, giving a 'starry sky' appearance to the tissue sections (Figure **13.6**). A starry sky appearance is also sometimes apparent on a film of a fine needle aspirate (Figure **13.7**).

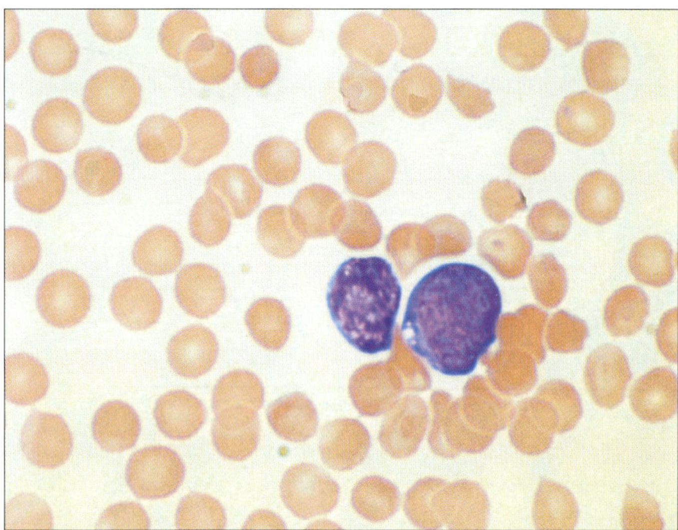

Figure 13.1 Peripheral blood film in Burkitt's lymphoma showing two cells with strongly basophilic vacuolated cytoplasm. Romanowsky stain, x 100 objective.

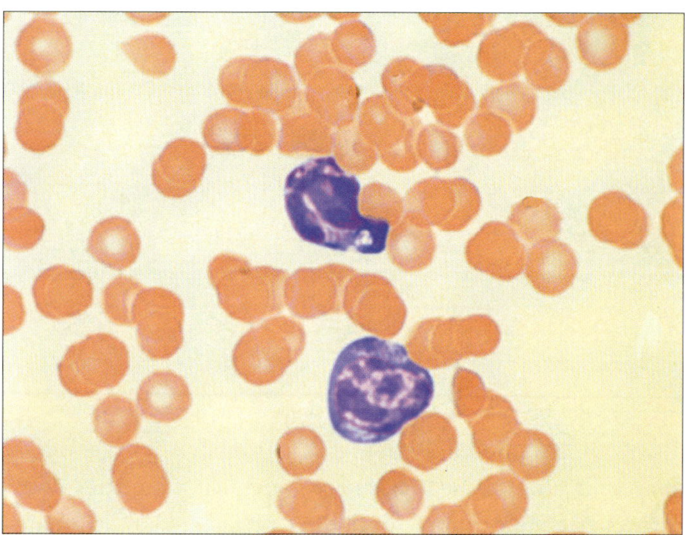

Figure 13.2 Peripheral blood film in Burkitt's lymphoma showing two cells with strongly basophilic cytoplasm and apoptotic nuclei. Romanowsky stain, x 100 objective.

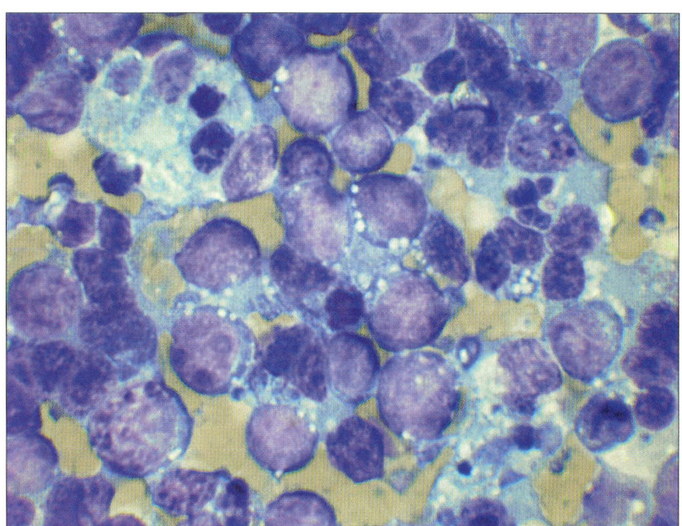

Figure 13.3 Film of fine needle aspirate from a patient with Burkitt's lymphoma showing lymphoma cells with strongly basophilic, heavily vacuolated cytoplasm. There are also several macrophages containing cellular debris. Romanowsky stain, x 100 objective. With thanks to Dr Julie McCarthy.

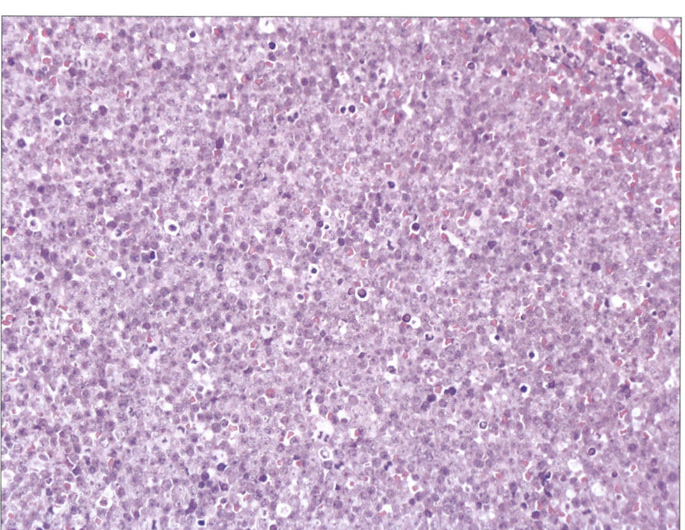

Figure 13.4 Section of a lymph node biopsy showing a diffuse infiltrate of lymphoma cells that show a high rate of apoptosis. H&E, x 40 objective.

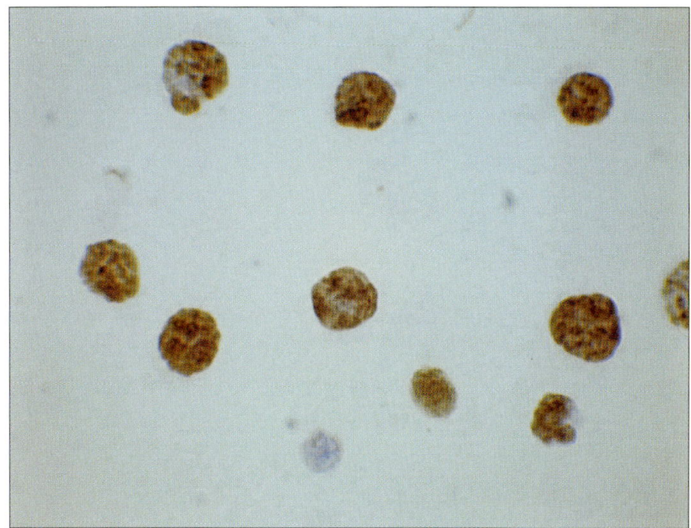

Figure 13.5 Film of fine needle aspirate from a patient with Burkitt's lymphoma showing that almost all cells are MIB1 positive. Immunoperoxidase stain, x 100 objective. With thanks to Dr Julie McCarthy.

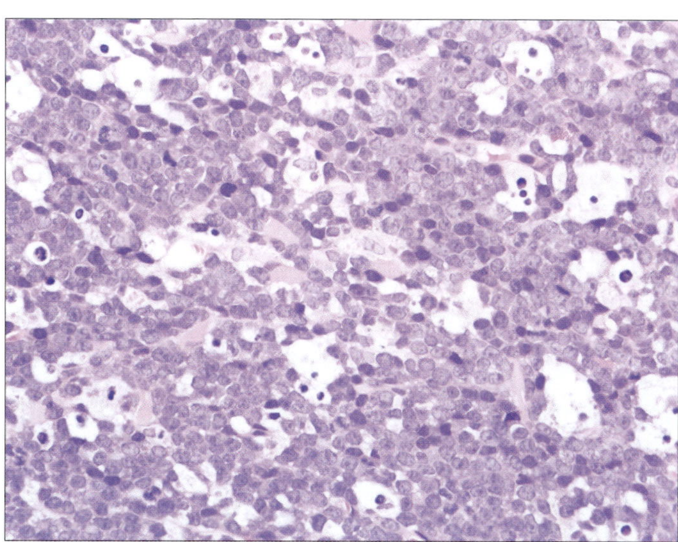

Figure 13.6 Section of a lymph node biopsy showing a diffuse infiltrate of lymphoma cells with interspersed macrophages creating a 'starry sky' appearance. H&E, x 60 objective.

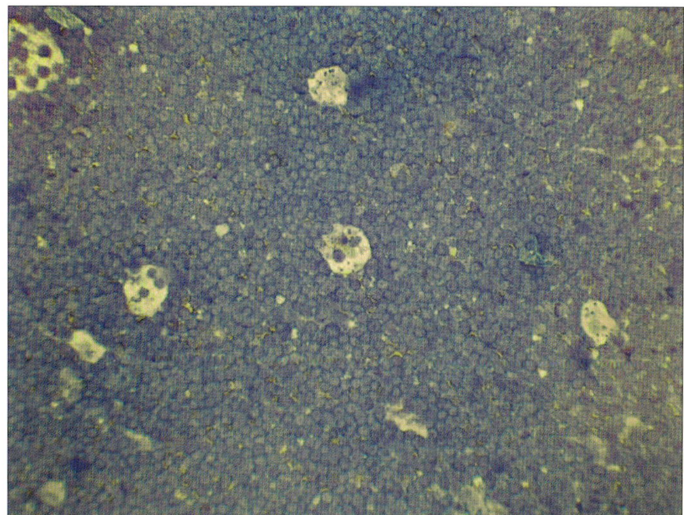

Figure 13.7 Film of fine needle aspirate from a patient with Burkitt's lymphoma showing a starry sky appearance. Romanowsky stain, x 10 objective. With thanks to Dr Julie McCarthy.

Immunophenotype

Because of the high rate of apoptosis, it is important that immunophenotyping is done rapidly. Lymphoma cells express monotypic surface membrane immunoglobulin (IgM) and B-cell associated antigens such as CD19, CD20, CD22 and CD79a (Figure **13.8**). CD10 is usually expressed [5, 6] (Figure **13.9**) and cytoplasmic μ chain is sometimes expressed. BCL6 is expressed whereas BCL2 is not [5, 6] (Figure **13.10**); BCL2 negativity can be diagnostically important. CD5 and CD23 are not expressed. Terminal deoxynucleotidyl transferase and CD34 are not usually expressed. There is over-expression of *TP53* (p53) and other tumour suppressor pathways are also disrupted [7].

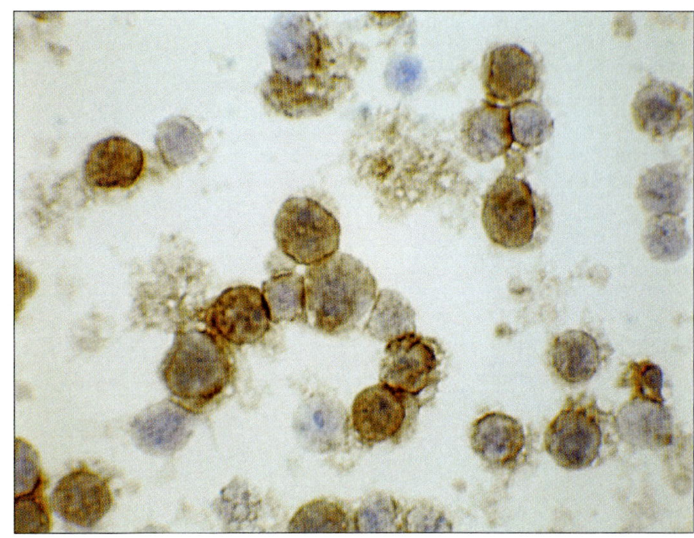

Figure 13.8 Film of fine needle aspirate from a patient with Burkitt's lymphoma showing that cells express CD79a. Immunoperoxidase stain, x 100 objective. With thanks to Dr Julie McCarthy.

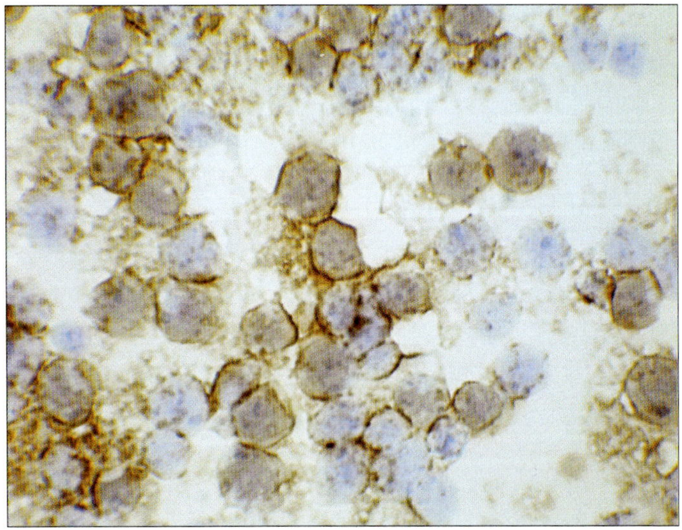

Figure 13.9 Film of fine needle aspirate from a patient with Burkitt's lymphoma showing that cells express CD10. Immunoperoxidase stain, x 100 objective. With thanks to Dr Julie McCarthy.

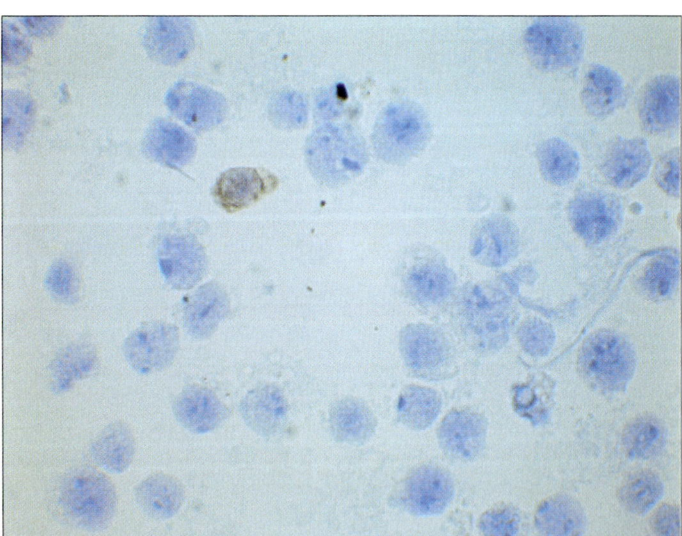

Figure 13.10 Film of fine needle aspirate from a patient with Burkitt's lymphoma showing that cells do not express BCL2. Immunoperoxidase stain, x 100 objective. With thanks to Dr Julie McCarthy.

Cytogenetic and molecular genetic abnormalities

The characteristic cytogenetic abnormality, present in the majority of cases, is t(8;14)(q24;q32), leading to dysregulation of the *MYC* oncogene when it is translocated from chromosome 8 and is juxtaposed to the *IGH* gene, on chromosome 14 (Figure **13.11**). In a minority of cases there is either t(2;8)(p12;q24) or t(8;22)(q24;q11), leading to dysregulation of *MYC* as a result of translocation of either the *IGK* gene from 2p12 or the *IGL* gene from 22q11 to chromosome 8. These genes encode kappa (κ) and lambda (λ) immunoglobulin light chains so that the mechanism of dysregulation of *MYC* is similar in the three translocations. There is often mutation of the *MYC* gene as well as translocation. Detection of translocations can be achieved by standard cytogenetic analysis or by fluorescence *in situ* hybridization (FISH). For FISH analysis, a break-apart probe is preferred since it permits detection of all three translocations. The precise breakpoints differ at a molecular level between EBV-associated cases and other cases. EBV-associated cases show more mutated $IG_{V}H$ genes and evidence of antigen selection [8].

Diagnosis and differential diagnosis

Burkitt's lymphoma is readily suspected if L3 morphology is observed but confirmation by genetic analysis is needed since cases of B-lineage, and less often T-lineage, ALL can have very similar cytological features. Histological diagnosis is usually straightforward in endemic cases but in some sporadic and HIV-related cases there are atypical features (plasmacytoid differentiation or cellular pleomorphism). The differential diagnosis includes diffuse large B-cell lymphoma and HIV-related lymphomas other than Burkitt's lymphoma. Burkitt's type transformation of other B-cell lymphomas, e.g. follicular lymphoma, should also be considered in the differential diagnosis [9]. In atypical cases, demonstration of involvement of *MYC* and consideration of the immunophenotype and the proliferative fraction are essential to make a diagnosis of Burkitt's lymphoma or atypical/Burkitt-like lymphoma.

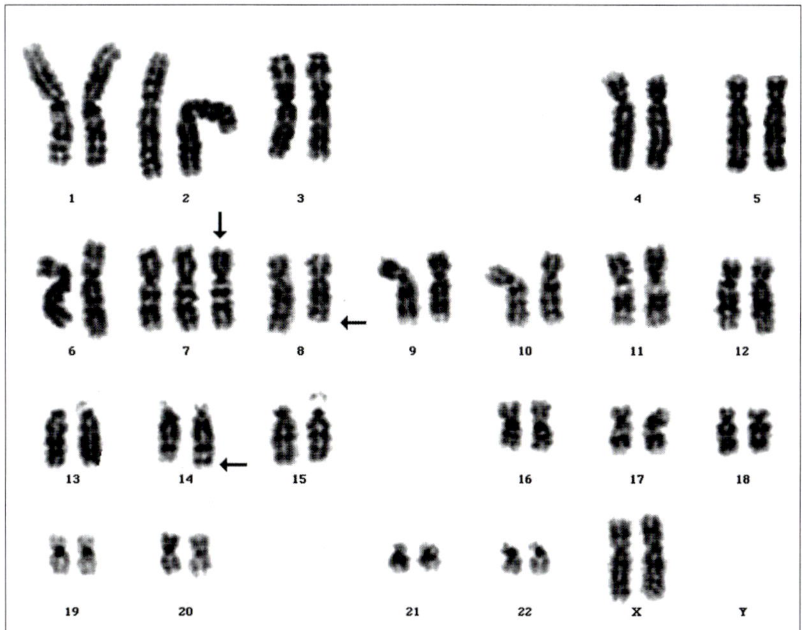

Figure 13.11 Karyogram from a patient with Burkitt's lymphoma showing t(8;14)(q24;q32) and trisomy 7. The arrows indicate the supernumerary chromosome 7 and the two chromosomes involved in the translocation. With thanks to Dr John Swansbury.

Prognosis

Although this tumour is highly aggressive it is potentially curable in the majority of appropriately treated patients. Poor prognostic factors include advanced stage, high lactate dehydrogenase and bone marrow or central nervous system involvement.

Treatment

Burkitt's lymphoma requires intensive multi-agent chemotherapy with specific regimes that include cyclophosphamide and anthracyclines. Treatment is more intensive but briefer than that for ALL.

References

1. Jaffe ES, Diebold J, Harris NL, Muller-Hermelink HK, Flandrin G and Vardiman JW (1999). Burkitt's lymphoma: a single disease with multiple variants. The World Health Organization classification of neoplastic diseases of the hematopoietic and lymphoid tissues. *Blood*, **93**, 1124.
2. Diebold J, Jaffe ES, Raphael M and Warnke RA (2001). Burkitt lymphoma. *In* Jaffe ES, Harris NL, Stein H and Vardiman JW (Eds). *World Health Organization Classification of Tumours: Pathology and Genetics of Tumours of Haematopoietic and Lymphoid Tissues*, IARC Press, Lyon, pp. 181–184.
3. Hummel M, Bentink S, Berger H, Klapper W, Wessendorf S, Barth TFE *et al.* (2006). A biologic definition of Burkitt's lymphoma from transcriptional and genomic profiling. *N Engl J Med*, **354**, 2419–2430.
4. Dave SS, Fu K, Wright GW, Lam LT, Kluin P, Boerma E-J *et al.* (2006). Molecular diagnosis of Burkitt's lymphoma. *N Engl J Med*, **354**, 2431–2442.
5. Dogan A, Bagdi E, Munson P and Isaacson PG (2000). CD10 and BCL-6 expression in paraffin sections of normal lymphoid tissue and B-cell lymphomas. *Am J Surg Pathol*, **24**, 846–852.
6. Nakamura N, Nakamine H, Tamaru J, Nakamura S, Yoshino T *et al.* (2002). The distinction between Burkitt lymphoma and diffuse large B-cell lymphoma with c-myc rearrangement. *Mod Pathol*, **15**, 771–776.
7. Lindstrom MS and Wiman KG (2002). Role of genetic and epigenetic changes in Burkitt lymphoma. *Semin Cancer Biol*, **12**, 381–387.
8. Bellan C, Lazzi S, Hummel M, Palumno N, de Santi M, Amato T *et al.* (2005). Immunoglobulin gene analysis reveals 2 distinct cells of origin for EBV-positive and EBV-negative Burkitt lymphomas. *Blood*, **106**, 1031–1036.
9. Karsan A, Gascoyne RD, Coupland RW, Shepherd JD, Philips GL and Horsman DE (1993). Combination of t(14;18) and a Burkitt's type translocation in B-cell malignancies. *Leuk Lymphoma*, **10**, 433–441.

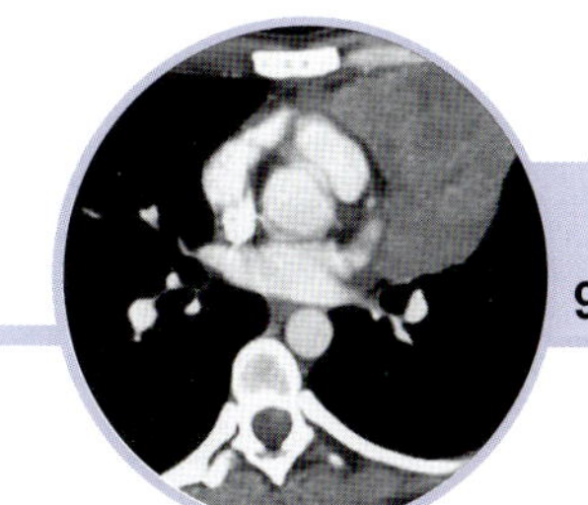

Chapter 14

Diffuse large B-cell lymphoma

The term diffuse large B-cell lymphoma (DLBCL) covers a rather heterogeneous group of lymphomas that are all characterized by diffuse tissue infiltration by large B-lineage lymphoma cells. Those that are related to human immunodeficiency virus (HIV) infection are dealt with separately (see Chapter 15). There are uncommon subtypes, including mediastinal (thymic) large B-cell lymphoma, primary effusion-associated lymphoma and intravascular B-cell lymphoma. The disease can be primarily nodal or extra-nodal and can occur *de novo* or represent transformation of a lower grade non-Hodgkin's lymphoma, of nodular lymphocyte predominant Hodgkin's disease or of chronic lymphocytic leukaemia (known as Richter's syndrome).

Clinical features

Patients may present with localized or generalized lymphadenopathy (Figure **14.1**) or with extra-nodal disease at a great variety of sites. In advanced disease there may be hepatomegaly, splenomegaly and involvement of central nervous system or bone marrow, with or without circulating lymphoma cells. Mediastinal large B-cell lymphoma [1] presents as a thymic mass (Figures **14.2**–**14.5**), primary effusion lymphoma with pleural or pericardial effusion or ascites (usually in an HIV-positive patient) [2] and intravascular B-cell lymphoma with multiorgan symptoms [3].

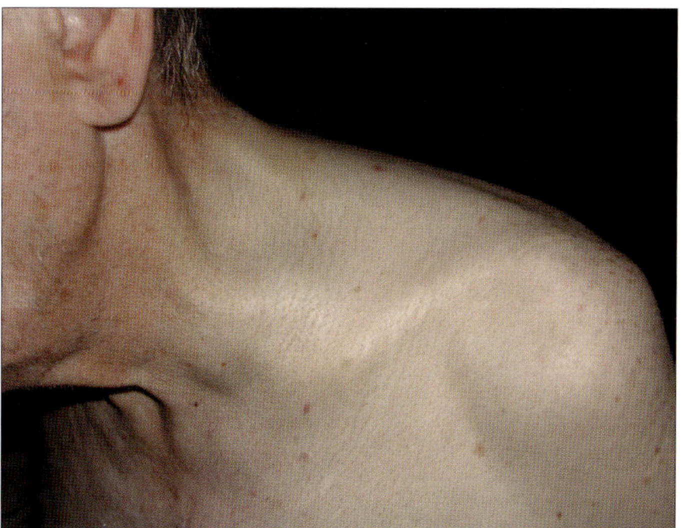

Figure 14.1 Clinical photograph showing cervical lymphadenopathy in a patient with diffuse large B-cell lymphoma (T-cell rich B-cell lymphoma).

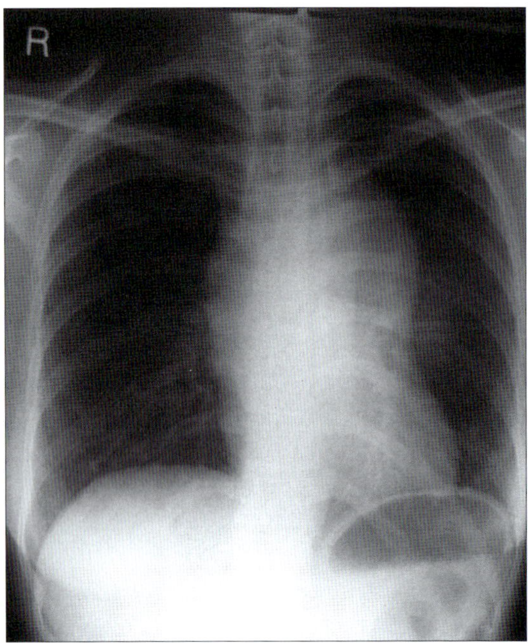

Figure 14.2 Pre-treatment chest radiograph in a patient with mediastinal (thymic) large B-cell lymphoma.

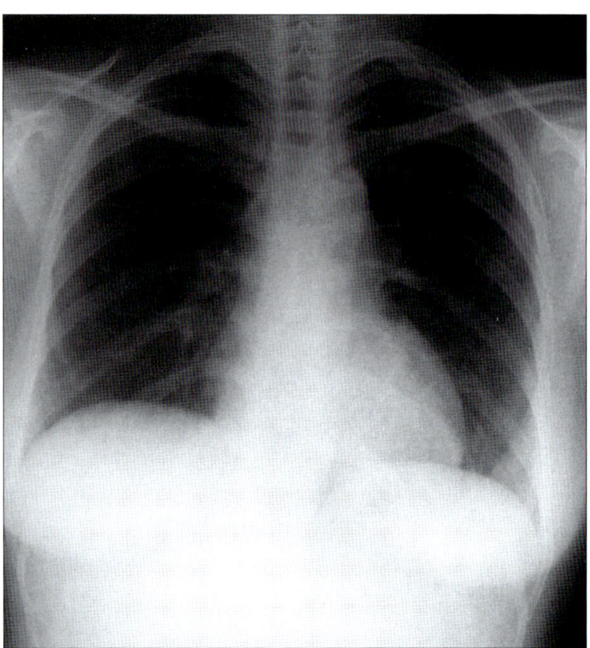

Figure 14.3 Post-treatment chest radiograph in a patient with mediastinal (thymic) large B-cell lymphoma (same patient as Figure **14.2**).

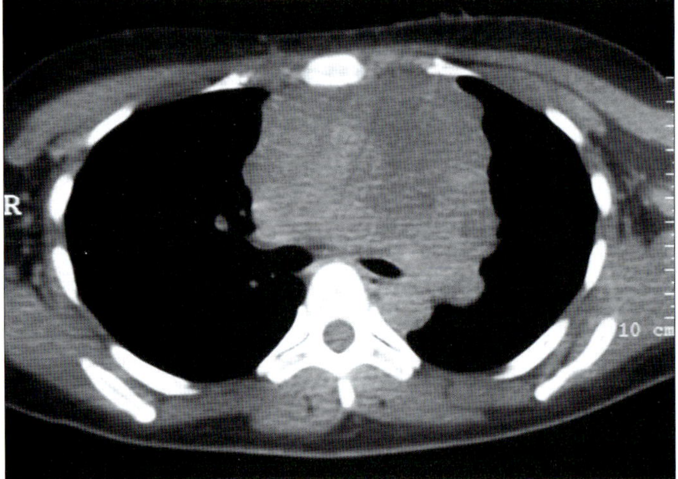

Figure 14.4 CT scan in another patient with mediastinal (thymic) large B-cell lymphoma.

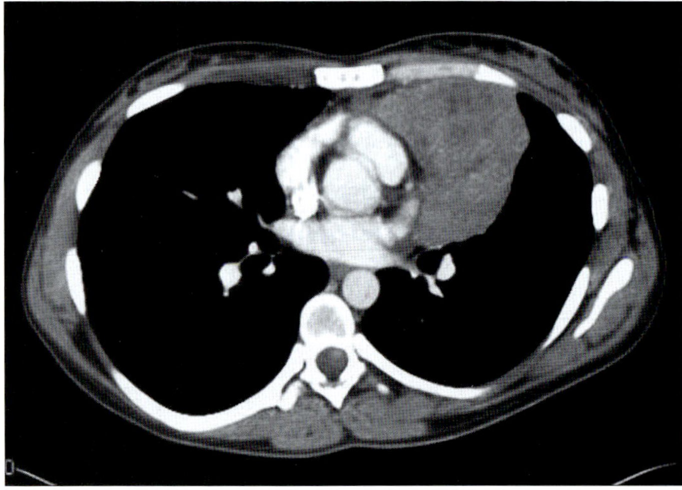

Figure 14.5 CT scan in a patient with mediastinal (thymic) large B-cell lymphoma (same patient as Figure **14.4**).

Haematological and pathological features

In the minority of patients with peripheral blood involvement, the lymphoma cells have a diameter that exceeds that of three erythrocytes (Figure **14.6**). They are usually pleomorphic, and may have large nucleoli and irregular or cleft nuclei [4] (Figure **14.7**). Sometimes cytoplasmic basophilia is prominent and a Golgi zone may be apparent.

Bone marrow infiltration is usually random focal with cohesive infiltrates of large lymphoma cells. In other patients there is infiltration by lymphoma cells with associated T cells or macrophages with these reactive cells sometimes dominating the histological picture. In some patients trephine biopsy reveals a low-grade lymphoma with, or more

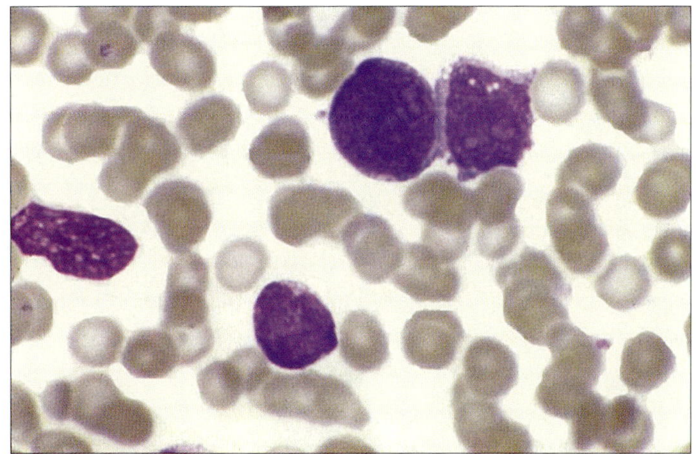

Figure 14.6 Peripheral blood film showing large lymphoma cells with prominent nucleoli. Romanowsky stain, x 100 objective.

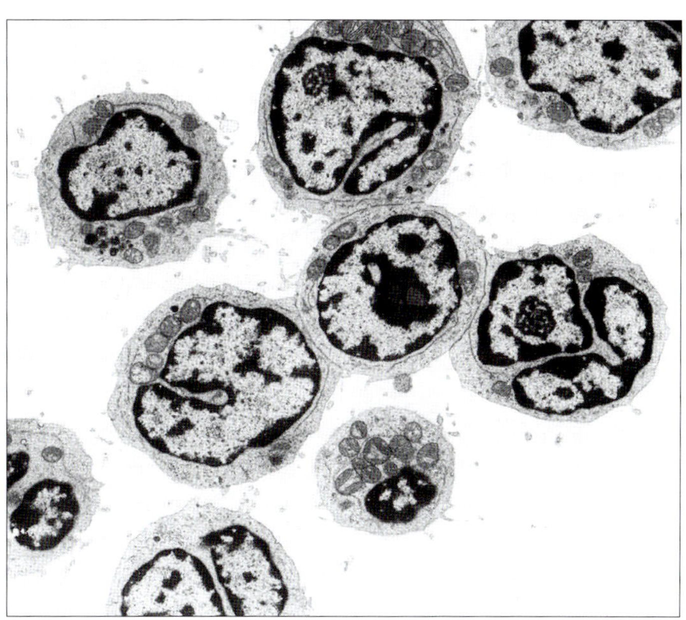

Figure 14.7 Ultrastructural examination showing pleomorphic large lymphoma cells, some with irregular nuclei and some with large nucleoli. Lead nitrate and uranyl acetate stain.

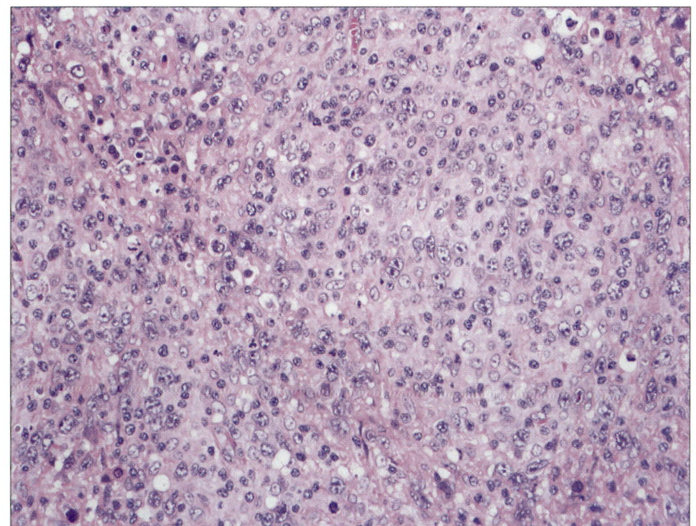

Figure 14.8 Section of lymph node biopsy showing a diffuse infiltrate by pleomorphic nucleolated large lymphoma cells. H&E, x 20 objective.

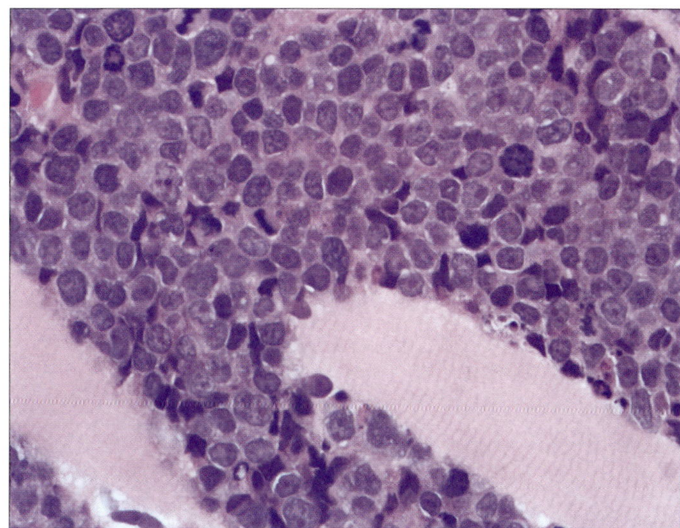

Figure 14.9 Section of lymph node biopsy showing a diffuse infiltrate by large lymphoma cells; several mitotic figures are apparent. H&E, x 100 objective.

often without, infiltration by large cell lymphoma; this is usually indicative of evolution from a preceding subclinical low-grade lymphoma. In intra-vascular large cell lymphoma, lymphoma cells may be seen within bone marrow sinusoids.

Lymph nodes are usually effaced by a diffuse infiltrate of large lymphoma cells, with or without an associated population of inflammatory cells (Figures **14.8–14.10**). In some patients lymph node involvement is focal, interfollicular or sinusoidal. Morphological variants include centroblastic (multiple membrane-bound nucleoli), immunoblastic (single large central nucleolus) and anaplastic DLBCL.

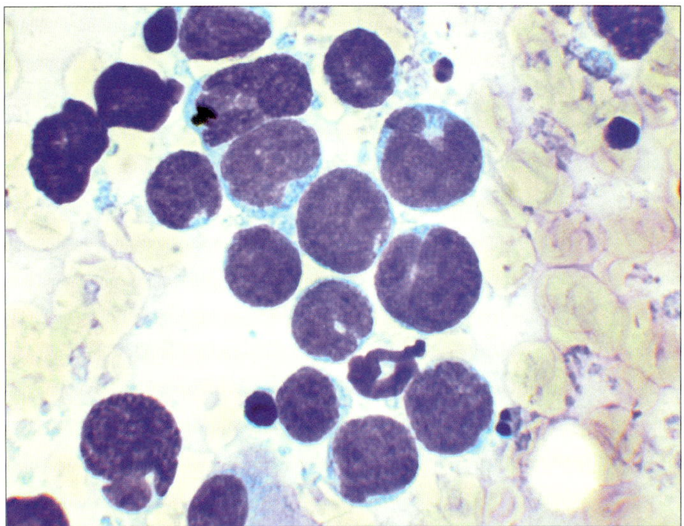

Figure 14.10 Film of fine needle aspirate showing pleomorphic large lymphoma cells. Romanowsky stain, x 100 objective. With thanks to Dr Julie McCarthy.

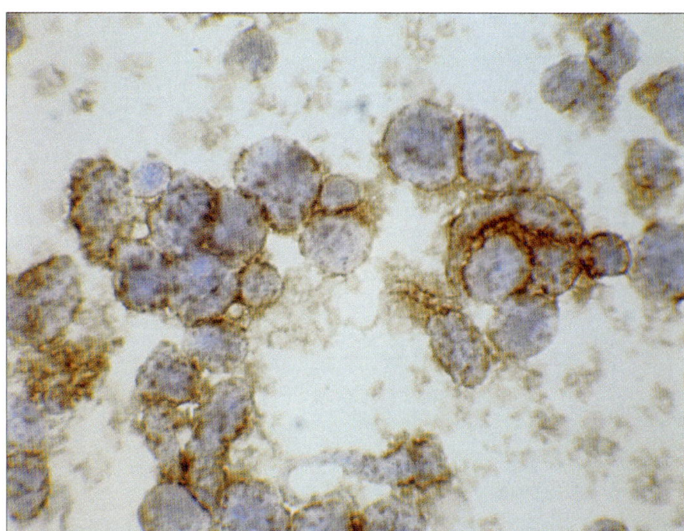

Figure 14.11 Film of fine needle aspirate showing that the lymphoma cells express CD20 (same case as Figure **14.10**). Immunoperoxidase, x 100 objective. With thanks to Dr Julie McCarthy.

Immunophenotype

Lymphoma cells usually express monotypic surface membrane immunoglobulin and express B-cell associated antigens such as CD19, CD20, CD22, CD79a and CD79b (Figures **14.11** and **14.12**). Cases with plasmacytic differentiation may have cytoplasmic immunoglobulin. On immunohistochemistry there is expression of CD20, CD79a and PAX5. Other antigens, such as CD5, CD10 (Figure **14.13**), CD23, BCL2 (Figure **14.14**), BCL6, IRF4 and TP53, are expressed in only some cases; cases with anaplastic morphology usually express CD30. The proliferation fraction (Ki67 or MIB1 reactivity) (Figure **14.15**) is usually around 30–40% of cells but may be higher, sometimes even exceeding 90%. Differences in immunophenotype are apparent between those with a germinal centre and those with an 'activated B-cell' gene expression pattern (see below). Germinal centre-type DLBCL usually expresses CD10 and BCL6 but not IRF4. Activated B-cell-type DLBCL usually expresses BCL6 and IRF4 but not CD10 (*Table 14.1*).

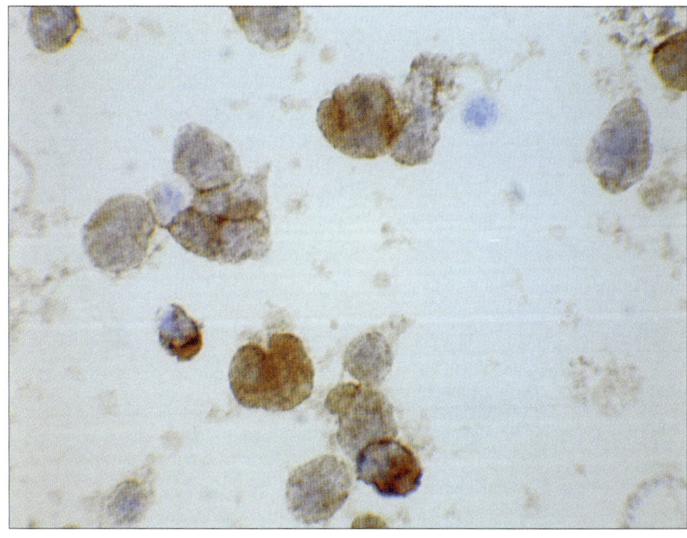

Figure 14.12 Film of fine needle aspirate showing that the lymphoma cells express CD79a (same case as Figure **14.10**). Immunoperoxidase, x 100 objective. With thanks to Dr Julie McCarthy.

Cytogenetic and molecular genetic abnormalities

Cytogenetic and molecular genetic analysis indicate the heterogeneity of this category of lymphoma. Among cytogenetic abnormalities that may be found are t(14;18)(q32;q21) and chromosomal rearrangements with a 3q27 breakpoint such as t(3;14)(q27;q32). The former translocation dysregulates *BCL2* and the latter group

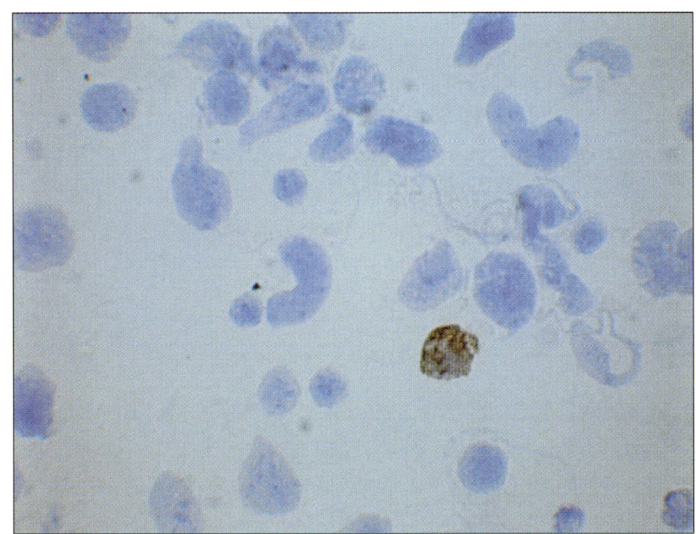

Figure 14.13 Film of fine needle aspirate showing that the lymphoma cells do not express CD10 (same case as Figure **14.10**). Immunoperoxidase, x 100 objective. With thanks to Dr Julie McCarthy.

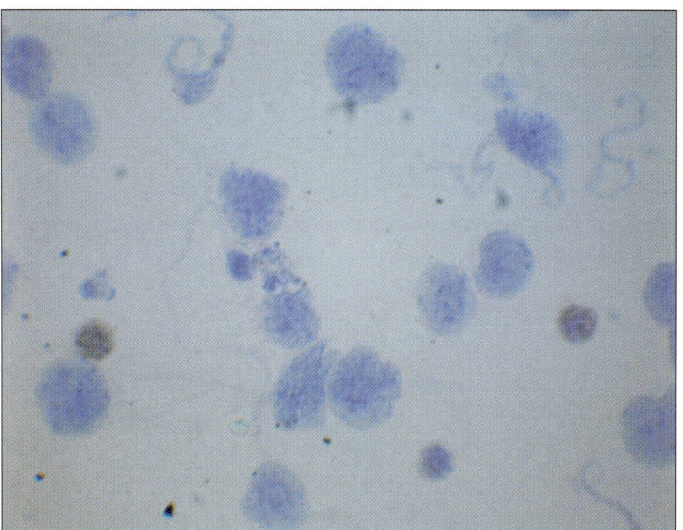

Figure 14.14 Film of fine needle aspirate showing that the lymphoma cells do not express BCL2 (same case as Figure **14.10**). Immunoperoxidase, x 100 objective. With thanks to Dr Julie McCarthy.

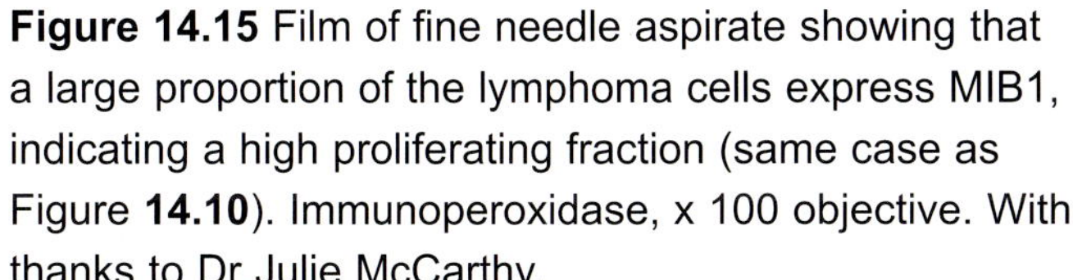

Figure 14.15 Film of fine needle aspirate showing that a large proportion of the lymphoma cells express MIB1, indicating a high proliferating fraction (same case as Figure **14.10**). Immunoperoxidase, x 100 objective. With thanks to Dr Julie McCarthy.

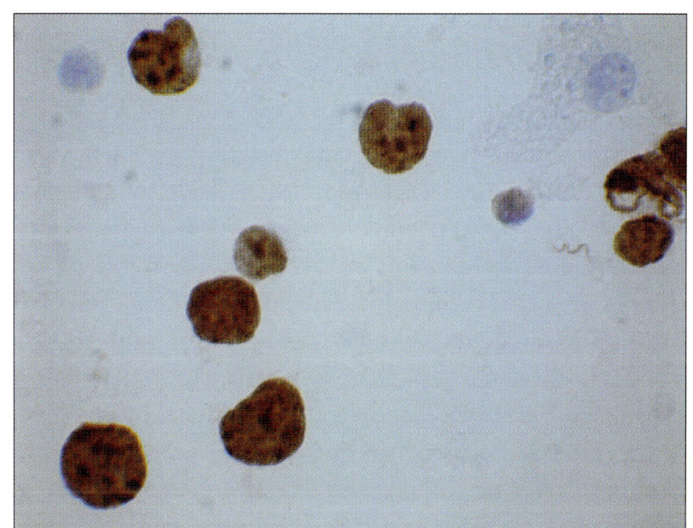

Table 14.1 Comparison of germinal centre type and 'activated B-cell' type of diffuse large B-cell lymphoma

Germinal centre type	*'Activated B-cell' type*
Usually CD10+, BCL6+	Usually CD10–, BCL6+, IRF4+
Sometimes CD10–, BCL6+, IRF4–	Sometimes CD10–, BCL6–, IRF4+
Better prognosis	Worse prognosis

dysregulate *BCL6*. Cytogenetic abnormalities are often complex. Microarray analysis permits the division of cases into three groups characterized as follicular centre phenotype, activated B-cell phenotype and 'other' [5, 6]. Cytogenetic/molecular genetic analysis to exclude Burkitt's lymphoma is indicated if lymphoma cells are BCL2 negative and the proliferation fraction is very high.

Diagnosis and differential diagnosis

The differential diagnosis includes large cell lymphoma of T lineage. In patients with peripheral blood involvement, distinction from large cell lymphoma of T lineage is not possible on morphology alone. In some patients circulating lymphoma cells resemble those of either plasmablastic plasma cell leukaemia or acute monoblastic leukaemia.

On histological sections differential diagnosis includes T-cell lymphoma.

Prognosis

This lymphoma is potentially curable with five-year survival rates of around 60% when treatment is with combination chemotherapy and immunotherapy. Adverse prognostic factors, for patients treated with anthracycline-based combination chemotherapy, include advanced stage disease, high lactate dehydrogenase, older age and worse performance status (all combined into the International Prognostic Index), an activated B-cell rather than germinal centre gene expression pattern, lack of a germinal centre immunophenotype (a germinal centre phenotype being defined as CD10 positive, BCL6 positive), t(14;18) in those with a germinal centre immunophenotype, *BCL2* expression in those with a non-germinal centre phenotype and overall, t(8;14)(q24;q32), 3q27 rearrangement and over-expression of *TP53* (p53) or p21 [5, 7–9].

Treatment

Treatment of advanced disease is with combination chemotherapy plus immunotherapy, e.g. 6–8 courses of the CHOP regime (cyclophosphamide, doxorubicin, vincristine and prednisone or prednisolone) plus rituximab (an anti-CD20 monoclonal antibody). Patients with more localized disease (stage I and non-bulky stage II) can be treated with fewer courses of combination chemotherapy (e.g. three courses of CHOP) followed by involved field radiotherapy. The role of radio-immune conjugates, of dose intensification in rituximab-containing regimes and of maintenance rituximab remain to be evaluated.

References

1. Aisenberg AC (1999). Primary large cell lymphoma of the mediastinum. *Semin Oncol*, **26**, 251–258.
2. Cesarman E, Chang Y, Moore PS, Said JW and Knowles DM (1995). Kaposi's sarcoma-associated herpesvirus-like DNA sequences in AIDS-related body-cavity-based lymphomas. *N Engl J Med*, **332**, 1186–1191.
3. Gatter KC and Warnke RA (2001). Intravascular large B-cell lymphoma. *In* Jaffe ES, Harris NL, Stein H and Vardiman JW (Eds). *World Health Organization Classification of Tumours: Pathology and Genetics of Tumours of Haematopoietic and Lymphoid Tissues*, IARC Press, Lyon, pp. 177–178.
4. Bain BJ, Matutes E, Robinson D, Lampert IA, Brito-Babapulle V, Morilla R and Catovsky D (1991). Leukaemia as a manifestation of large cell lymphoma. *Br J Haematol*, **77**, 301–310.
5. Alizadeh AA, Eisen MB, Davis RE, Ma C, Lossos IS, Rosenwald A *et al.* (2000). Distinct types of diffuse large cell B-cell lymphoma identified by gene expression profiling. *Nature*, **403**, 503–511.
6. Wright G, Tan B, Rosenwald A, Hurt EH, Wiestner A and Staudt LM (2003). A gene expression-based method to distinguish clinically subgroups of diffuse large B cell lymphoma. *Proc Natl Acad Sci USA*, **100**, 9991–9996.
7. The International Non-Hodgkin's Lymphoma Prognostic Factors Project (1993). A predictive model for aggressive non-Hodgkin's lymphoma. *New Engl J Med*, **329**, 987–994.
8. Barrans SL, Carter I, Owen RG, Davies FE, Patmeore RD, Haynes AP *et al.* (2002). Germinal center phenotype and bcl-2 expression combined with the International Prognostic Index improves patient risk stratification in diffuse large B-cell lymphoma. *Blood*, **99**, 1136–1143.
9. Lossos IS, Jones CD, Warnke R, Natkunam Y, Kaizer H, Zehnder JL *et al.* (2001). Expression of a single gene, BCL-6, strongly predicts survival in patients with diffuse large B-cell lymphoma. *Blood*, **98**, 945–951.

Chapter 15

AIDS-related and other immunodeficiency-related lymphomas

The appearance and worldwide spread of the human immunodeficiency virus (HIV) have been associated with a steep rise in the incidence of lymphoma in HIV-infected individuals, with lymphoma being an acquired immune deficiency syndrome (AIDS)-defining event in an infected person [1, 2]. The increased incidence is particularly in non-Hodgkin's lymphoma (NHL) and, to a lesser extent, in Hodgkin's disease. The increased lymphoma incidence is attributable to (i) a high rate of infection with oncogenic viruses such as Epstein–Barr virus (EBV) and human herpesvirus 8 (HHV8), previously known as Kaposi's sarcoma-associated herpesvirus (KSHV), (ii) a high rate of opportunistic infections leading to chronic stimulation of the immune system and (iii) failure of immune surveillance. The incidence of NHL is increased about 100-fold and of Hodgkin's disease (Hodgkin lymphoma) about sixfold.

There is also an increased incidence of NHL in patients with congenital or iatrogenic immune deficiency [3, 4]. Most iatrogenic cases follow immunosuppressive therapy for haemopoietic or solid organ transplantation or methotrexate treatment for autoimmune disease. Some immune deficiency diseases, e.g. ataxia-telangiectasia, have an increased incidence of lymphoma resulting from defective DNA repair rather than from the immune deficiency.

The lymphomas that are increased in incidence in HIV infection are summarized in *Table 15.1*, together with known

Table 15.1 Lymphomas that are increased in incidence in HIV-infected individuals

Type of lymphoma	*Percentage of cases of HIV-associated lymphoma*	*Known aetiological factors*
Diffuse large B-cell lymphoma (systemic)	25–35	EBV in some cases, particularly those with immunoblastic histological features
Diffuse large B-cell lymphoma (intracerebral)	25–35	EBV
Primary effusion lymphoma	5	EBV and HHV8
Plasmablastic lymphoma of oral cavity	Uncommon	EBV in more than 50% of cases
Burkitt's lymphoma	30–50	EBV in about 30% of cases
Extranodal marginal B-cell lymphoma of MALT type	Uncommon	Bacterial infection
Peripheral T-cell lymphoma	Uncommon	HIV (very rarely)
Hodgkin's disease (classical)		EBV

EBV, Epstein–Barr virus; HIV, human immunodefficiency virus; HHV8, human herpesvirus 8; MALT, mucosa-associated lymphoid tissue aetiological factors for specific subtypes. Certain lymphomas show a very strong correlation with HIV positivity, specifically primary effusion lymphoma [5] and plasmablastic lymphoma of the oral cavity.

Clinical features

The clinical features are those usually associated with lymphoma but the disease is more rapidly progressive and often presents at a more advanced stage. Extra-nodal disease is considerably more common than among other cases of lymphoma and unusual sites may be involved, e.g. oral cavity and pleural and peritoneal cavities. In addition to the usual clinical features of lymphoma, there are specific clinical features associated with individual lymphomas – intracerebral lymphoma, primary effusion lymphoma and mucosa-associated lymphoid tissue (MALT)-type lymphoma of the lungs. Cases of Burkitt's lymphoma and Hodgkin's disease often present with stage IV disease. Some patients have other features of AIDS, with the diagnosis having already been established. In others lymphoma is the presenting feature of AIDS. Because of the common aetiological factor, HHV8, patients with primary effusion lymphoma may also have multicentric Castleman's disease or Kaposi's sarcoma.

Haematological and pathological features

Because of the usual presentation at an advanced stage, Burkitt's lymphoma may be diagnosed from the blood film and both Burkitt's lymphoma and Hodgkin's disease from trephine biopsy. Other lymphomas are usually diagnosed from biopsy of lymph nodes or extra-nodal sites.

The haematological and pathological features are similar to those usually associated with the specific lymphomas but disease may be more widespread and histological features may vary from those of NHL not associated with HIV [2]. Diffuse large B-cell lymphoma (Figures **15.1** and **15.2**) is centroblastic in about 90% of cases and immunoblastic, often with plasmacytoid features, in about 10%. Intracerebral diffuse large B-cell lymphoma is usually immunoblastic. Burkitt's lymphoma (Figure **15.3**) may be histologically atypical, being more pleomorphic than is otherwise usual. There is also a variant of Burkitt's lymphoma, showing plasmacytoid differentiation, which is specifically associated with HIV infection; it is more often EBV positive than cases with classical histology. Primary effusion lymphoma (Figure **15.4**) shows moderately pleomorphic medium to large cells, which may be immunoblastic, plasmablastic or anaplastic, with large prominent nucleoli and basophilic cytoplasm. Hodgkin's disease usually shows histological features associated with poor prognosis, being mixed cellularity or lymphocyte-depleted in type. Immunohistochemical detection of EBV LMP1 (latent membrane protein 1) and detection of EBER (Epstein–Barr virus-encoded RNA) by *in situ* hybridization can be useful in diagnosis.

Immunophenotype

The immunophenotype is that usually associated with the given type of lymphoma.

The immunophenotype of plasmablastic lymphoma of the oral cavity is CD20–, cytoplasmic immunoglobulin (CyIg)+ and CD138+.

The immunophenotype of primary effusion lymphoma is CD45+, CD19–, CD20–, CD79a–, CD138+ (B-cell lineage being supported by *IGH* analysis). There may be expression of epithelial membrane antigen (EMA) and activation markers such as CD30, CD38 and CD71. Surface membrane immunoglobulin (SmIg) may be positive or negative. Cytoplasmic Ig is expressed in about one-fifth of cases. HHV8 latent nuclear antigen 1 (LNA1) is expressed in the nucleus but EBV LMP1 is not expressed [6].

Cytogenetic and molecular genetic abnormalities

The cytogenetic and molecular genetic abnormalities found are those expected in the individual lymphomas. Demonstration of a clonal cytogenetic or molecular genetic abnormality can be useful when it is not clear if a patient has a lymphoma or a polyclonal potentially prelymphomatous disorder. However, sometimes a clonal rearrangement of *IGH*, *TCRB* or *TCRG* is a marker of an expanded but non-lymphomatous clone of cells. Clonality can also be demonstrated in EBV-associated lymphomas by analysis of the long terminal repeats of the episomal form of the virus.

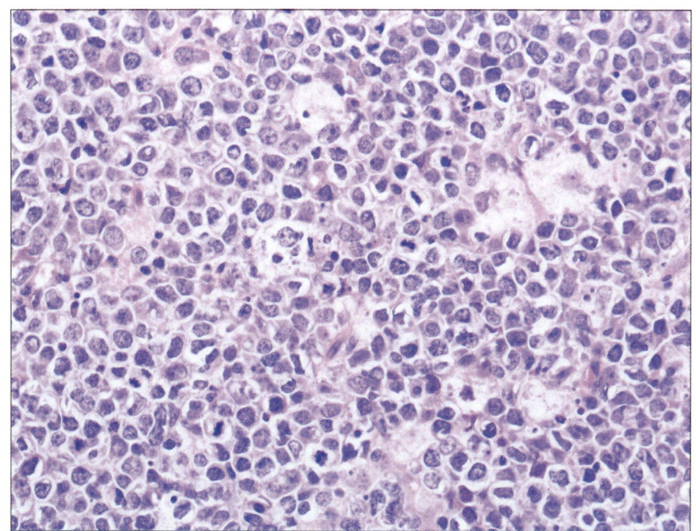

Figure 15.1 Section of lymph node biopsy in diffuse large B-cell lymphoma in an HIV-positive patient. H&E, x 60 objective.

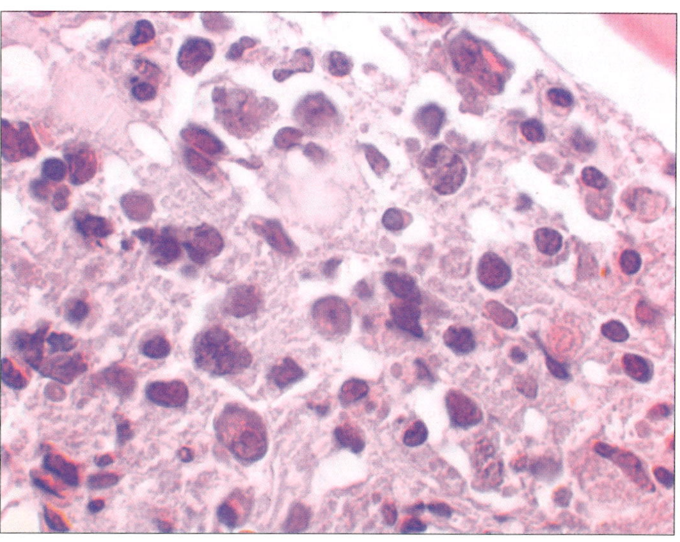

Figure 15.2 Section of trephine biopsy section in diffuse large B-cell lymphoma in an HIV-positive patient. H&E, x 100 objective.

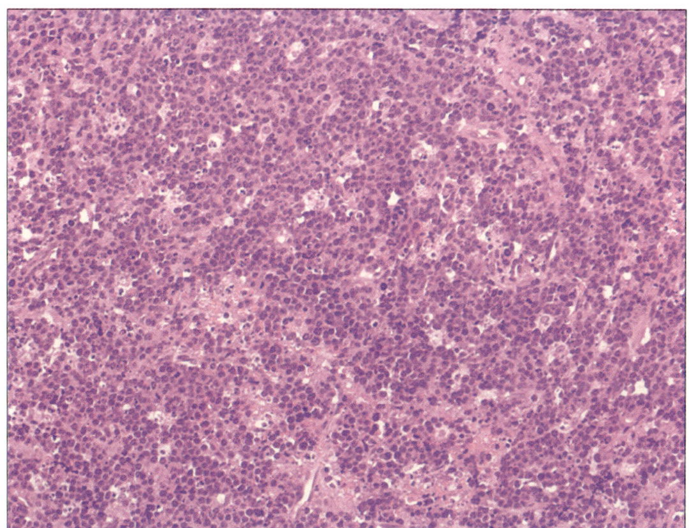

Figure 15.3 Section of lymph node biopsy showing Burkitt's lymphoma in an HIV-positive patient. H&E, x 10 objective.

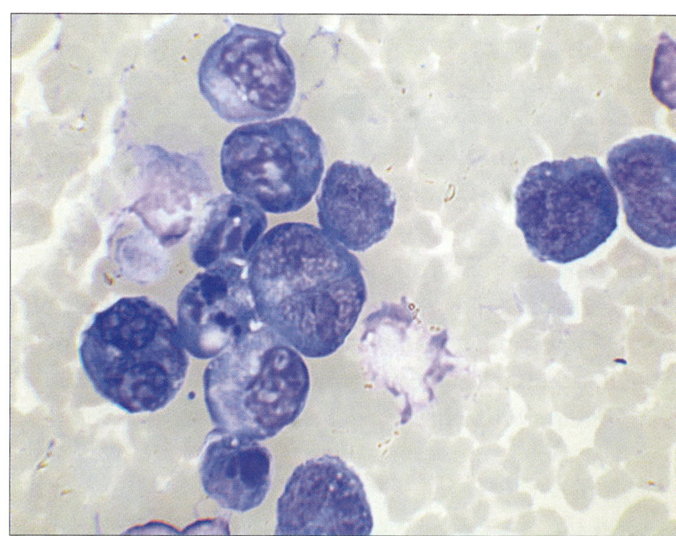

Figure 15.4 Film of pericardial fluid from an HIV-positive patient with a primary effusion lymphoma. Romanowsky stain, x 100 objective. With thanks to Dr Julie McCarthy.

Diagnosis and differential diagnosis

The differential diagnosis includes pre-lymphomatous conditions such as post-transplant lymphoproliferative disorder, which is often EBV-driven and may evolve from a polyclonal to an oligoclonal proliferation with overt lymphoma developing in some patients. Polyclonal lymphoproliferative disorders also occur in HIV infection and in primary immune defects.

Prognosis

The prognosis is much worse than in HIV-negative patients but, if the patient is also given effective anti-retroviral treatment, some long remissions and even cures are achieved. Prognosis is related to the specific diagnosis (Burkitt's lymphoma has a better outcome than diffuse large B-cell lymphoma while primary effusion lymphoma has a particularly unfavourable prognosis), the severity of the immune deficiency, the age of the patient and the stage of the disease.

Treatment

Treatment of AIDS-related cases must be a combination of conventional treatment directed at the lymphoma and highly-active anti-retroviral therapy [7]. Treatment is more difficult than in other patients because of poor bone marrow reserve and a high probability of opportunistic infections during treatment. In lymphomas resulting from immunosuppressive therapy the prognosis is improved if immunosuppressive drugs can be reduced or stopped.

References

1. Bain BJ (1998). Lymphomas and reactive lymphoid lesions in HIV infection. *Blood Reviews*, **12**, 154–162.
2. Raphael M, Borsich B and Jaffe ES (2001). Lymphomas associated with infection by the human immune deficiency virus (HIV). *In* Jaffe ES, Harris NL, Stein H and Vardiman JW (Eds). *World Health Organization Classification of Tumours: Pathology and Genetics of Tumours of Haematopoietic and Lymphoid Tissues*, IARC Press, Lyon, pp. 260–263.
3. Borisch B, Raphael M, Swerdlow SH and Jaffe ES (2001). Lymphoproliferative diseases associated with primary immune disorders. *In* Jaffe ES, Harris NL, Stein H and Vardiman JW (Eds). *World Health Organization Classification of Tumours: Pathology and Genetics of Tumours of Haematopoietic and Lymphoid Tissues*, IARC Press, Lyon, pp. 257–259.
4. Harris NL, Swerdlow SH, Frizzera G and Knowles DM (2001). Post-transplant lymphoproliferative disorders. *In* Jaffe ES, Harris NL, Stein H and Vardiman JW (Eds). *World Health Organization Classification of Tumours: Pathology and Genetics of Tumours of Haematopoietic and Lymphoid Tissues*, IARC Press, Lyon, pp. 264–269.
5. Nador RG, Cesarman E, Chadburn A, Dawson DB, Ansari MQ, Sald J and Knowles DM (2004). Primary effusion lymphoma: a distinct clinicopathologic entity associated with the Kaposi's sarcoma-associated herpes virus. *Blood*, **88**, 645–656.
6. Banks PM and Warnke RA (2001). Primary effusion lymphoma. *In* Jaffe ES, Harris NL, Stein H and Vardiman JW (Eds). *World Health Organization Classification of Tumours of Haematopoietic and Lymphoid Tissues*, IARC Press, Lyon, pp. 179–180.
7. Mounier N, Spina M, Gabarre J, Raphael M, Rizzardini G, Golfier JB *et al.* (2006). AIDS-related non-Hodgkin lymphoma: final analysis of 485 patients treated with risk-adapted intensive chemotherapy. *Blood*, **107**, 3832–3840.

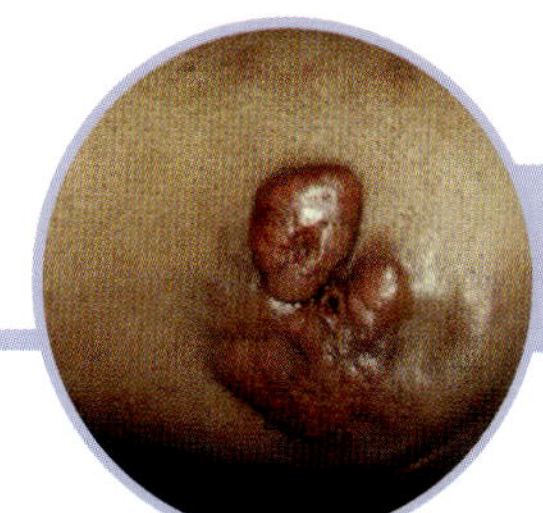

Chapter 16

Adult T-cell leukaemia/lymphoma

Adult T-cell leukaemia/lymphoma (ATLL) is a unique lymphoproliferative disorder [1–4] that develops only in individuals who are chronic carriers of the retrovirus, human T-cell lymphotropic virus I (HTLV-I) [5, 6]. The interval between acquiring the virus and developing the lymphoma is usually 30–60 years with the life-time risk of developing ATLL being of the order of 2% for women and 6% for men. Since only a minority of HTLV-I carriers develop ATLL it is clear that there must be co-factors that contribute to development of the condition; the nature of these remains unknown although *Strongyloides stercoralis* infection has been suspected. HTLV-I can also cause polymyositis, arthritis, uveitis and HTLV-I-associated myelopathy (also known as tropical spastic paraparesis). In addition it leads to immunosuppression, which is responsible for an increased incidence of infective dermatitis, *Pneumocystis jiroveci* (previously known as *Pneumocystis carinii*) pneumonia, *Strongyloides stercoralis* hyperinfection and virus-related tumours (e.g. carcinoma of the cervix, Kaposi's sarcoma and hepatoma related to hepatitis viruses). Because of the distribution of HTLV-I, ATLL is distributed unevenly throughout the world. The best-recognized endemic areas are Japan (particularly the island of Kyushu) and the Caribbean but, in fact, there are likely to be more cases in South America and Africa, where carriers of the virus are even more numerous. Endemic cases have also been observed in Eastern Europe. Cases are found in Europe and North America, among migrants from endemic areas.

Clinical features

About 10–20% of individuals who develop ATLL present with lymphoma without involvement of the peripheral blood or bone marrow. The other 80–90% have leukaemic manifestations. There is usually lymphadenopathy (Figure **16.1**) and there may be hepatomegaly, splenomegaly and skin infiltration (papules, nodules and plaques) (Figure **16.2**). A minority of patients have pleural effusions, ascites or infiltration of lung, liver, gastrointestinal tract, leptomeninges or brain (Figure **16.3**). Hypercalcaemia is a common clinical feature, either at presentation or during disease progression; it may be associated with lytic bone lesions and is the result of stimulation of osteoclasts by cytokines secreted by the neoplastic cells. Hypercalcaemia can lead to dehydration and renal impairment. The clinical course is usually acute but smouldering and chronic forms of the disease are recognized.

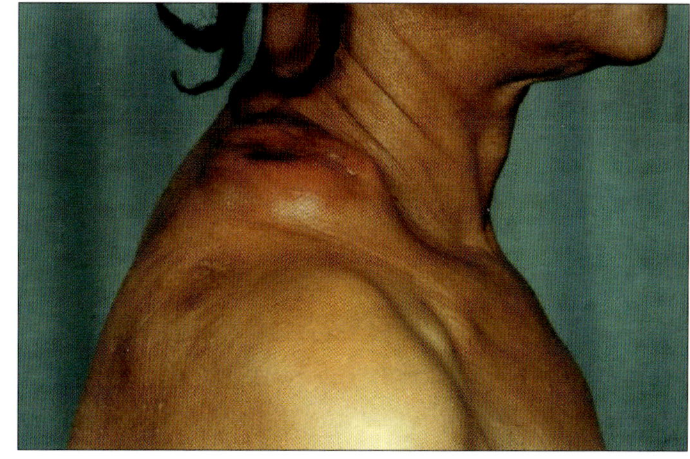

Figure 16.1 Clinical photograph showing lymphadenopathy and skin infiltration.

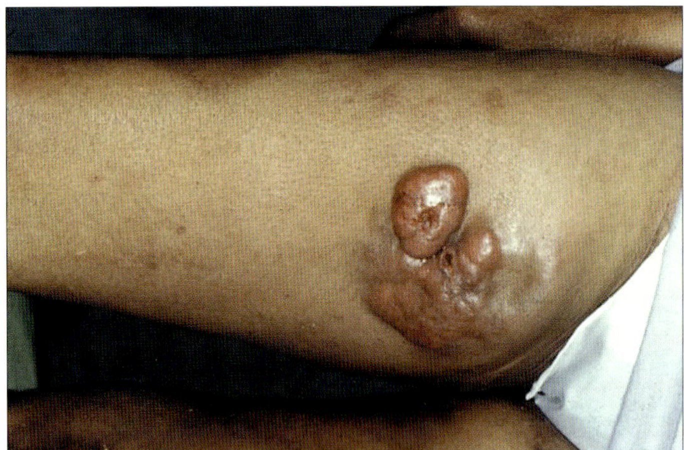

Figure 16.2 Clinical photograph showing skin infiltration.

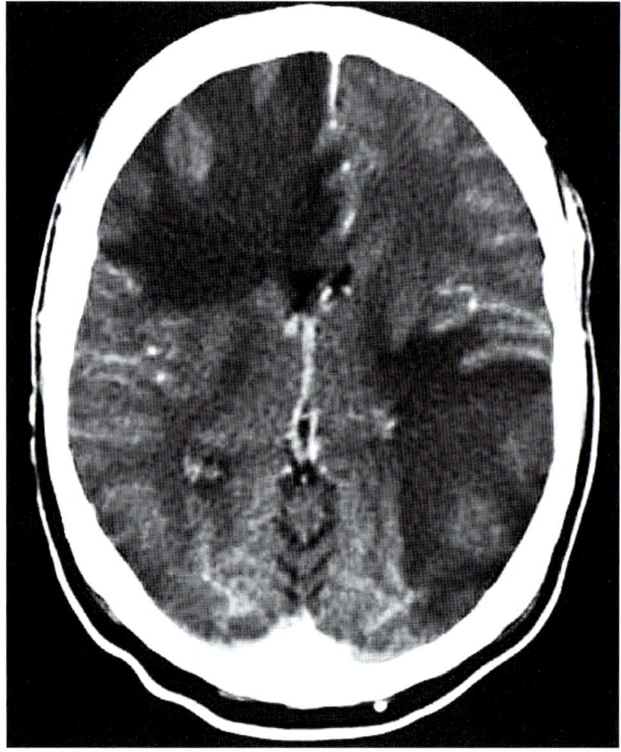

Figure 16.3 CT scan of the brain showing cerebral infiltration.

Haematological and pathological features

Leukaemic cells are distinctive, being medium sized pleomorphic cells with irregular nuclei, which may be convoluted or deeply lobulated. Nucleoli are often present and some have a blastic chromatin pattern. The cytoplasm is often basophilic. A variable number of 'flower cells' are present (Figures **16.4** and **16.5**). There may be reactive eosinophilia and neutrophilia. The extent of bone marrow infiltration (Figure **16.6**) is often much less than would be anticipated from the number of leukaemic cells in the peripheral blood. In trephine biopsy sections, the pattern of infiltration is most often interstitial. Increased osteoclasts with bone resorption may be apparent. Lymph node infiltration (Figure **16.7**) may be diffuse or there may be an expanded paracortex or sinusoidal infiltration [7, 8]. Skin infiltration (Figure **16.8**) may be not only in the dermis, including perivascular infiltration, but also within the epidermis (Pautrier's microabscesses), thus resembling Sézary syndrome.

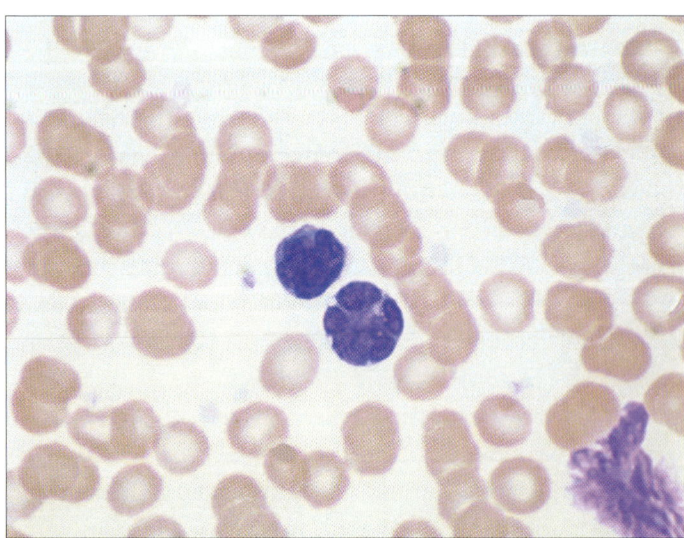

Figure 16.4 Peripheral blood film showing two lymphoma cells, one of which is a 'flower cell'. Romanowsky stain, x 100 objective.

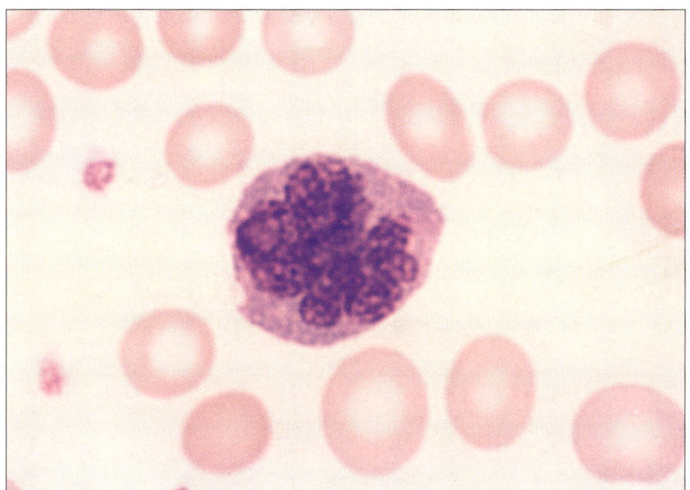
Figure 16.5 Peripheral blood film showing a 'flower cell'. Romanowsky stain, x 100 objective (detail).

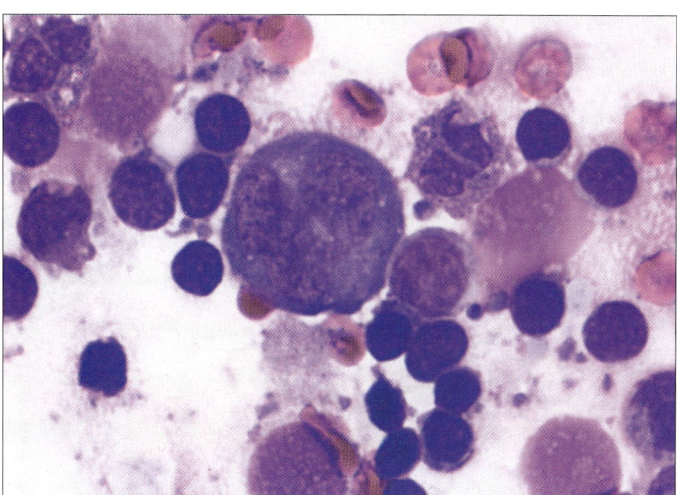
Figure 16.6 Bone marrow aspirate film showing numerous small lymphoma cells and one very large lymphoma cell with an irregular nucleus and deeply basophilic cytoplasm. Romanowsky stain, x 100 objective.

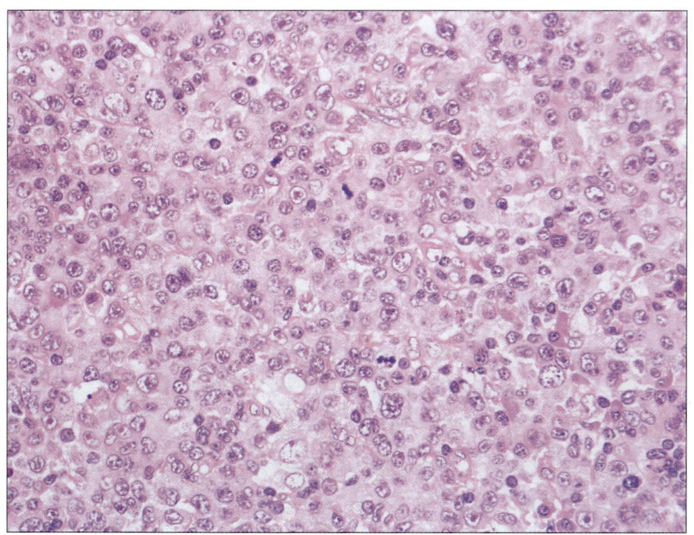
Figure 16.7 Section of a lymph node biopsy showing pleomorphic lymphoma cells. H&E, x 60 objective.

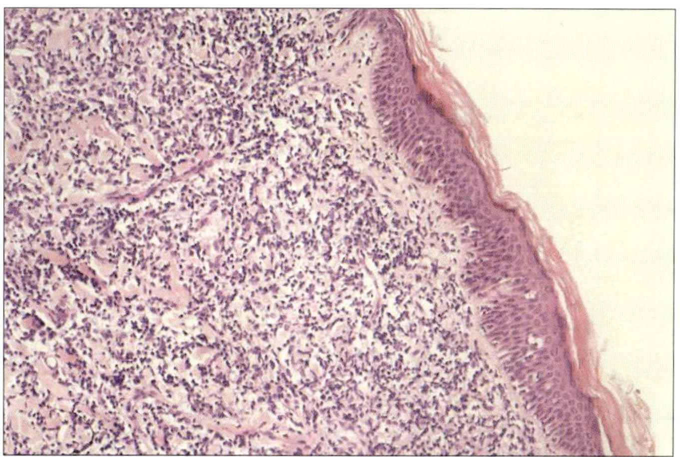
Figure 16.8 Section of a skin biopsy showing a predominantly dermal infiltrate. H&E, x 10 objective.

Immunophenotype

The immunophenotype is that of a mature T cell, usually expressing CD2, CD3 and CD5 but lacking CD7 expression (Figures **16.9** and **16.10**). Neoplastic cells are usually CD4 positive but in a minority of cases there is expression of either CD8 alone or of both CD4 and CD8. HLA-DR is usually expressed and CD38 may be expressed.

The most distinctive feature of the immunophenotype is the strong expression of CD25, the receptor for interleukin 2 (Figure **16.11**). Such expression is usual but not universal. Immunocytochemical stains can demonstrate the presence of the causative virus (Figure **16.12**).

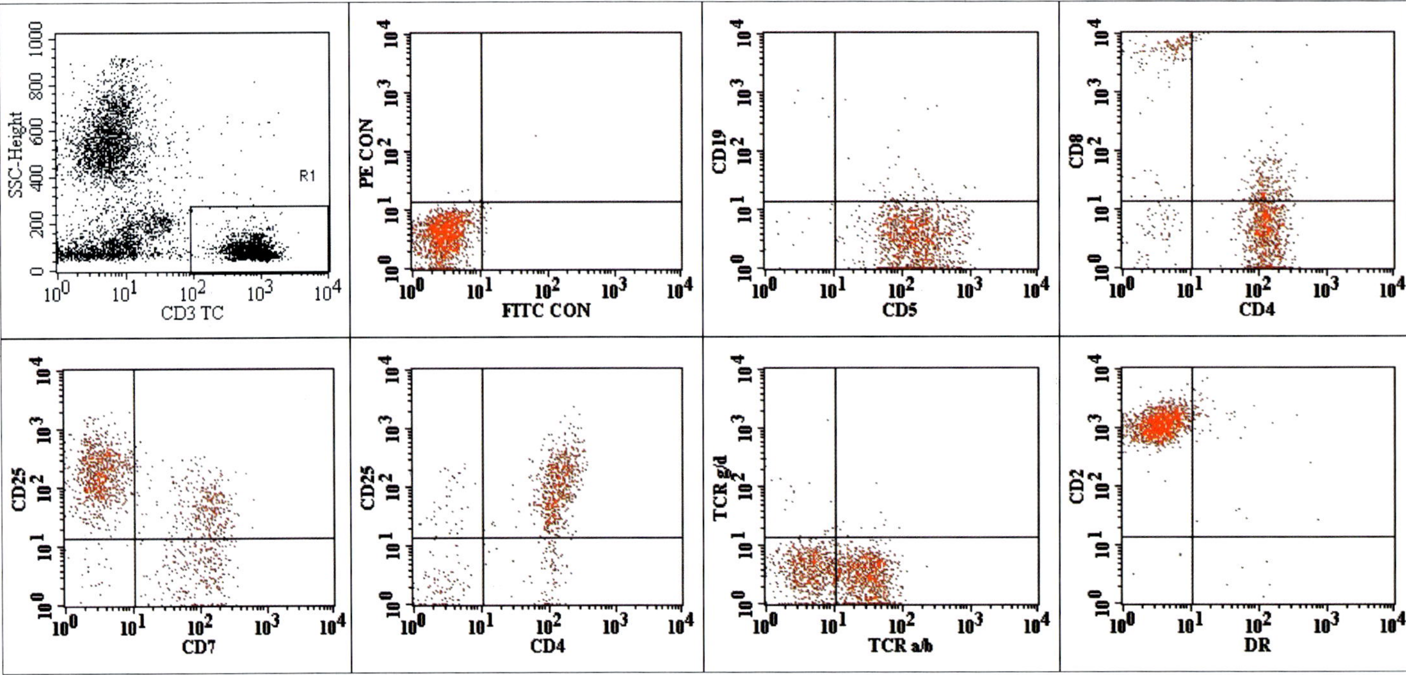

Figure 16.9 Peripheral blood flow cytometry immunophenotyping in ATLL following gating on CD3-positive cells. In addition to CD3, cells express CD2, CD4, CD5, CD25 and TCR αβ but do not express CD7, CD8 or TCR γδ. CD16 and CD52 were also expressed. With thanks to Mr Ricardo Morilla.

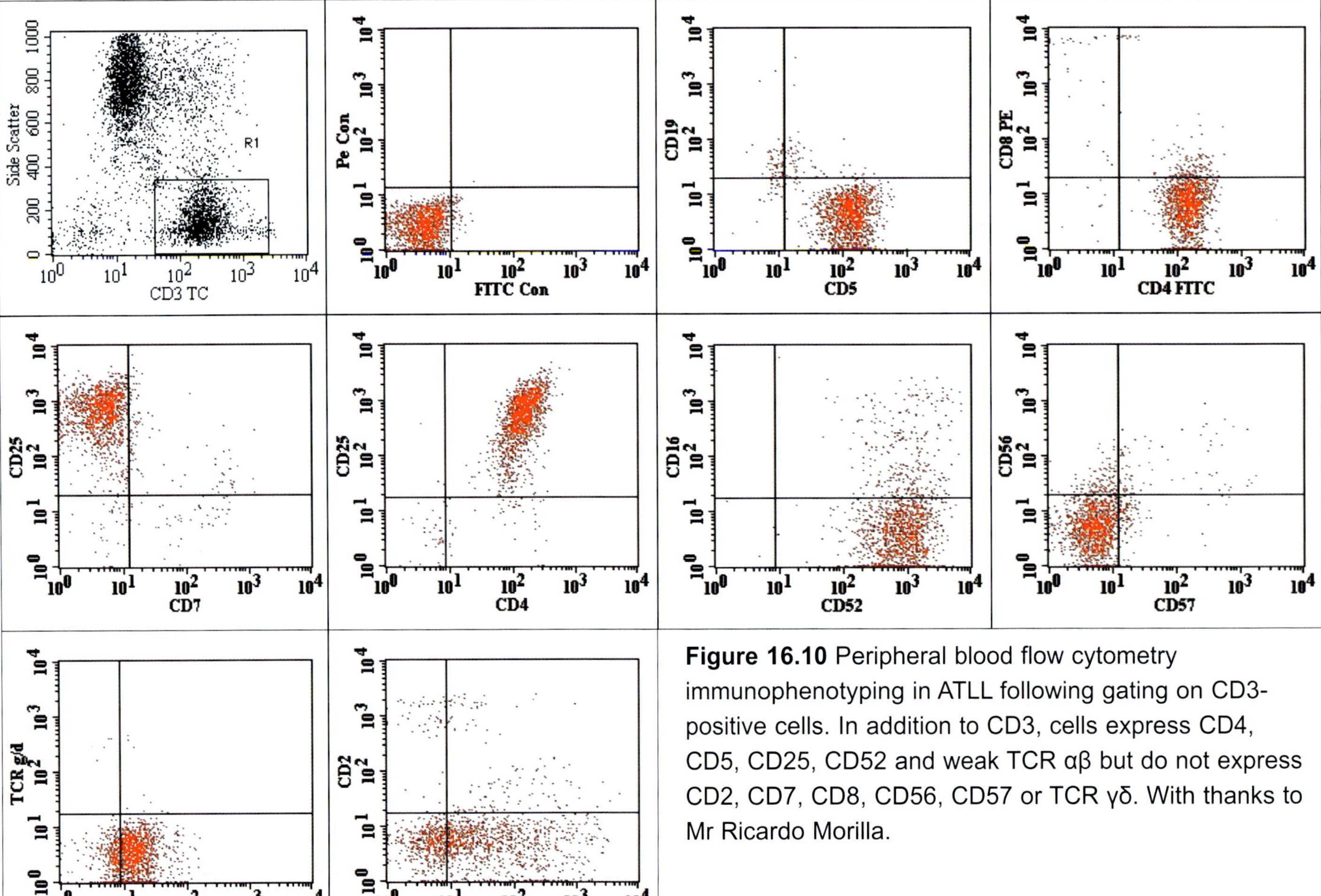

Figure 16.10 Peripheral blood flow cytometry immunophenotyping in ATLL following gating on CD3-positive cells. In addition to CD3, cells express CD4, CD5, CD25, CD52 and weak TCR αβ but do not express CD2, CD7, CD8, CD56, CD57 or TCR γδ. With thanks to Mr Ricardo Morilla.

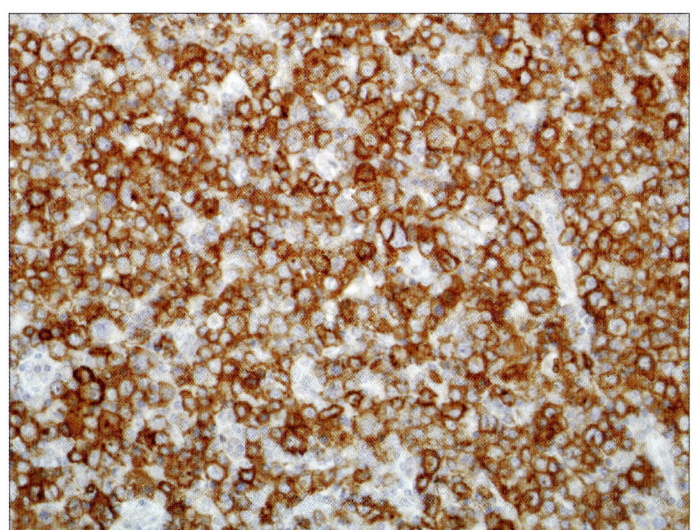

Figure 16.11 Section of lymph node biopsy in adult T-cell leukaemia/lymphoma showing that cells express CD25. Immunoperoxidase, x 40 objective.

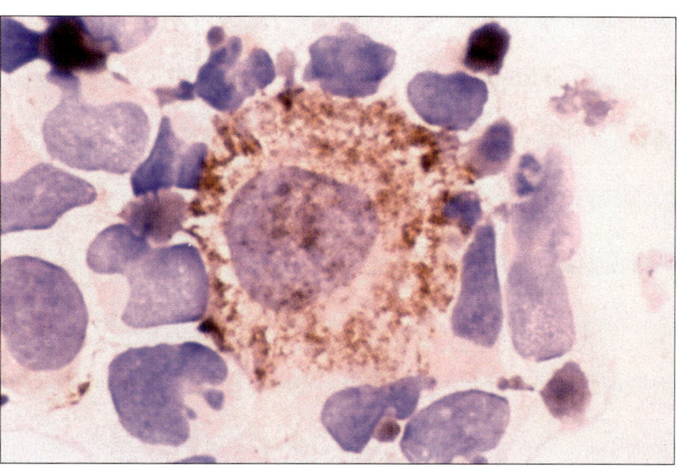

Figure 16.12 HTLV-I expression by a lymphoma cell with a McAb against the P19 HTLV-I protein. Cells have been cultured for 48 hours. Immunoperoxidase, x 100 objective.

Cytogenetic and molecular genetic abnormalities

There is no specific cytogenetic or molecular genetic abnormality [9]. Recurrent abnormalities include +3, +7, +21, monosomy X, chromosome Y deletion and abnormalities of chromosomes 6 (6q-) and 14 (translocations with a 14q32 or 14q11 breakpoint). Complex cytogenetic abnormalities are often present. Mutations of tumour-suppressing genes, *CDKN2A* (p16), *CDKN2B* (p15) and *TP53* (p53), may be found in the acute and lymphomatous forms of ATLL. T-cell receptor genes are rearranged and clonality can also be demonstrated by showing that there is monoclonal integration of HTLV-I.

Diagnosis and differential diagnosis

Diagnosis is made by detection of typical cytological and immunophenotypic features in a patient who has antibodies to HTLV-I. The differential diagnosis includes other T-cell leukaemias and lymphomas, particularly cutaneous lymphomas, which can also have convoluted and deeply lobulated nuclei. Diagnosis is usually more straightforward in patients with leukaemic manifestations. The histological features are less distinctive than the cytological features. Because of the non-specific lymph node histology, the diagnosis can be easily missed on lymph node biopsy if ATLL is not included in the differential diagnosis.

Prognosis

Prognosis is poor, the median survival being less than one year. Adverse prognostic factors include poor performance status, leucocytosis, high lactate dehydrogenase, high β2-microglobulin, high serum soluble CD25, high serum neuron-specific enolase, hypercalcaemia and a high proliferation fraction.

Treatment

The two main approaches to treatment are combination chemotherapy and a combination of zidovudine and interferon [4, 10]. Antibodies to CD25, including radiolabelled antibodies, have also been used.

References

1. Shimomaya M (1991). Diagnostic criteria and clinical subtypes of ATLL. A report from the Lymphoma Study Group (1984-87). *Br J Haematol*, **79**, 428–437.
2. Mahieux R and Gessain A (2003). HTLV-1 and associated adult T-cell leukemia/lymphoma. *Rev Clin Exp Hematol*, 7, 336–361.
3. Nicot C (2005). Current views in HTLV-I-associated adult T-cell leukemia/lymphoma. *Am J Hematol*, **78**, 232–239.
4. Taylor GP and Matsuoka M (2005). Natural history of adult T-cell leukemia/lymphoma and approaches to therapy. *Oncogene*, **24**, 6047–6057.
5. Yamaguchi K (1994). Human T-lymphotropic virus type I in Japan. *Lancet*, **343**, 213–216.
6. Iwanaga R, Ohtani K, Hayashi T and Nakamura M (2001). Molecular mechanisms of cell cycle progression induced by the oncogene product Tax of human T-cell leukemia virus type I. *Oncogene*, **20**, 2055–2067.
7. Lennert K, Kikuchi M, Sato E, Suchi T, Stansfeld AG, Feller AC *et al.* (1985). HTLV-positive and -negative T-cell lymphomas. Morphological and immunohistochemical differences between European and HTLV-positive Japanese T-cell lymphomas. *Int J Cancer*, **35**, 65–72.
8. Ohshima K, Suzumiya J, Sato K, Kanda M, Sugihara M, Haraoka S *et al.* (1998). Nodal T-cell lymphoma in an HTLV-1 endemic area: proviral HTLV-1 DNA, histological classification and clinical evaluation. *Br J Haematol*, **101**, 703–711.
9. Fifth International Workshop on Chromosomes in Leukemia–lymphoma (1987). Correlation of chromosome abnormalities with histologic and immunologic characteristics in non-Hodgkin's lymphoma and adult T-cell leukemia-lymphoma. *Blood*, **70**, 1554–1564.
10. Matutes E, Taylor GP, Cavenagh J, Pagliuca A, Bareford D, Domingo A *et al.* (2001). Interferon alpha and zidovudine therapy in adult T-cell leukaemia lymphoma: response and outcome in 15 patients. *Br J Haematol*, **113**, 779–784.

Chapter 17

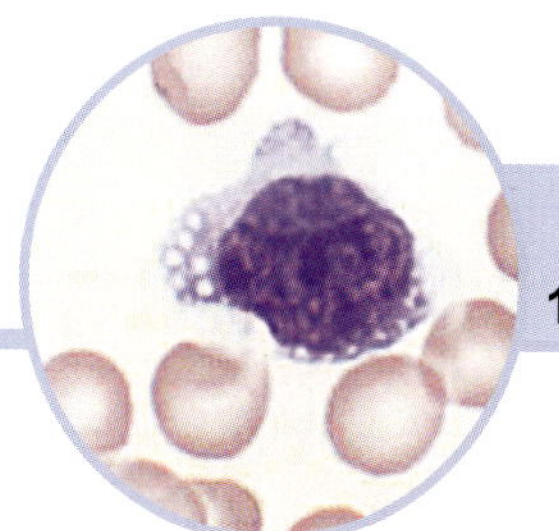

Mycosis fungoides and Sézary syndrome

Mycosis fungoides and Sézary syndrome (SS) are primary cutaneous T-cell lymphomas [1–4]. Mycosis fungoides is characterized by cutaneous disease without circulating lymphoma cells necessarily being present whereas the diagnosis of SS requires the presence of circulating neoplastic cells. In the World Health Organization/European Organization for Research and Treatment of Cancer (WHO-EORTC) classification these are two distinct types of primary cutaneous T-cell lymphoma [4]. Although the pathogenic role of HTLV-I has been entertained, a large multinational study has ruled out the involvement of this retrovirus in mycosis fungoides and SS.

Clinical features

Mycosis fungoides affects mainly older adults. It is a slowly progressive condition characterized by cutaneous patches, plaques and, finally, tumours as a result of infiltration of the skin by lymphoma cells with cerebriform nuclei. Transformation to a large T-cell lymphoma can occur.

Sézary syndrome is a disease of the elderly, characterized by erythroderma and circulating Sézary cells with characteristic cerebriform nuclei.

Haematological and pathological features

The peripheral blood is usually normal in mycosis fungoides but circulating lymphoma cells may be present in later stages. Skin biopsy (Figures **17.1–17.3**) shows epidermotropism in the early stages with formation of intraepidermal Pautrier's microabscess in some but not all cases [4].

By definition, circulating Sézary cells (Figures **17.4–17.6**) are required for the diagnosis of SS. Suggested minimum diagnostic criteria of the International Society for

Figure 17.1 Skin biopsy in mycosis fungoides. H&E, x 4 objective.

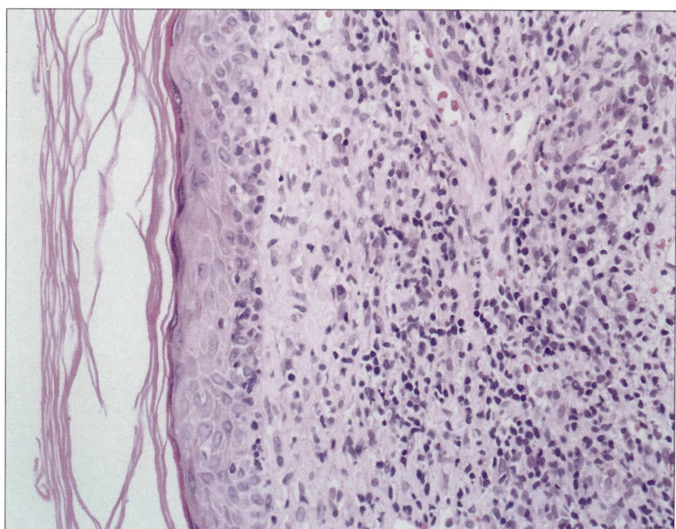

Figure 17.2 Skin biopsy in mycosis fungoides; at higher power the infiltration of lymphocytes into the epidermis is apparent. H&E, x 40 objective.

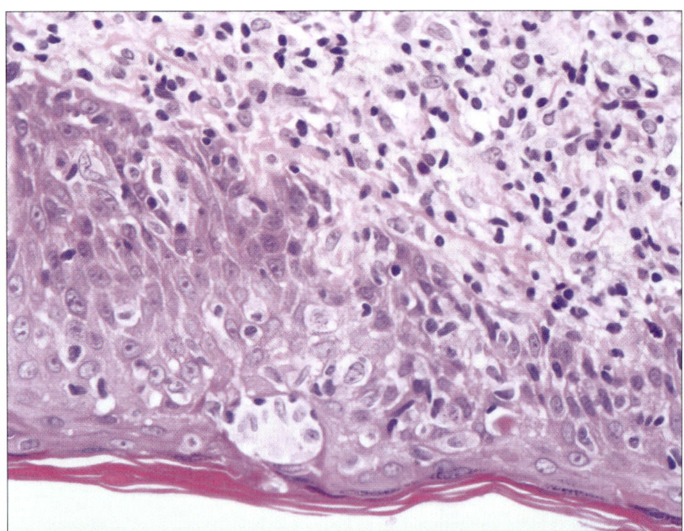

Figure 17.3 Skin biopsy in mycosis fungoides; several Pautrier's microabscesses are apparent. H&E, x 60 objective.

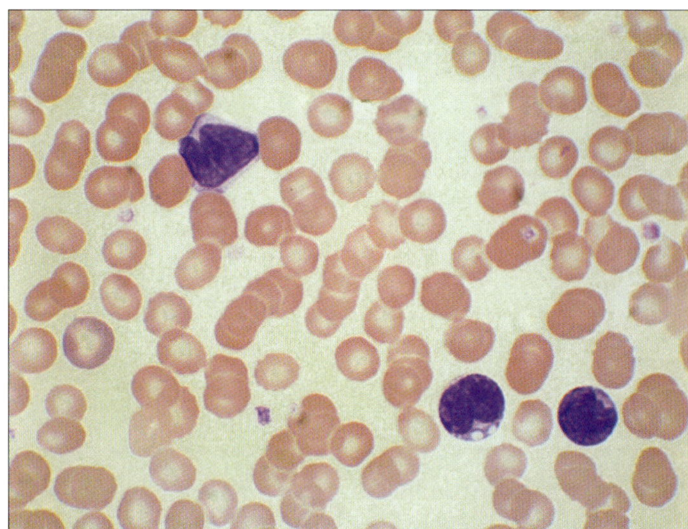

Figure 17.4 Peripheral blood film in SS showing neoplastic cells with lobulated and grooved nuclei; one cell is vacuolated. Romanowsky, x 100 objective.

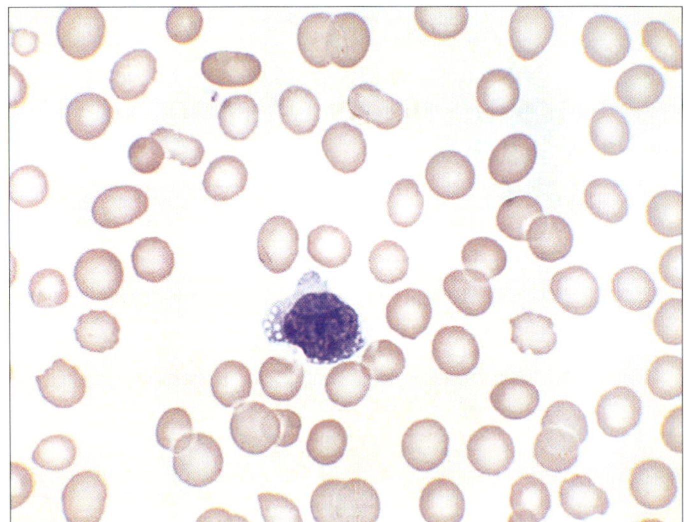

Figure 17.5 Peripheral blood film in SS showing a neoplastic cell with vacuoles ringing the nucleus. Romanowsky, x 100 objective.

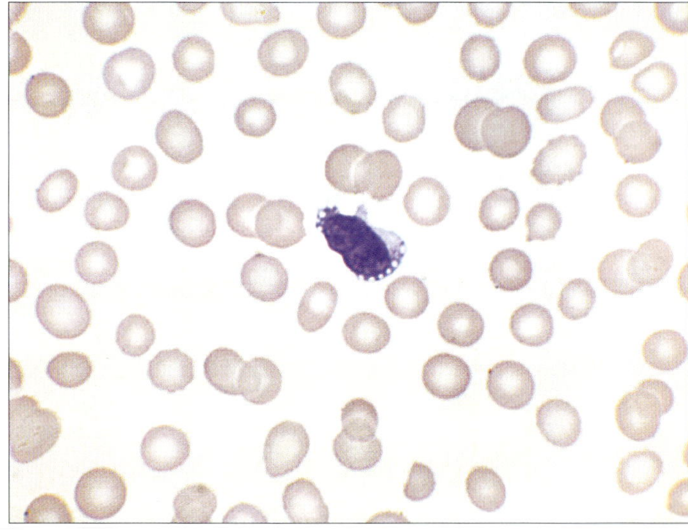

Figure 17.6 Peripheral blood film in SS showing a neoplastic cell with vacuoles ringing the nucleus (same patient as Figure **17.5**). Romanowsky, x 100 objective.

Cutaneous Lymphomas are one of the following: an absolute Sézary cell count of at least 1×10^9/l, relevant immunophenotypic abnormalities (see below) or demonstration of a T-cell clone by molecular or cytogenetic studies [4]. Sézary cells may be either small or large. Individual patients may have mainly small cells, mainly large cells or a mixture of both. Transformation from small cell disease to large cell disease can occur [5]. Sézary cells are characterized by a deeply convoluted or cerebriform nucleus. In small cells the cytoplasm is scanty and the nucleus appears to have a grooved surface. Larger cells have more cytoplasm and nuclei may appear cerebriform or lobulated. In both variants, nuclei may be hyperchromatic and cytoplasmic vacuoles may encircle the nucleus (see Figures **17.5** and **17.6**). The characteristic nuclear form is most readily observed on ultrastructural examination (Figures **17.7** and **17.8**). Skin histology resembles that of mycosis fungoides; sometimes microabscesses are absent although single lymphoma cells are present in the epidermis.

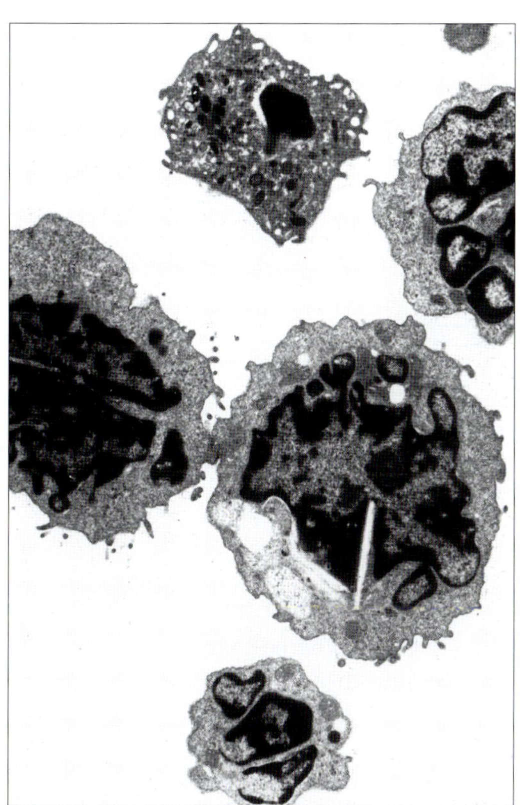

Figure 17.7 Ultrastructural features in SS. Lead nitrate and uranyl acetate stain.

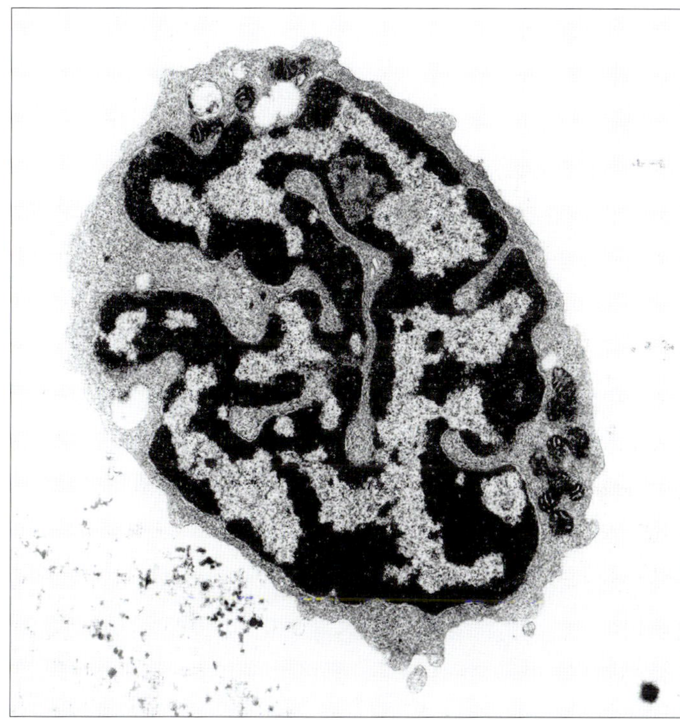

Figure 17.8 Ultrastructural features in SS; the nucleus has a serpentine configuration characteristic of Sézary cells. Lead nitrate and uranyl acetate stain.

Immunophenotype

The cells of mycosis fungoides usually express CD3 and CD4 but not CD8. There may be loss of pan-T antigens such as CD2, CD3, CD5 and CD7.

Sézary cells have a similar phenotype. Suggested immunophenotypic criteria for the presence of an abnormal clone in the peripheral blood are a CD4:CD8 positive ratio of more than 10 or loss of one or more of the pan-T antigens, CD2, CD3, CD4, CD5 and CD7 (Figures **17.9** and **17.10**).

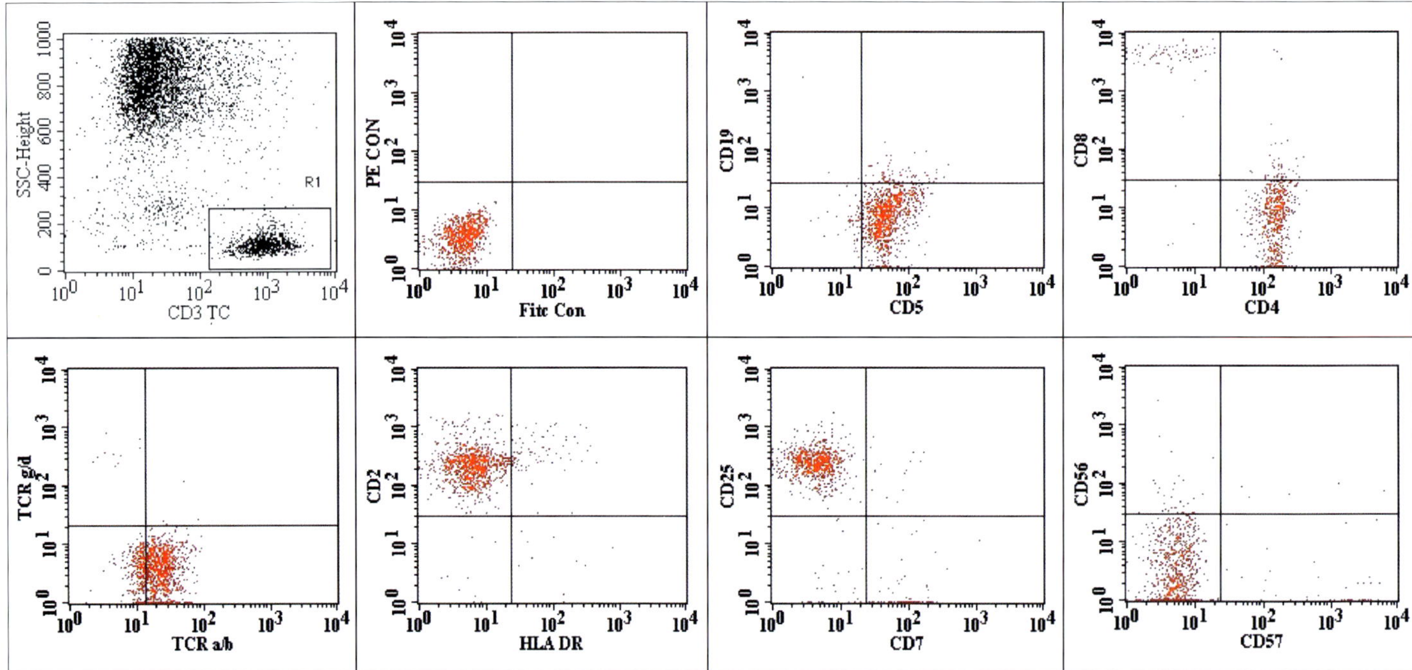

Figure 17.9 Flow cytometry immunophenotyping in a patient with SS, following gating on CD3-positive cells. In addition to CD3, the cells express CD2, CD4, CD5, CD25 and TCR αβ; they do not express CD7, CD8, CD56, CD57, HLA-DR or TCR γδ. The expression of CD25 is not usual. With thanks to Mr Ricardo Morilla.

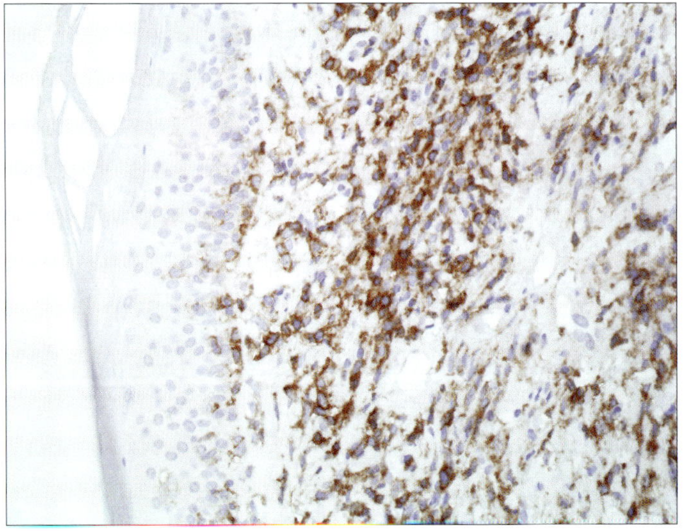

Figure 17.10 Section of skin biopsy in mycosis fungoides (same patient and same magnification as Figure **17.2**) confirming that CD4-positive cells are infiltrating both the dermis and the epidermis. Immunoperoxidase, x 40 objective.

Cytogenetic and molecular genetic abnormalities

Cytogenetic abnormalities may be present in mycosis fungoides but there is no specific associated abnormality [6]. Molecular genetic lesions may include mutation in tumour suppressor genes, *CDKN2B* (p15), *CDKN2A* (p16) and *TP53*.

Complex karyotypes are common in SS and, in the large cell variant, hyperdiploidy is characteristic. *JUNB* may be amplified. Rearrangement of T-cell receptor genes or other clonal molecular or cytogenetic abnormalities provide evidence on which the diagnosis can be based. Demonstration of aneuploidy is also useful to confirm the diagnosis [7].

Similar chromosomal abnormalities are seen in mycosis fungoides and Sézary syndrome, indicating a relationship between the two conditions.

Diagnosis and differential diagnosis

The differential diagnosis of mycosis fungoides and SS includes both benign conditions (e.g. reactive erythroderma) and other cutaneous lymphomas. Sézary syndrome needs to be distinguished from Sézary-like leukaemia, which is more closely related to T-lineage prolymphocytic leukaemia, and also from adult T-cell leukaemia/lymphoma.

Prognosis

The clinical course of mycosis fungoides is usually chronic with survival differing little from age-matched controls but when lymph node effacement, visceral involvement or large cell transformation occurs the prognosis is much worse. Sézary syndrome has a much worse prognosis than mycosis fungoides with median survivals of 2–4 years.

Treatment

Mycosis fungoides confined to the skin is treated by skin-directed therapy such as topical chlormethine (nitrogen mustard) or a psoralen plus ultraviolet light (PUVA); advanced and disseminated disease is treated with combination chemotherapy.

Treatments applied in SS include extracorporeal photopheresis, low-dose chemotherapy, pentostatin, alemtuzumab, systemic corticosteroids and PUVA.

References

1. Bazarbachi A, Soriano V, Pawson R, Vallejo A, Moudgil T, Matutes E *et al.* (1997). Mycosis fungoides and Sézary syndrome are not associated with HTLV-I infection: an international study. *Br J Haematol*, **98**, 927–933.
2. Matutes E (2002). Chronic T-cell lymphoproliferative disorders. *Rev Clin Exp Hematol*, **6**, 401–420.
3. Matutes E (2005). T-cell lymphoproliferative disorders. *In* Hoffbrand AV, Catovsky D, and Tuddenham GD (Eds). *Postgraduate Haematology*, 5th edition, Blackwell, Oxford, pp. 644–661.
4. Willemze R, Jaffe ES, Burg G, Cerroni L, Berti E, Swerdlow SH *et al.* (2005). WHO-EORTC classification for cutaneous lymphomas. *Blood*, **105**, 3768–3785.
5. Diamandidou E, Colome-Grimmer M, Fayad L, Duvic M and Kurzrock R (1998). Transformation of mycosis fungoides/Sézary syndrome: clinical characteristics and prognosis. *Blood*, **92**, 1150–1159.
6. Thangavelu M, Finn WG, Yelavarthi KK, Roenigk HH, Samuelson E, Peterson L *et al.* (1997). Recurrent structural chromosome abnormalities in peripheral blood lymphocytes from patients with mycosis fungoides/Sézary syndrome. *Blood*, **89**, 3371–3377.
7. Wang S, Li N, Heald P, Fisk JM, Fadare O, Howe JG *et al.* (2004). Flow cytometric DNA ploidy analysis of peripheral blood from patients with Sézary syndrome: detection of aneuploid neoplastic T cells in the blood is associated with large cell transformation in tissue. *Am J Clin Pathol*, **122**, 774–782.

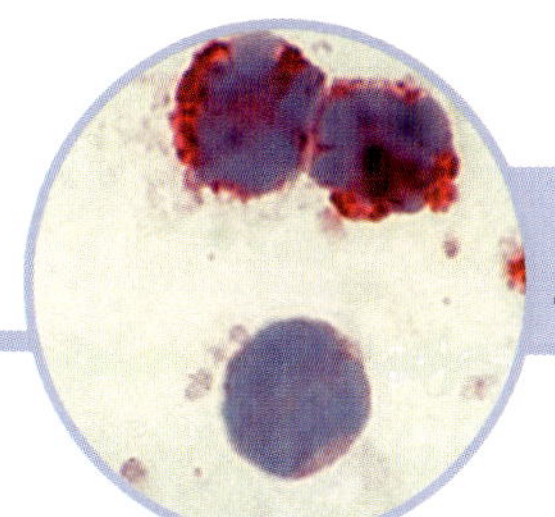

Chapter 18

Large granular lymphocyte leukaemia

Large granular lymphocyte leukaemia (LGLL) may be of T lineage or natural killer (NK) lineage [1]. The former is dealt with in this section. It is mainly a disease of the elderly. There is no relationship to human lymphotropic viruses I and II [2].

Clinical features

Some diagnoses are incidental. Other patients present with symptoms resulting from cytopenia, e.g. infection as a result of neutropenia. Lymphadenopathy is quite uncommon. Splenomegaly is more common. Some patients have associated rheumatoid arthritis. Transformation to high-grade lymphoma is very rare [3].

Haematological and pathological features

There is an increase in large granular lymphocytes but the extent of this is very variable. The lymphocytes are very similar to normal large granular lymphocytes (Figure **18.1**). In some patients there is neutropenia, anaemia with macrocytosis, anaemia with a low reticulocyte count (associated with red cell aplasia), anaemia with a high reticulocyte count (associated with autoimmune haemolytic anaemia) or thrombocytopenia. The bone marrow aspirate contains a variable number of large granular lymphocytes and in those with a complicating autoimmune cytopenia may show 'maturation arrest' in the granulocyte series, megaloblastic or macronormoblastic erythropoiesis, erythroid hyperplasia, pure red cell aplasia and increased or,

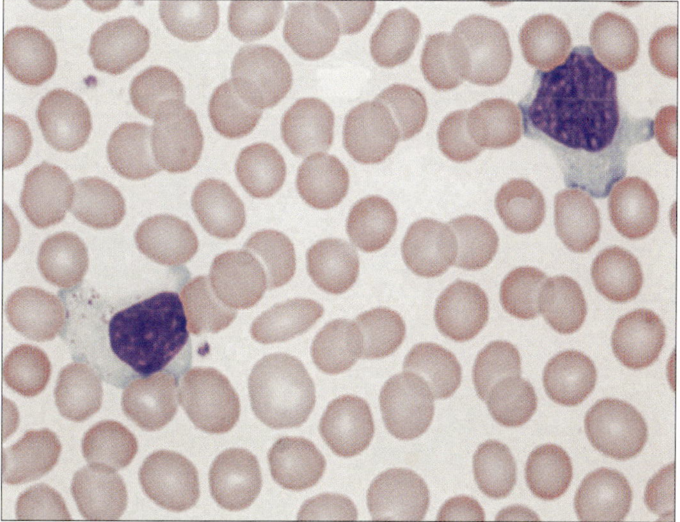

Figure 18.1 Peripheral blood film from a patient with large granular lymphocyte leukaemia of T lineage showing two large granular lymphocytes. Romanowsky, x 100 objective.

less often, reduced megakaryocytes. Myeloid cells may be dysplastic. On trephine biopsy sections the usual pattern is of interstitial infiltration, which may be quite subtle (Figures **18.2** and **18.3**). Infiltration within sinusoids and capillaries can also be a feature. There may be prominent lymphoid nodules composed of B cells and reactive T cells (Figures **18.2** and **18.4–18.6**).

The spleen (Figures **18.7** and **18.8**) shows red pulp infiltration and, in the white pulp, germinal centre hyperplasia with expanded mantle zones [4].

Some patients have hypergammaglobulinaemia and rheumatoid factor and anti-nuclear antibodies may be present. Hypogammaglobulinaemia is much less common. The direct anti-globulin test may be positive.

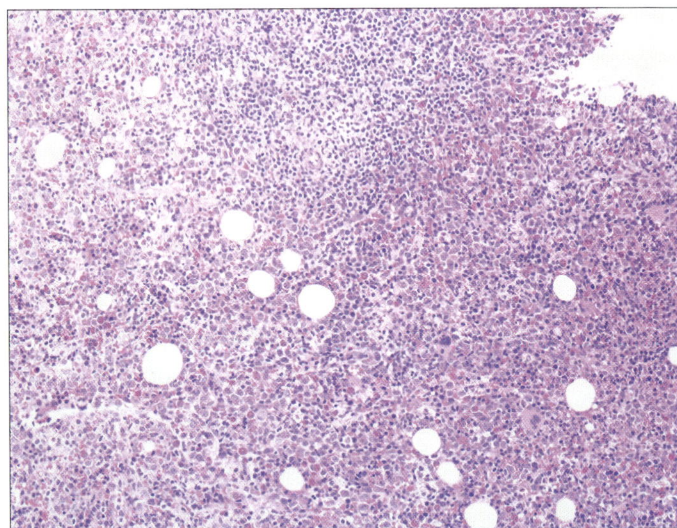

Figure 18.2 Bone marrow section in T-lineage large granular lymphocyte leukaemia showing a hypercellular bone marrow and an interstitial infiltrate with a reactive lymphoid nodule. H&E, x 20 objective.

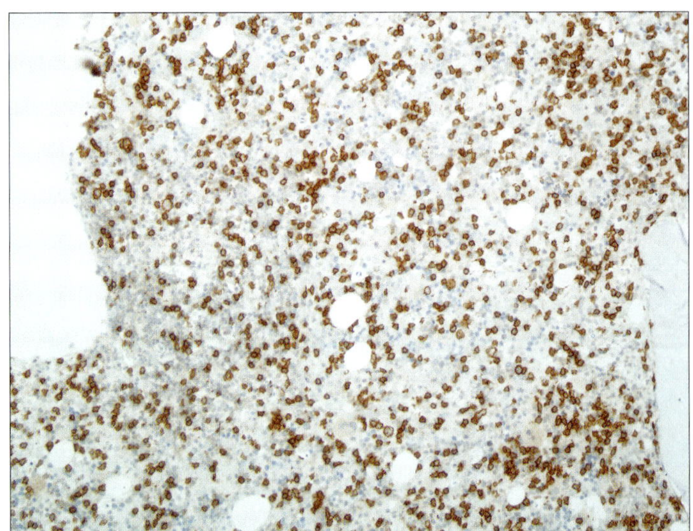

Figure 18.3 Bone marrow section in T-lineage large granular lymphocyte leukaemia showing an interstitial infiltrate by CD8-positive lymphocytes. Immunoperoxidase, x 20 objective.

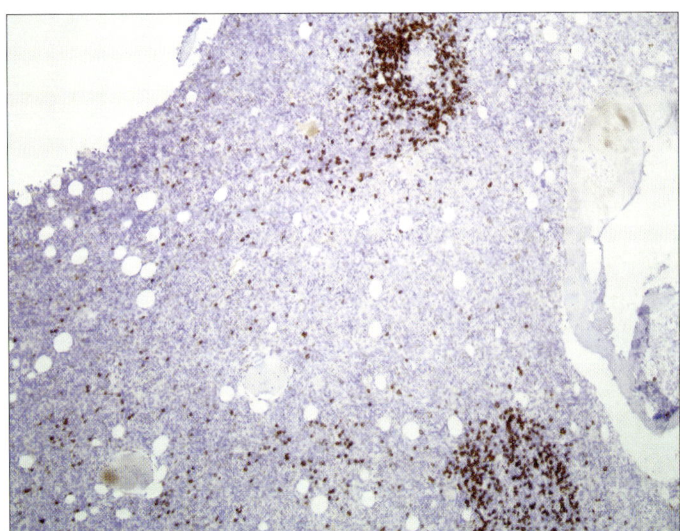

Figure 18.4 Bone marrow section in T-lineage large granular lymphocyte leukaemia showing CD20-positive lymphocytes in a reactive lymphoid nodule. Immunoperoxidase, x 10 objective.

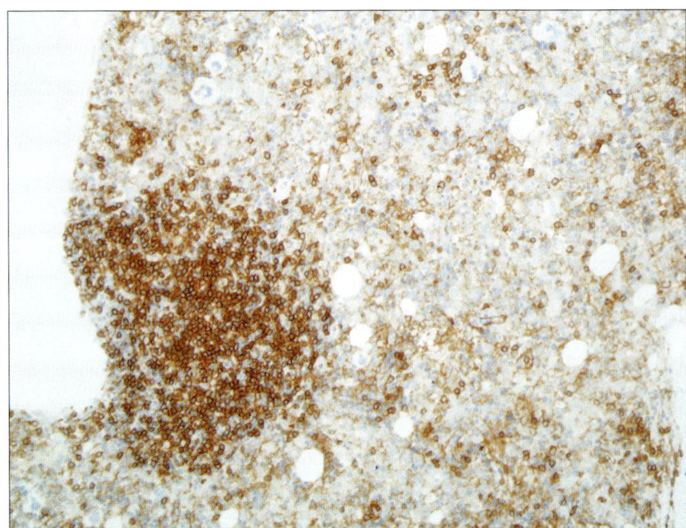

Figure 18.5 Bone marrow section in T-lineage large granular lymphocyte leukaemia showing CD4-positive lymphocytes in a reactive lymphoid nodule. Immunoperoxidase, x 20 objective.

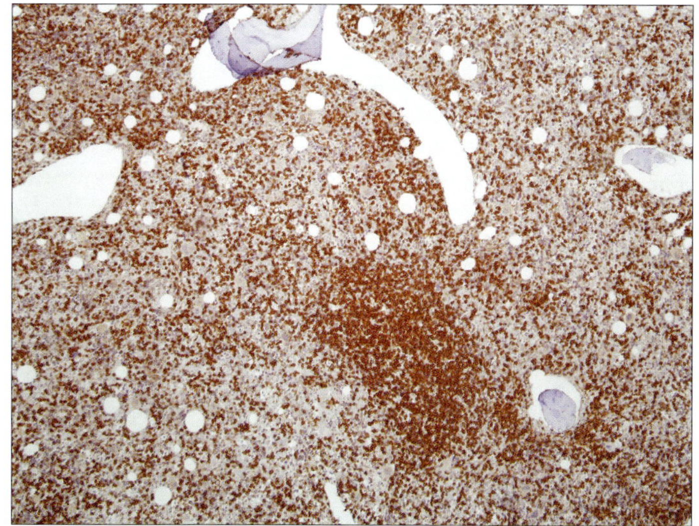

Figure 18.6 Bone marrow section in T-lineage large granular lymphocyte leukaemia showing CD3-positive lymphocytes. Immunoperoxidase, x 10 objective.

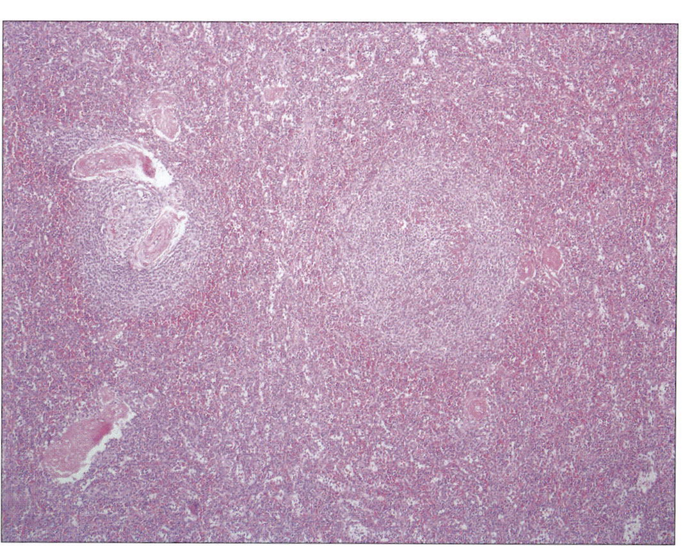

Figure 18.7 Spleen section in T-lineage large granular lymphocyte leukaemia showing red pulp infiltration. H&E, x 10 objective.

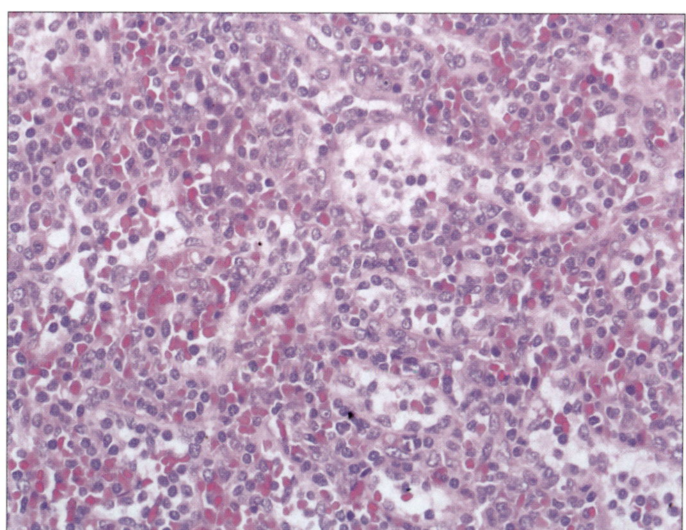

Figure 18.8 Spleen section in T-lineage large granular lymphocyte leukaemia showing interstitial infiltration. H&E, x 60 objective.

Immunophenotype

The neoplastic cells are T cells, expressing CD3 and usually CD2, CD8 and T-cell receptor (TCR) αβ (Figures **18.9** and **18.10**). Less often there is expression of CD4 rather than CD8 or expression of both CD4 and CD8; these cases often express NK-cell-associated antigens. Of the cytotoxic T-cell/NK-cell markers expression of CD57 and CD16 are most frequent. Sometimes there is expression of CD11b or CD56. CD56 expression has been related to more aggressive disease [5]. Perforin, TIA1 (Figure **18.11**) and CD158 (KIR, killer immunoglobulin-like receptor) may be expressed, the latter with a monoclonal pattern of expression of CD158a, CD158b or CD158e [6, 7]. Monoclonal antibodies directed at the variable chains of the TCR can also be useful to demonstrate clonality.

Cytogenetic and molecular genetic abnormalities

TCR receptor gene rearrangement is present, usually *TCRB* and sometimes *TCRG* [8]. There are no specific cytogenetic rearrangements recognized.

Diagnosis and differential diagnosis

The differential diagnosis includes other T-lineage leukaemias, NK-lineage leukaemia and a reactive increase in large granular lymphocytes (including that seen in hyposplenism and viral infections).

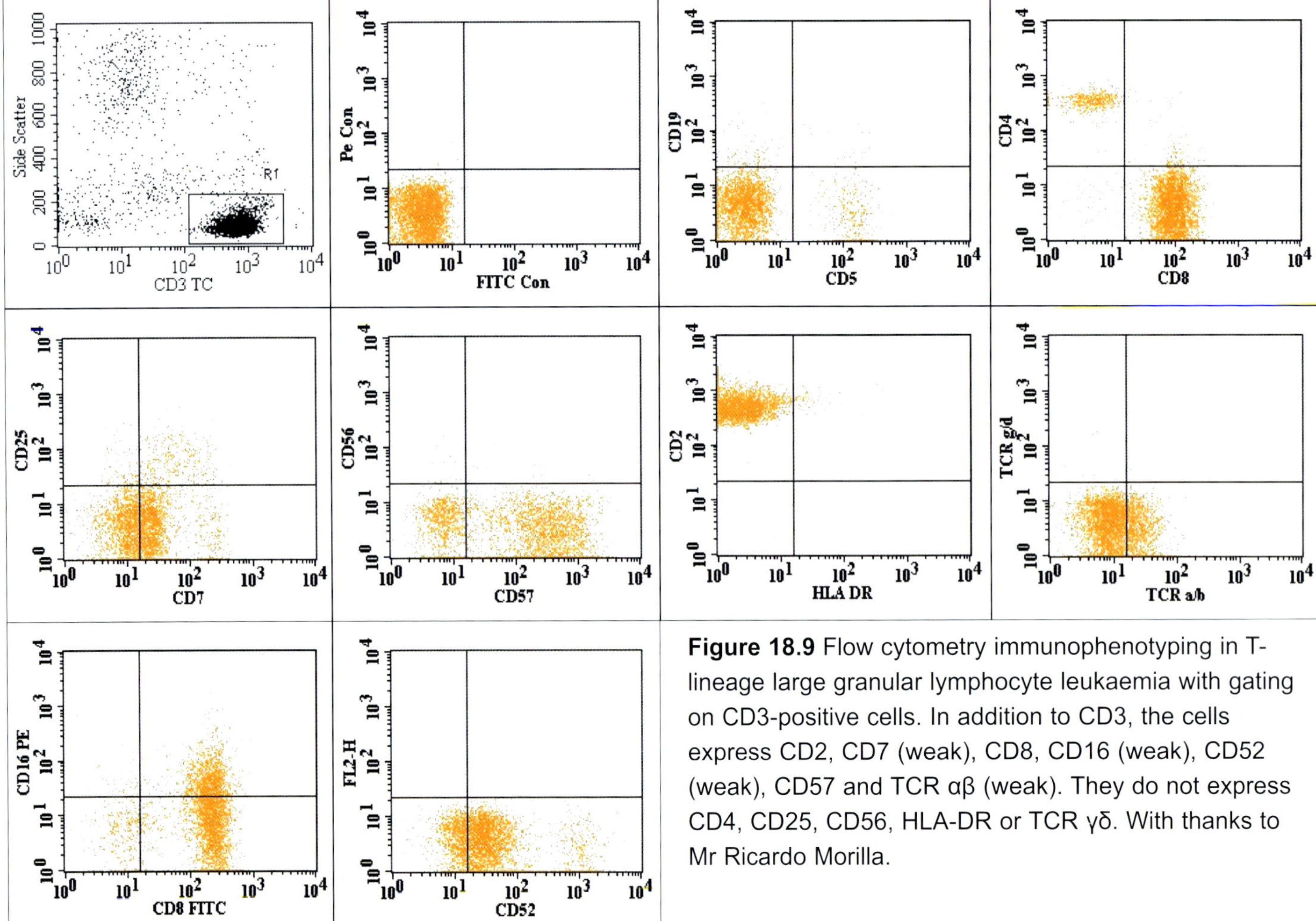

Figure 18.9 Flow cytometry immunophenotyping in T-lineage large granular lymphocyte leukaemia with gating on CD3-positive cells. In addition to CD3, the cells express CD2, CD7 (weak), CD8, CD16 (weak), CD52 (weak), CD57 and TCR αβ (weak). They do not express CD4, CD25, CD56, HLA-DR or TCR γδ. With thanks to Mr Ricardo Morilla.

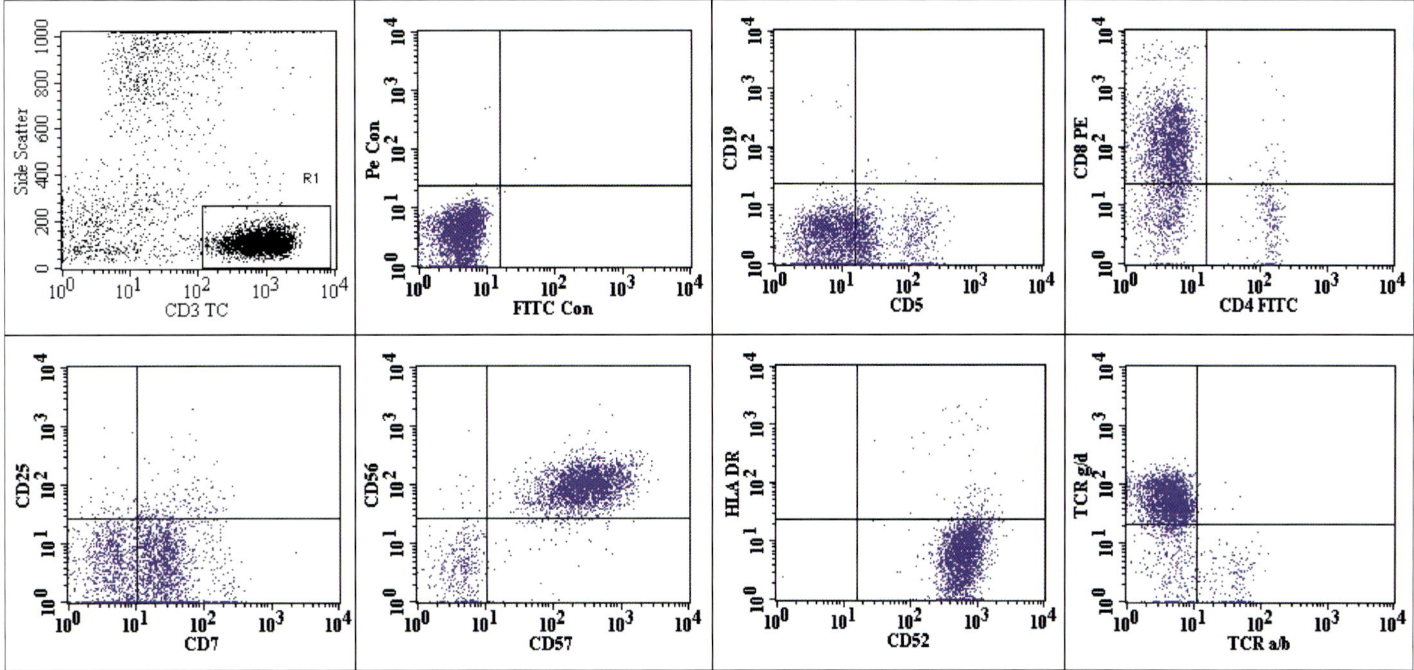

Figure 18.10 Flow cytometry immunophenotyping in T-lineage large granular lymphocyte with gating on CD3-positive cells. In addition to CD3, the cells express CD7 (weak), CD8, CD52, CD56, CD57 and TCR γδ. They do not express CD4, CD5, CD25, HLA-DR or TCR αβ. Expression of TCR γδ is uncommon. With thanks to Mr Ricardo Morilla.

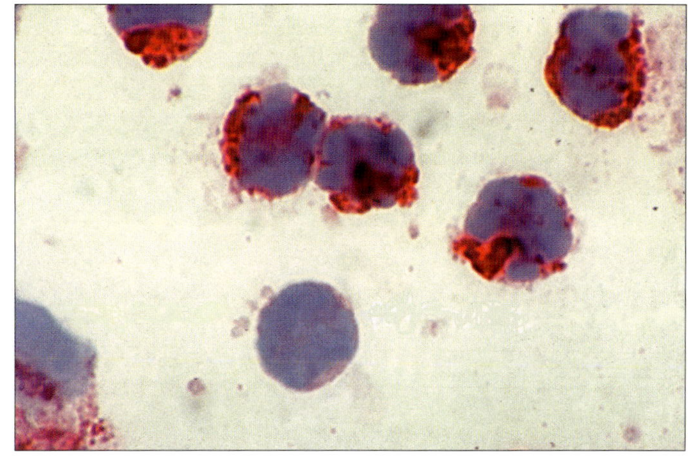

Figure 18.11 Cytospin of leukaemic cells in T-lineage large granular lymphocyte leukaemia showing expression of the cytotoxic granule protein, TIA1. Alkaline phosphatase-anti-alkaline phosphatase technique, x 100 objective.

Prognosis

The disease is indolent. Not all patients require treatment. Cases in which the cells express CD56 are more aggressive.

Treatment

Treatment options include methotrexate, cyclophosphamide, ciclosporin and prednisolone. Treatment may be aimed at autoimmune complications or at the underlying disease.

References

1. Lamy T and Loughran TP (2003). Clinical features of large granular lymphocyte leukemia. *Semin Hematol*, **40**,185–195.
2. Pawson R, Schulz TF, Matutes E and Catovsky D (1997). The human T-cell lymphotropic viruses types I/II are not involved in T prolymphocytic leukemia and large granular lymphocytic leukemia. *Leukemia*, **11**, 1305–1311.
3. Matutes E, Wotherspoon AC, Parker NE, Osuji N, Isaacson PG and Catovsky D (2001). Transformation of T-cell large granular lymphocyte leukaemia into a high-grade large T-cell lymphoma. *Br J Haematol*, **115**, 801–806.
4. Osuji N, Matutes E, Catovsky D, Lampert I and Wotherspoon A (2005). Histopathology of the spleen in T-cell large granular lymphocyte leukemia and T-cell prolymphocytic leukemia: a comparative review. *Am J Surg Pathol*, **29**, 935–941.
5. Gentile TC, Uner AH, Hutchison RE, Wright J, Ben-Ezra J, Russell EC and Loughran TP (1994). CD3+, CD56+ aggressive variant of large granular lymphocyte leukemia. *Blood*, **84**, 2315–2321.
6. Matutes E, Coelho E, Aguado MJ, Morilla R, Crawford A, Owusu-Ankomah K and Catovsky D (1996). Expression of TIA-1 and TIA-2 in T cell malignancies and T cell lymphocytosis. *J Clin Pathol*, **49**, 154–158.
7. Morice WG, Kurtin PJ, Leibson PJ, Tefferi A and Hanson CA (2003). Demonstration of aberrant T-cell and natural killer-cell antigen expression in all cases of granular lymphocytic leukaemia. *Br J Haematol*, **120**, 1026–1036.
8. Langerak AW, van den Beemd R, Wolvers-Tettero IL, Boor PP, van Lochen EG, Hooijkaas H and van Dongen JJ (2001). Molecular and flow cytometric analysis of the V repertoire for clonality assessment in mature TCR αβ T-cell proliferations. *Blood*, **98**, 167–173.

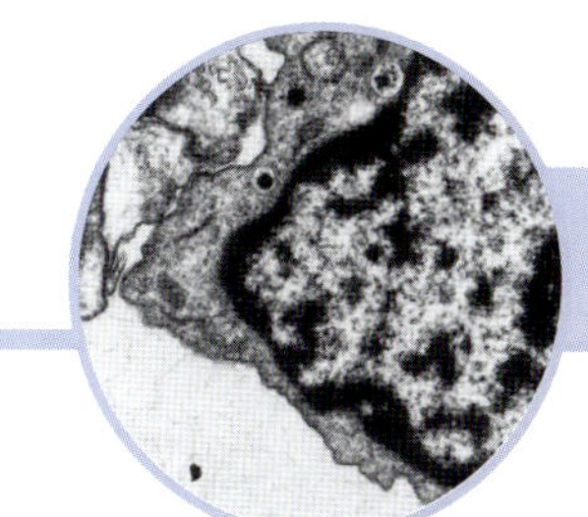

Chapter 19

Aggressive NK-cell leukaemia

Large granular lymphocyte leukaemia (LGLL) may be of T lineage or natural killer (NK) lineage. NK-cell leukaemia may be indolent or aggressive [1–4]. Recognition of indolent NK-cell leukaemia is complicated by the fact that markers of clonality have not been readily available and have often not been employed, leading to uncertainty as to whether the condition is reactive or leukaemic in nature. Recognition of aggressive cases is more straightforward and it is this group that has been designated aggressive NK-cell lymphoma in the World Health Organization (WHO) classification. Aggressive NK-cell lymphoma is more common in Far East Asia than in the West and there is a strong association with the Epstein–Barr virus.

Clinical features

Some cases are indolent while others have aggressive disease with constitutional symptoms and often abnormal coagulation. There may be hepatosplenomegaly and lymphadenopathy.

Haematological and pathological features

The number of circulating neoplastic cells may be low or high. Indolent cases have cells resembling normal large granular lymphocytes and similar to the neoplastic cells of T-lineage LGLL. Patients with aggressive disease have neoplastic cells that are more atypical than those of T-lineage LGLL (Figures **19.1**–**19.3**); they are granular lymphocytes that may be increased in size and have moderately basophilic cytoplasm or irregular or hyperchromatic nuclei. Anaemia, neutropenia and thrombocytopenia are common in patients with aggressive disease and in these patients the bone marrow shows not only infiltration but often also haemophagocytosis.

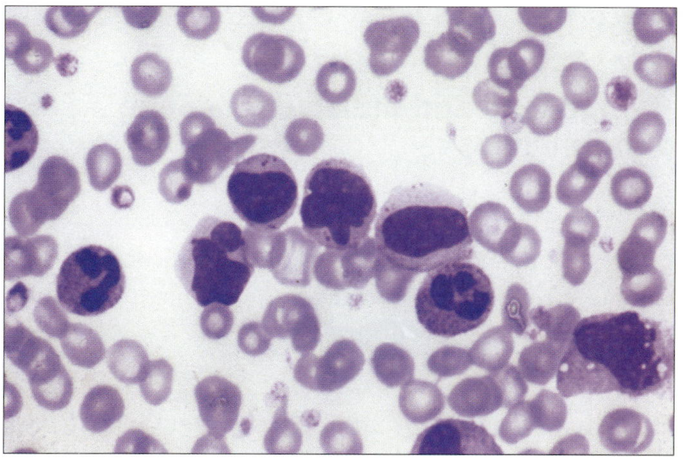

Figure 19.1 Peripheral blood film from a patient with NK-lineage large granular lymphocyte leukaemia showing atypical large granular lymphocytes, many of which are larger than their normal equivalent and have lobulated nuclei. Romanowsky, x 100 objective.

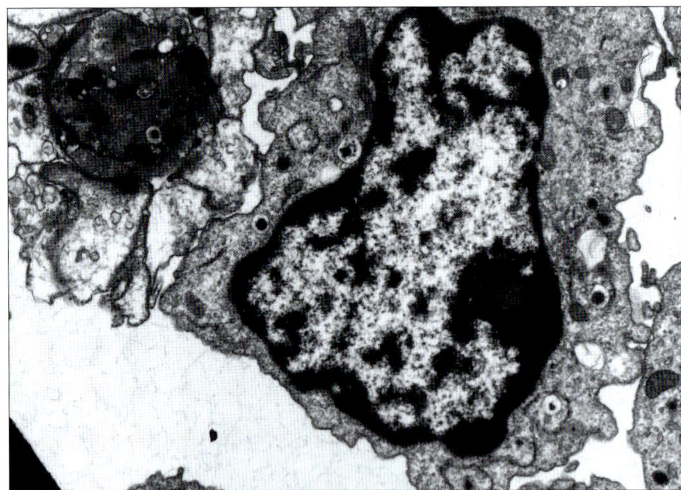

Figure 19.2 Ultrastructure of a neoplastic cell from a patient with NK-lineage large granular lymphocyte leukaemia showing cytoplasmic granules and a somewhat irregular nucleus with a nucleolus. Lead nitrate and uranyl acetate stain.

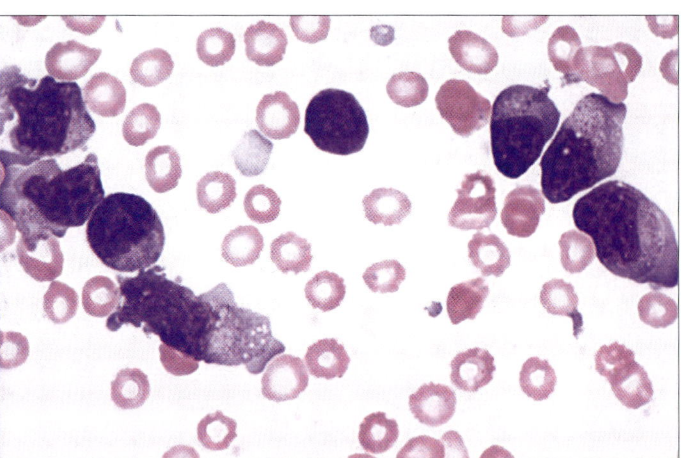

Figure 19.3 Bone marrow film from a patient with NK-lineage large granular lymphocyte leukaemia showing pleomorphic large granular lymphocytes, with irregular nuclei and nucleoli. Romanowsky, x 100 objective.

Immunophenotype

The neoplastic cells are NK cells, not expressing CD3 but usually expressing CD2, CD56 and CD94 [5–7]. CD11c and CD16 may be expressed but CD57 is usually negative. CD158 may be expressed with a monoclonal pattern of expression – CD158a, CD158b or CD158e restricted or CD158 not expressed [6]. On immunohistochemistry, expression of cytoplasmic CD3ε chain may be detected; it should be noted that polyclonal antibodies used to detect CD3 in tissue sections cross-react with the zeta chain of the CD3 expressed in NK cells, giving a false impression that CD3 is expressed.

Cytogenetic and molecular genetic abnormalities

T-cell receptor gene rearrangement is absent. Clonal cytogenetic abnormalities may be present but there are no specific cytogenetic rearrangements recognized. Chromosome 6 is not infrequently involved.

Diagnosis and differential diagnosis

The differential diagnosis includes a reactive increase in large granular lymphocytes and T-lineage LGLL. This condition needs to be distinguished from 'blastic NK cell leukaemia/lymphoma' [8], which is probably actually a neoplasm of plasmacytoid dendritic cells.

Prognosis

The disease may be either indolent or aggressive.

Treatment

Patients with indolent disease often do not require treatment. For those who do, treatment options are not well defined. Aggressive disease is usually treated with treatment regimes applicable either to high-grade non-Hodgkin's lymphoma or to acute lymphoblastic leukaemia.

References

1. Imamura N, Kusunoki Y, Kawa-Ha K, Yumura K, Hara J, Oda K *et al.* (1990). Aggressive natural killer cell leukaemia/lymphoma: report of four cases and review of the literature. Possible existence of a new clinical entity originating from the third lineage of lymphoid cells. *Br J Haematol*, **75**, 49–59.
2. Nakamura MC (2002). Natural killer cells and their role in disease. *Lab Med*, **33**, 278–282.
3. Matutes E and Osuji N (2004). Clinical and morphological features of natural killer (NK) cell disorders. *Haematologica*, **89**, Suppl. 1, 260–264.
4. Foucar K, Matutes E and Catovsky D (2004). T-cell large granular lymphocytic leukemia, T-cell prolymphocytic leukaemia and aggressive natural-killer cell leukemia/lymphoma. *In* Mauch PM, Armitage JO, Coiffier B, Dalla-Favera R and Harris NL (Eds). *Non-Hodgkins Lymphomas*, Lippincott Williams & Wilkins, Philadelphia, pp. 283–294.
5. Mori KL, Egashira M and Oshimi K (2001). Differentiation stage of natural killer cell lineage lymphoproliferative disorders based on phenotypic analysis. *Br J Haematol*, **115**, 225–228.
6. Morice WG, Kurtin PJ, Leibson PJ, Tefferi A and Hanson CA (2003). Demonstration of aberrant T-cell and natural killer-cell antigen expression in all cases of granular lymphocytic leukaemia. *Br J Haematol*, **120**, 1026–1036.
7. Epling-Burnette PK, Painter JS, Chaurasia P, Bai F, Wei S and Djeu JY (2004). Dysregulated NK receptor expression in patients with lymphoproliferative disease of granular lymphocytes. *Blood*, **103**, 3431–3439.
8. Suzuki R, Nakamura S, Suzumiya J, Ichimura K, Ichikawa M, Ogata K *et al.*; NK-cell Tumor Study Group (2005). Blastic natural killer cell lymphoma/leukemia (CD56-positive blastic tumor): prognostication and categorization according to anatomic sites of involvement. *Cancer*, **104**, 1022–1031.

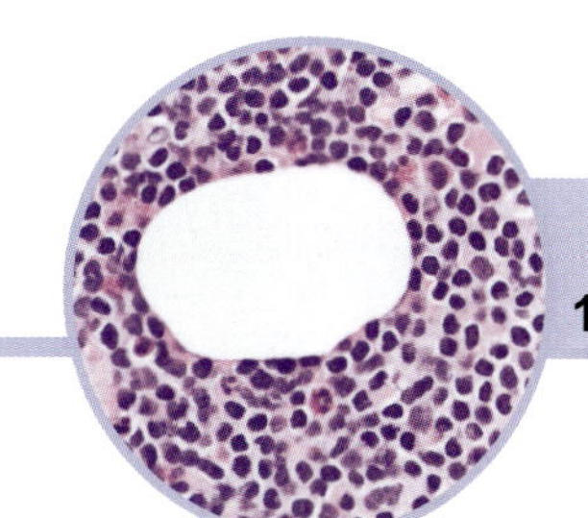

Chapter 20

T-cell prolymphocytic leukaemia

T-cell prolymphocytic leukaemia (T-PLL) is a clinicobiological entity that has no relationship to B-cell prolymphocytic leukaemia (B-PLL) other than some degree of similarity of cytological features [1, 2]. It is mainly a disease of the elderly. Ataxia telangiectasia predisposes [3]. There is no relationship to human lymphotropic viruses I or II [4].

Clinical features

Typical clinical features are lymphadenopathy, hepatomegaly and splenomegaly. Skin infiltration is present in about one-fifth of patients [5]. Serous effusions can occur. In most patients this is an aggressive disorder, although in a minority of patients the course is more indolent (smouldering T-PLL) [6].

Haematological and pathological features

The white cell count is usually high and anaemia and thrombocytopenia are common. Neoplastic cells can resemble those of B-PLL, being large with a round to oval nucleus, a moderate amount of cytoplasm and a prominent nucleolus; in some cases the nuclei are quite irregular (Figures **20.1**–**20.3**). In the small cell variant of T-PLL the cells are not much larger than those of chronic lymphocytic leukaemia but differ in that the cytoplasm is more basophilic and there are cytoplasmic blebs; nuclei are irregular and a nucleolus is apparent. In the small cell variant the nucleolus is smaller and much less prominent than in cases with larger cells. The two cytological variants represent the same disease. In addition the condition initially described as 'Sézary cell leukaemia', in which the cells are medium sized with a highly convoluted nucleus, is now seen as a variant of T-PLL.

Figure 20.1 Peripheral blood film in T-PLL showing small and medium sized cells with irregular nuclei and nucleoli. Romanowsky, x 60 objective.

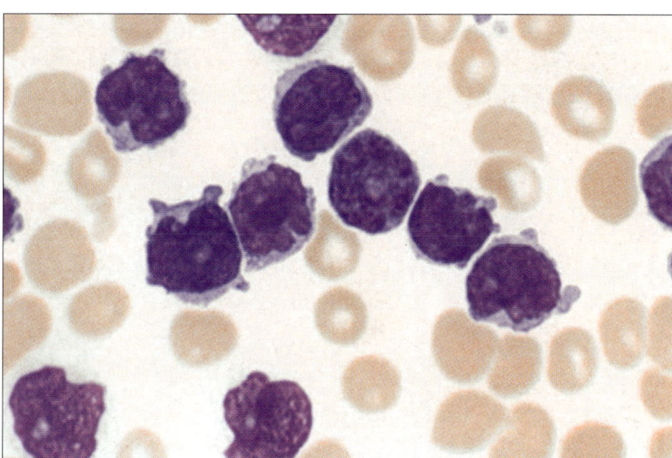

Figure 20.2 Peripheral blood film in T-PLL showing medium sized cells with basophilic cytoplasm and irregular nuclei with nucleoli. Romanowsky, x 100 objective.

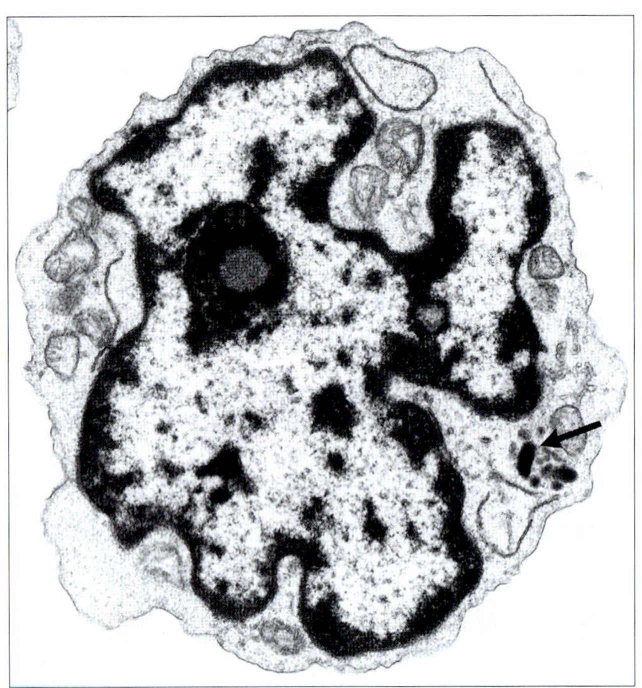

Figure 20.3 Ultrastructure of a T-PLL cell showing an irregular nucleus with a prominent nucleolus. The arrow shows electron-dense granules, a feature of T-PLL and not B-PLL. Lead nitrate and uranyl acetate stain.

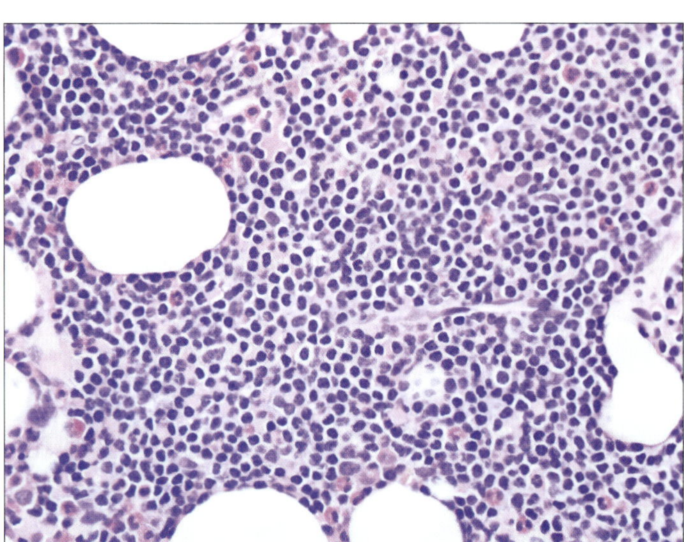

Figure 20.4 Section of bone marrow trephine biopsy specimen showing heavy interstitial infiltration. H&E, x 60 objective.

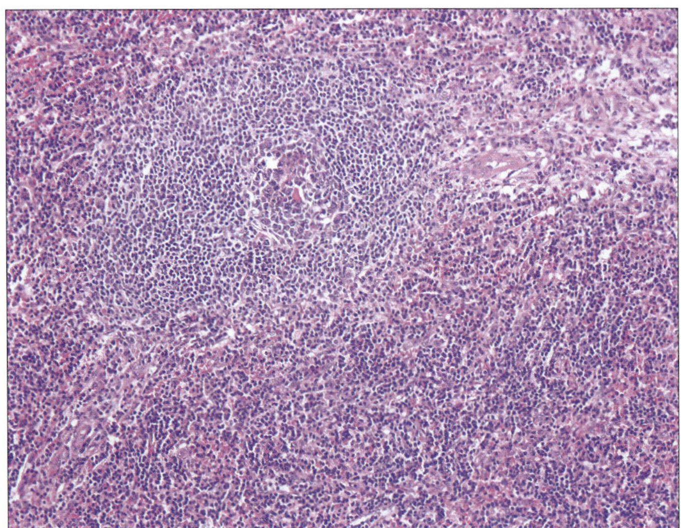

Figure 20.5 Section of spleen showing infiltration of red and white pulp. H&E, x 20 objective.

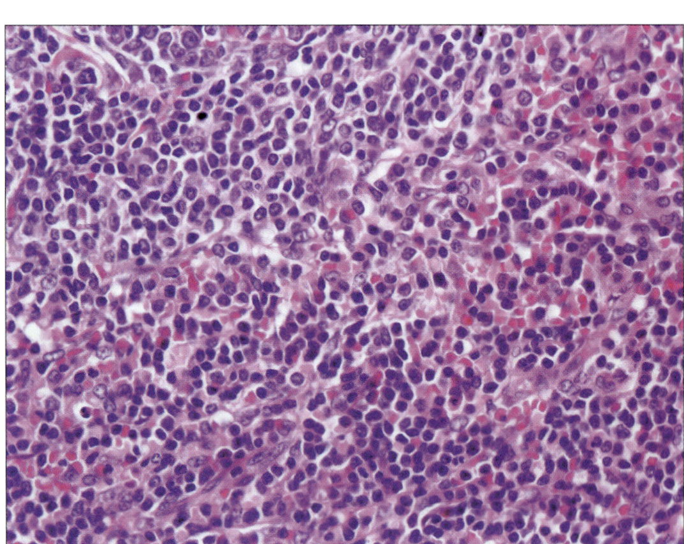

Figure 20.6 Section of spleen showing infiltration of red and white pulp. H&E, x 60 objective.

Bone marrow infiltration is variable, sometimes heavy interstitial and sometimes diffuse (Figure **20.4**). Spleen histology shows marked infiltration of the red pulp with invasion of the white pulp and splenic capsule [7] (Figures **20.5** and **20.6**). Skin infiltration is in the dermis, preferentially around the skin appendages, without epidermotropism (Figure **20.7**). Lymph node infiltration is preferentially paracortical with sparing of the follicles but may become diffuse.

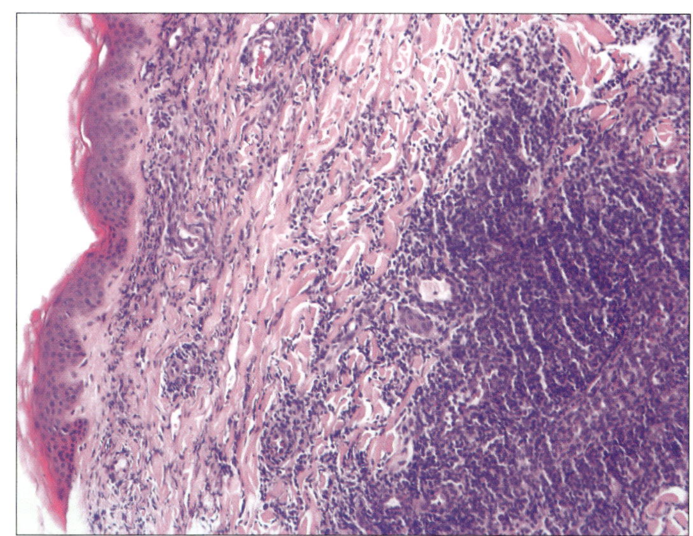

Figure 20.7 Section of skin biopsy showing lymphoid dermal infiltration. H&E, x 20 objective.

Immunophenotype

The immunophenotype is that of a mature T cell. CD2, CD3 and CD5 are expressed (Figures **20.8** and **20.9**). In contrast to other T-lineage lymphoproliferative disorders, CD7 is often strongly expressed (expression is stronger than in normal T lymphocytes) [2]. CD3 expression may be absent (20% of cases) and when expressed, is weaker than in normal lymphocytes; cases that lack surface membrane expression nevertheless show cytoplasmic expression. In most cases the leukaemic cells are CD4-positive but in a significant minority (about one-fifth of patients) they co-express CD4 and CD8 and in another 15% they are CD4 negative and CD8 positive. With the exception of T-PLL, the co-expression of CD4 and CD8 is quite uncommon in neoplastic conditions of mature T cells. CD1a and terminal deoxynucleotidyl transferase are negative.

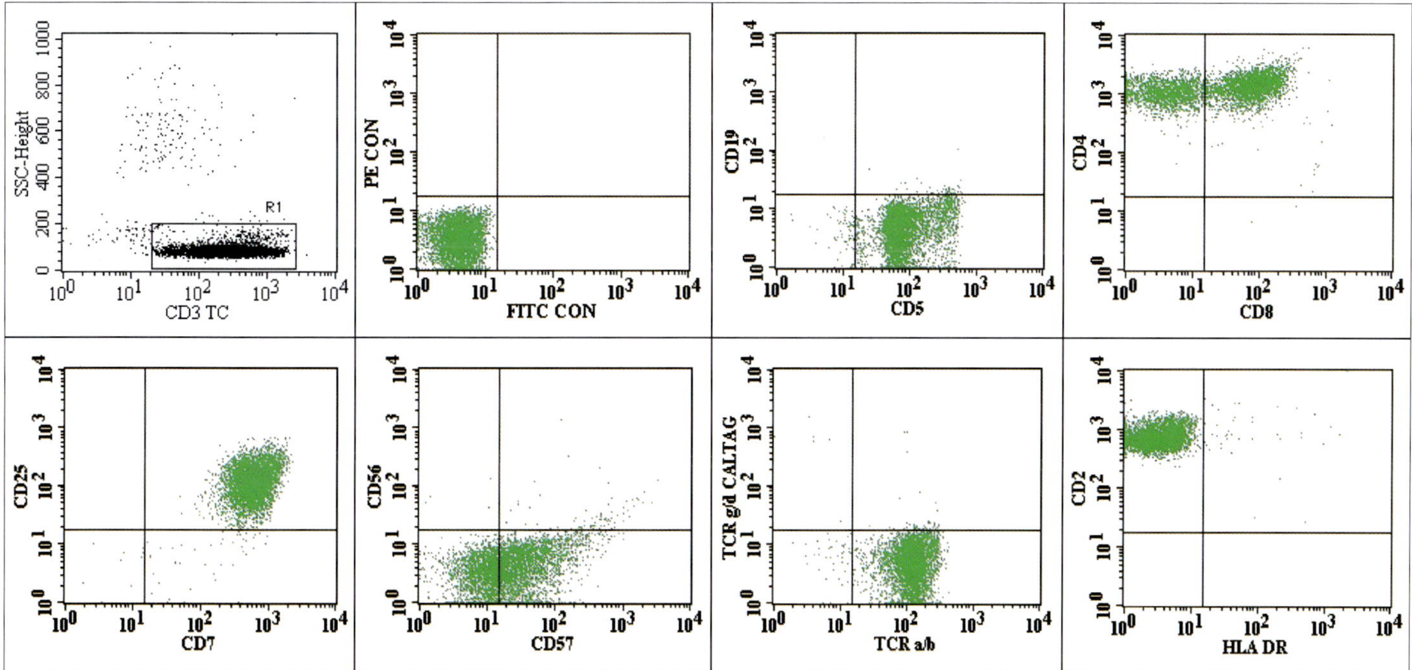

Figure 20.8 Flow cytometry immunophenotyping with gating on CD3-positive cells. In addition to CD3, cells express CD2, CD4, CD5, CD7, CD8 (subpopulation), CD25, CD57 (weak) and TCR αβ. They do not express CD56, HLA-DR or TCR γδ. With thanks to Mr Ricardo Morilla.

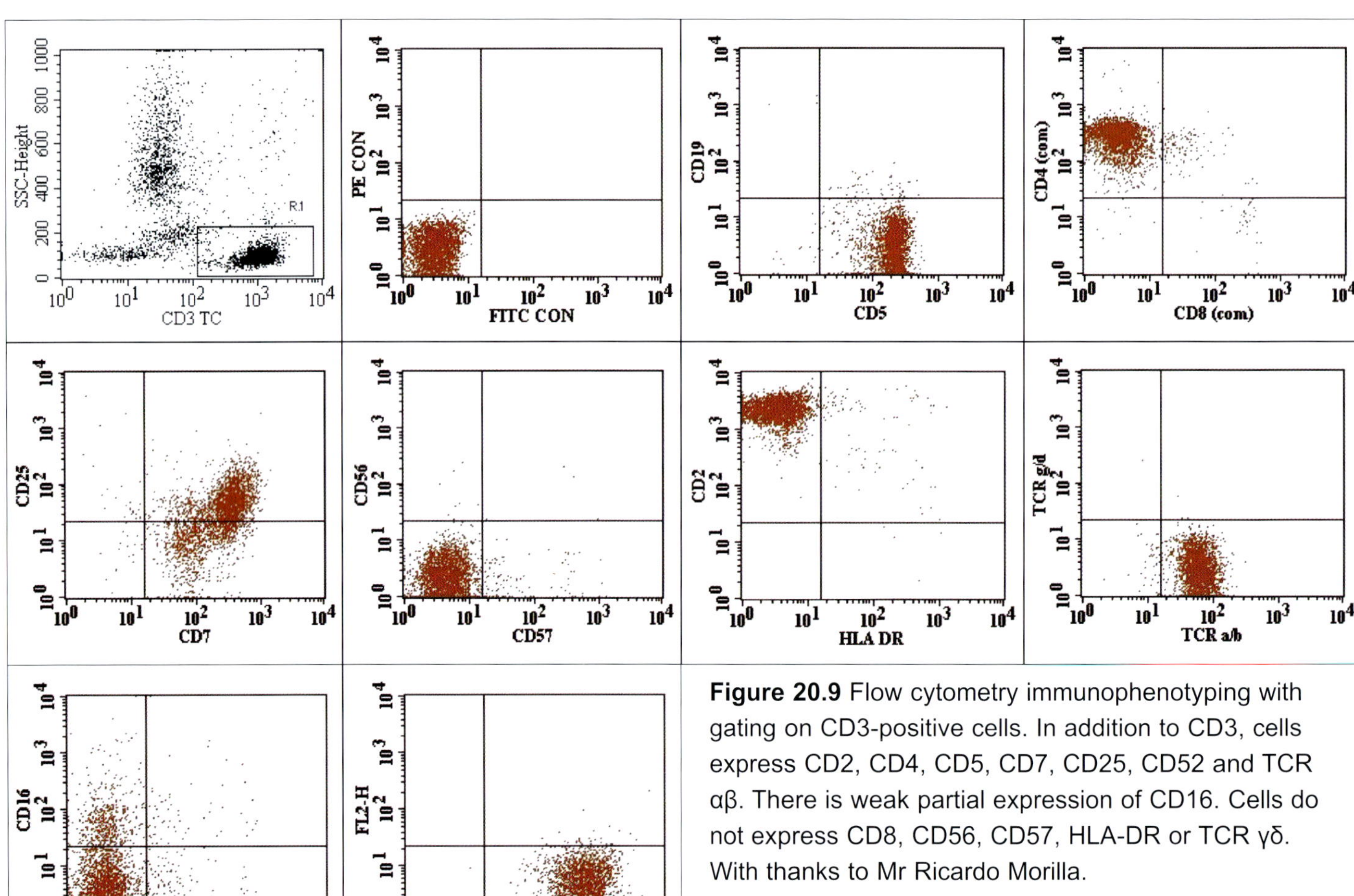

Figure 20.9 Flow cytometry immunophenotyping with gating on CD3-positive cells. In addition to CD3, cells express CD2, CD4, CD5, CD7, CD25, CD52 and TCR αβ. There is weak partial expression of CD16. Cells do not express CD8, CD56, CD57, HLA-DR or TCR γδ. With thanks to Mr Ricardo Morilla.

Cytogenetic and molecular genetic abnormalities

About three-quarters of cases of T-PLL show either inv(14)(q11q32) (Figure **20.10**) or t(14;14)(q11;q32) [8]. These chromosomal rearrangements involve the *TCRA* and *TCRD* loci at 14q11 and two oncogenes, *TCL1* and *TCL1b*, at 14q32.1 [9]. Less common but recurring translocations are t(X;14)(q28;q11) (Figure **20.11**) and t(X;7)(q28;q35), in which the *MTCP1* gene at Xq28 (which is homologous to *TCL1*) is dysregulated by proximity to the *TCRA* and *TCRD* loci and the *TCRB* gene respectively. Dysregulation of *MTCP1* can also result from fusion of this gene with the *TCRB* gene as a result of t(X;7)(q28;q35). Chromosome 8 abnormalities can occur as a second event. The *ATM* gene at 11q23, the gene involved in ataxia telangiectasia, may be mutated or lost as a result of an 11q23 deletion (both detected by molecular analysis) [10].

Diagnosis and differential diagnosis

The differential diagnosis includes B-PLL, Sézary syndrome and chronic lymphocytic leukaemia. A careful consideration of both the cytology and the immunophenotype permits the distinction.

Prognosis

Prognosis is poor. With the exception of patients with the indolent variant, survival is usually less than one year.

Treatment

Responses to chemotherapy are usually brief. The most effective agent is the anti-CD52 monoclonal antibody, alemtuzumab, but relapse occurs unless it is possible to consolidate with high dose therapy and stem cell transplantation [11]. Pentostatin is sometimes useful.

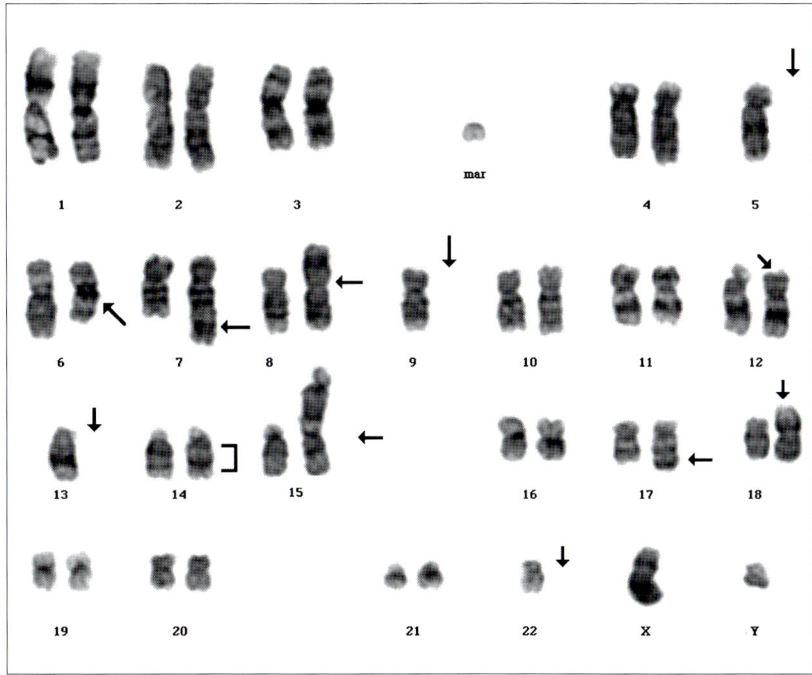

Figure 20.10 Karyogram of a patient with T-PLL with a complex karyotype including inv(14)(q11q32). The arrows indicate missing or abnormal chromosomes. With thanks to Dr John Swansbury.

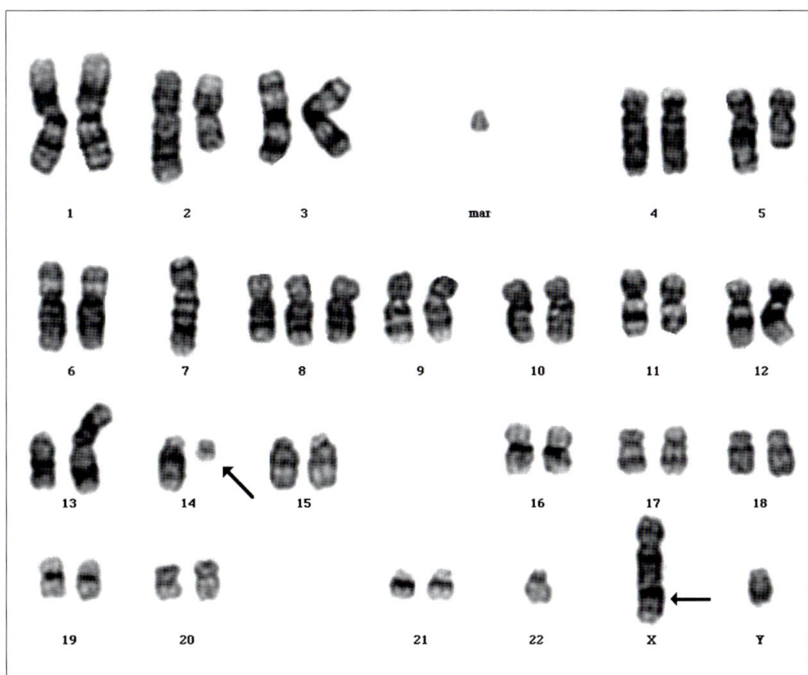

Figure 20.11 Karyogram of a patient with T-PLL with t(X;14)(q28;q11) and a marker chromosome. The arrows indicate the chromosomes involved in the translocation. With thanks to Dr John Swansbury.

References

1. Matutes E, Brito-Babapulle V, Swansbury J, Ellis J, Morilla R, Dearden C, Sempere A and Catovsky D (1991). Clinical and laboratory features of 78 cases of T-prolymphocytic leukemia. *Blood*, **78**, 3269–3274.
2. Matutes E (1998). T-cell prolymphocytic leukemia. *Cancer Control*, **5**, 19–24.
3. Taylor AM, Metcalfe JA, Thick M and Mak YF (1996). Leukemia and lymphoma in ataxia telangiectasia. *Blood*, **87**, 423–438.
4. Pawson R, Schulz TF, Matutes E and Catovsky D (1997). The human T-cell lymphotropic viruses types I/II are not involved in T prolymphocytic leukemia and large granular lymphocytic leukemia. *Leukemia*, **11**, 1305–1311.
5. Mallett RB, Matutes E, Catovsky D, MacLennan K, Mortimer PS and Holden CA (1994). Cutaneous infiltration in T-cell prolymphocytic leukaemia. *Br J Dermatol*, **132**, 263–266.
6. Garand R, Goasguen J, Brizard A, Buisine J, Charpentier A, Claisse JF *et al.* (1998). Indolent course as a relatively frequent presentation in T-prolymphocytic leukaemia. Groupe Francais d'Hematologie Cellulaire. *Br J Haematol*, **103**, 488–494.
7. Osuji N, Matutes E, Catovsky D, Lampert I and Wotherspoon A (2005). Histopathology of the spleen in T-cell large granular lymphocyte leukemia and T-cell prolymphocytic leukemia: a comparative review. *Am J Surg Pathol*, **29**, 935–941.
8. Brito-Babapulle V, Pomfret M, Matutes E and Catovsky D (1987). Cytogenetic studies on prolymphocytic leukemia. II. T cell prolymphocytic leukemia. *Blood*, **70**, 926–931.
9. Pekarsky U, Hallas C and Croce CM (2001). Molecular basis of mature T-cell leukemia. *JAMA*, **286**, 2308–2314.
10. Yuille MA, Coignet LJ, Abraham SM, Yaqub F, Luo L, Matutes E *et al.* (1998). ATM is usually rearranged in T-cell prolymphocytic leukaemia. *Oncogene*, **16**, 789–796. Erratum in: *Oncogene*, 1998, **16**, 2955.
11. Dearden CE, Matutes E, Cazin B, Tjonnfjord GE, Parreira A, Nomdedeu B *et al.* (2001). High remission rate in T-cell prolymphocytic leukaemia with CAMPATH-1H. *Blood*, **98**, 1721–1726.

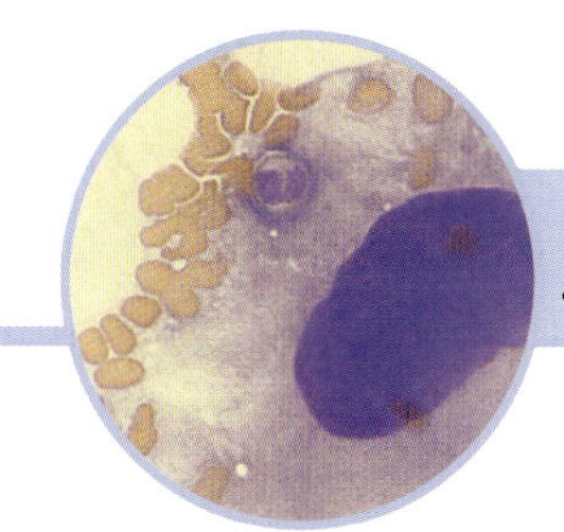

Chapter 21

Multiple myeloma

Multiple myeloma is a plasma cell neoplasm that is usually associated with synthesis of a monoclonal immunoglobulin (paraprotein), a monoclonal immunoglobulin light chain (Bence–Jones protein) or both [1–4]. In a minority of cases, multiple myeloma is non-secretory. Disease is mainly medullary (i.e. within the bone marrow cavity) but extra-medullary lesions also occur (extra-medullary plasmacytoma). In the World Health Organization (WHO) classification, multiple myeloma is designated 'plasma cell myeloma'.

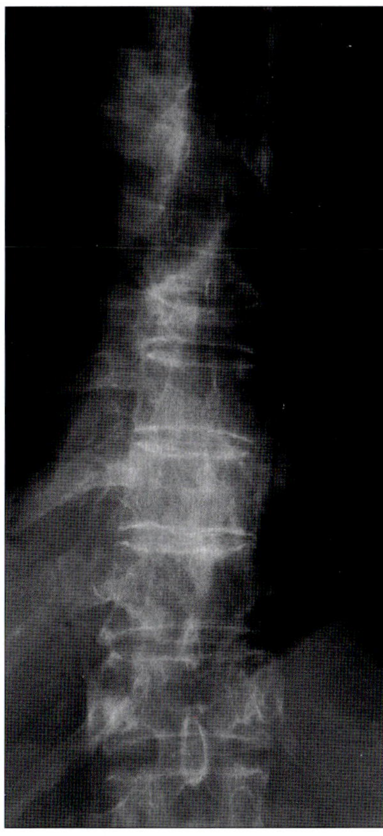

Figure 21.1 Vertebral collapse in multiple myeloma.

Clinical features

Clinical features can be the direct effect of the proliferation of plasma cells (e.g. pathological fracture, spinal cord compression) (Figure **21.1**), can result from marrow infiltration (anaemia) or can be caused directly by the paraprotein (hyperviscosity) or the Bence–Jones protein (renal failure). Some cases are complicated by amyloidosis, the amyloid being formed from altered light chains.

Haematological and pathological features

Anaemia is usual. Thrombocytopenia occurs less often. A blood film characteristically shows increased rouleaux formation (Figure **21.2**) and increased background staining

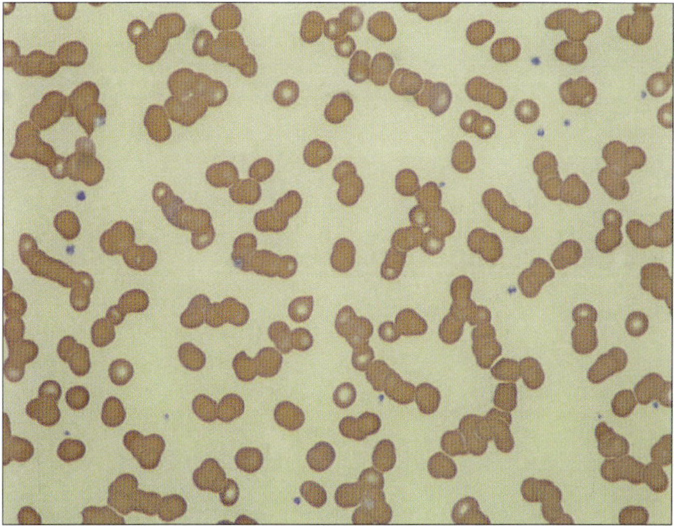

Figure 21.2 Peripheral blood film in multiple myeloma showing increased rouleaux formation. Romanowsky, x 50 objective.

(a blue tinge to the blood film), as a result of the presence of a paraprotein; patients with synthesis of Bence–Jones protein only or with non-secretory myeloma lack this feature. The erythrocyte sedimentation rate is characteristically elevated in patients with a serum paraprotein. Sometimes there are circulating neoplastic cells. When these are numerous the designation plasma cell leukaemia is used (Figure **21.3**).

Biochemical tests often show renal impairment and hypercalcaemia. There may be hyperuricaemia. Serum β2-microglobulin is increased and this may relate to the myeloma activity or to renal impairment. A paraprotein is

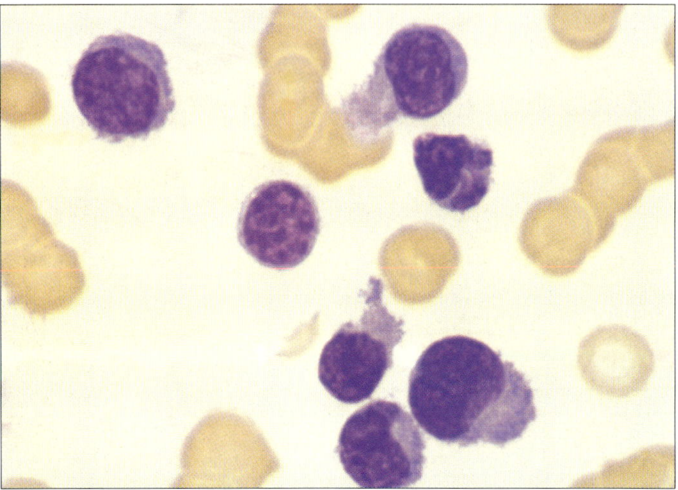

Figure 21.3 Peripheral blood film in plasma cell leukaemia showing lymphocytes and pleomorphic plasmacytoid lymphocytes. Romanowsky, x 100 objective.

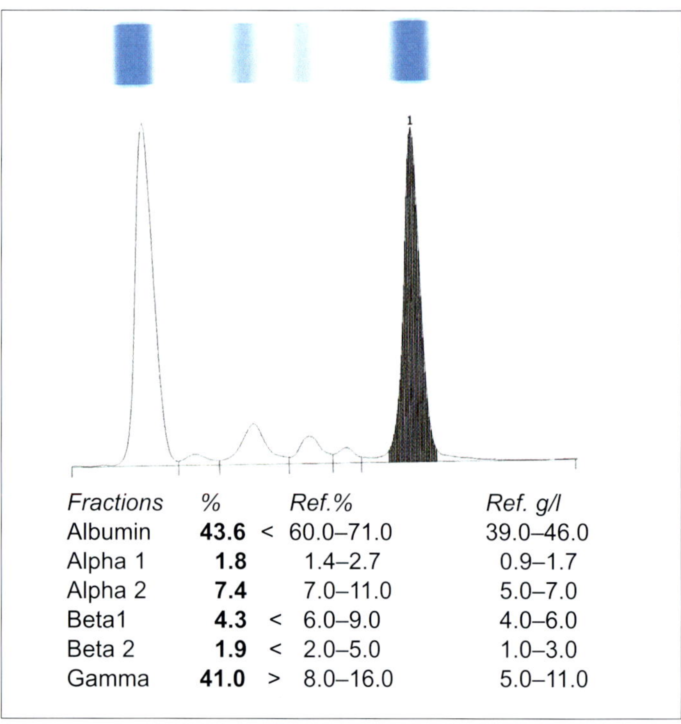

Fractions	*%*		*Ref.%*	*Ref. g/l*
Albumin	**43.6**	<	60.0–71.0	39.0–46.0
Alpha 1	**1.8**		1.4–2.7	0.9–1.7
Alpha 2	**7.4**		7.0–11.0	5.0–7.0
Beta1	**4.3**	<	6.0–9.0	4.0–6.0
Beta 2	**1.9**	<	2.0–5.0	1.0–3.0
Gamma	**41.0**	>	8.0–16.0	5.0–11.0

Figure 21.4 Serum protein electrophoretic pattern in multiple myeloma showing a prominent paraprotein band in the gamma region on an electrophoretic strip (top) and by densitometric scanning (middle). The < and > signs indicate if a percentage is above or below the reference range. With thanks to Miss Carol Hughes.

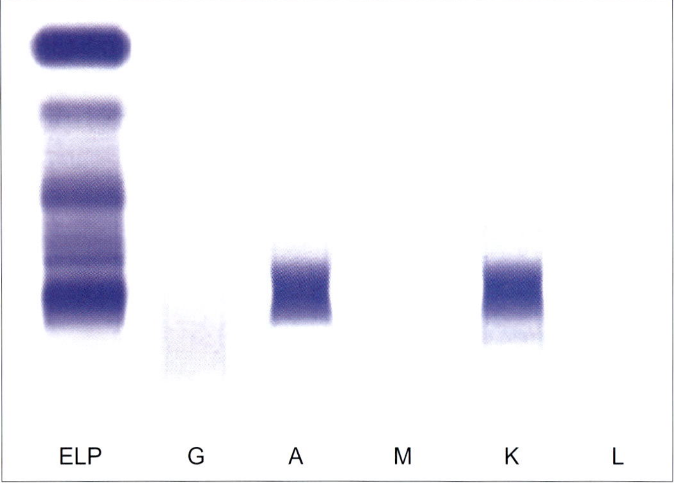

Figure 21.5 Serum protein electrophoresis showing a prominent paraprotein band in the gamma region (left) identified as an IgA κ paraprotein by immunofixation (right). With thanks to Miss Carol Hughes.

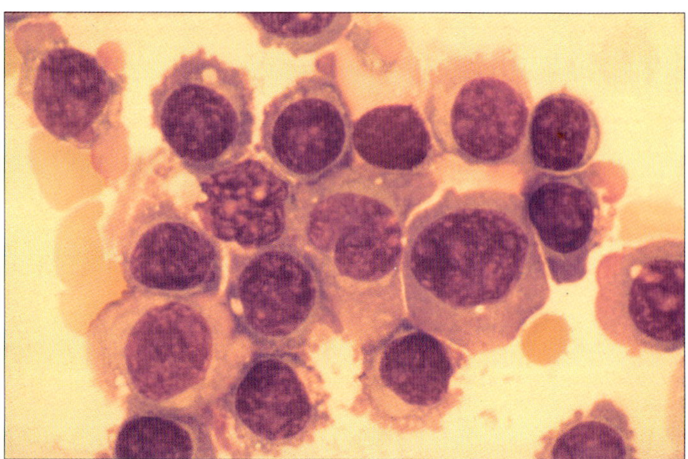

Figure 21.6 Bone marrow aspirate film in plasma cell leukaemia showing abnormal plasma cells, some with prominent Golgi zones. Romanowsky, x 100 objective.

often present in the serum (Figures **21.4** and **21.5**) and Bence–Jones protein in the urine. In patients with renal failure, Bence–Jones protein may be detected in the serum.

A bone marrow aspirate shows myeloma cells in quite variable numbers; the degree of cytological atypia is also variable. Because of the focal nature of the infiltrate, an aspirate may show as few as 10% of myeloma cells. More typically the neoplastic cells constitute from 30% to more than 90% of bone marrow nucleated cells. Myeloma cells may be morphologically similar to normal plasma cells with a low nucleocytoplasmic ratio, an eccentric nucleus and a well-developed Golgi zone. In other patients the myeloma cells show morphological abnormalities such as increased size, bi- or multi-nuclearity with nuclei of disparate sizes, the presence of nucleoli, a high nucleocytoplasmic ratio, non-condensed chromatin (plasmablastic morphology) or gigantism (Figures **21.6–21.11**). In other patients the predominant neoplastic cells are plasmacytoid lymphocytes

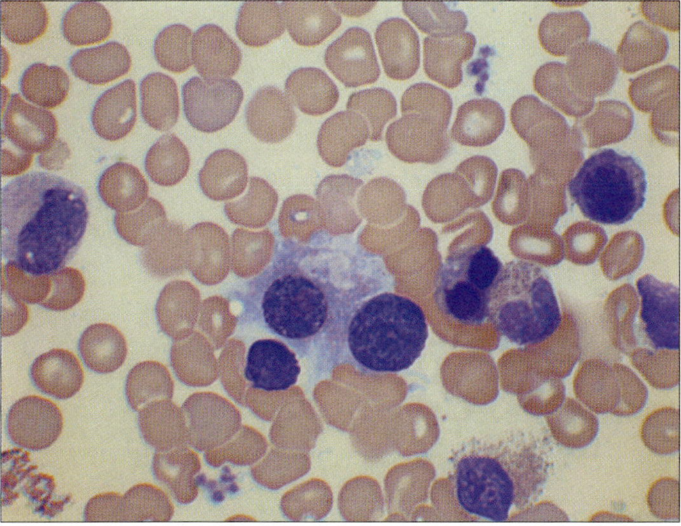

Figure 21.7 Bone marrow aspirate film in multiple myeloma showing a binucleated myeloma cell with disparate nuclei. Romanowsky, x 100 objective.

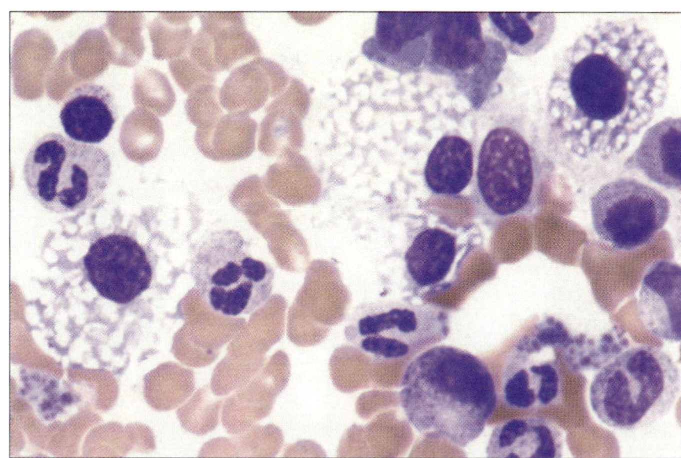

Figure 21.8 Bone marrow aspirate film in multiple myeloma showing heavily vacuolated myeloma cells. Romanowsky, x 100 objective.

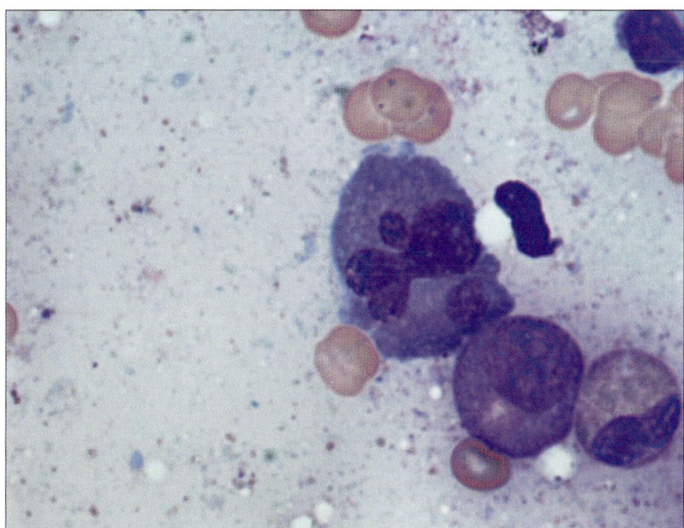

Figure 21.9 Bone marrow aspirate film in multiple myeloma showing a myeloma cell with a bizarrely shaped nucleus. Romanowsky, x 100 objective.

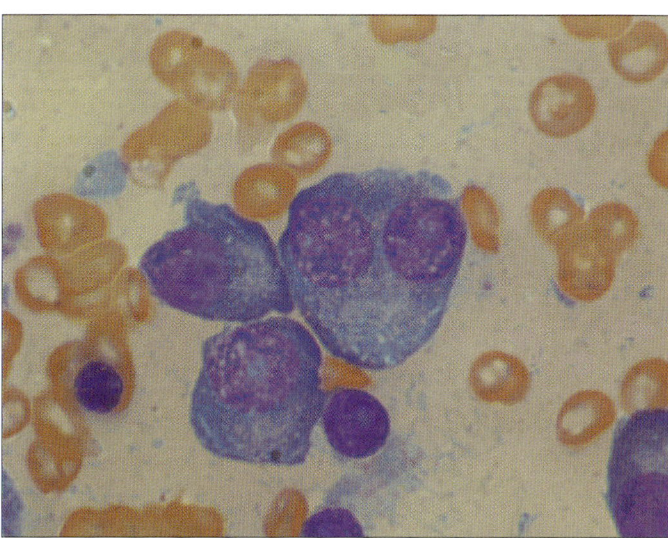

Figure 21.10 Bone marrow aspirate film in multiple myeloma showing myeloma cells, one binucleate, with prominent nucleoli. Romanowsky, x 100 objective.

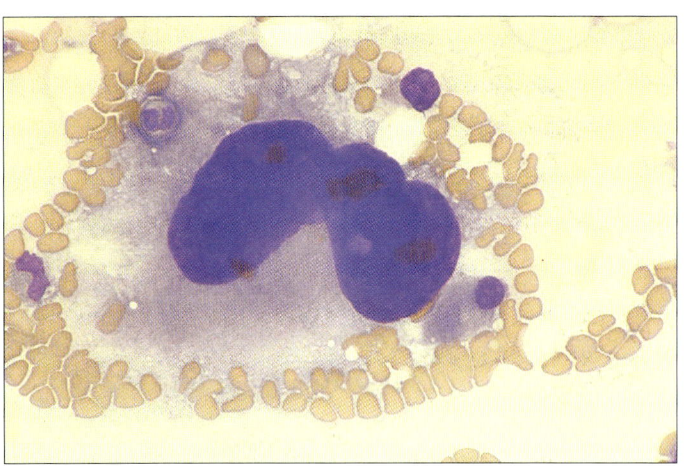

Figure 21.11 Bone marrow aspirate film in multiple myeloma showing a giant myeloma cell. Romanowsky, x 60 objective.

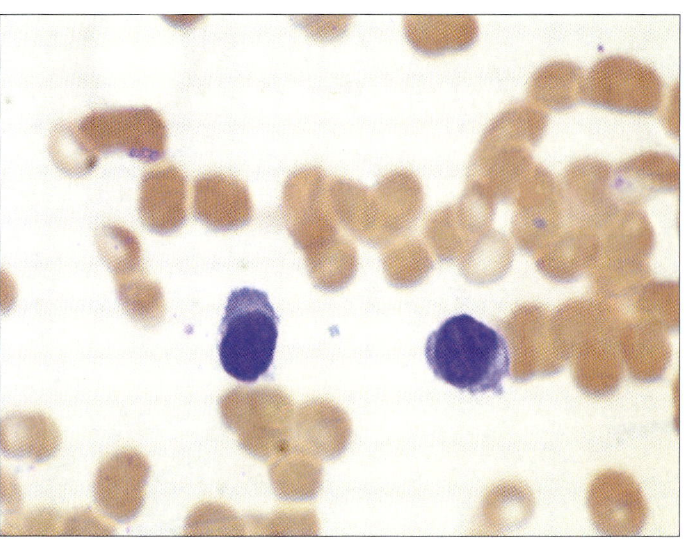

Figure 21.12 Bone marrow aspirate film in multiple myeloma showing two plasmacytoid lymphocytes. Romanowsky, x 100 objective.

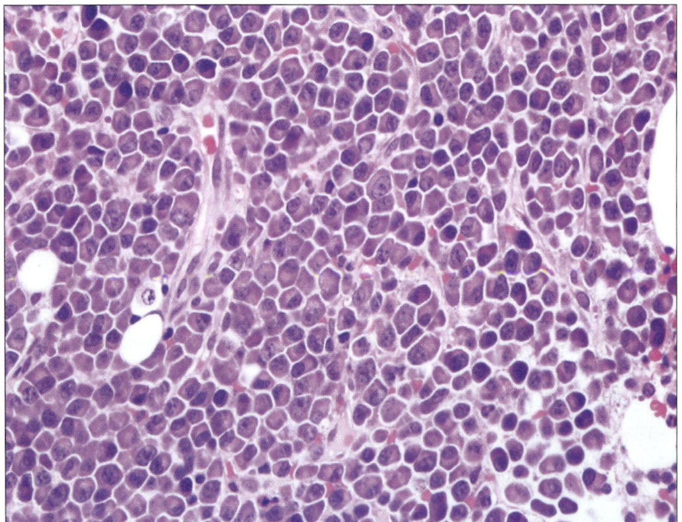

Figure 21.13 Bone marrow trephine biopsy section in multiple myeloma showing sheets of myeloma cells. H&E, x 60 objective.

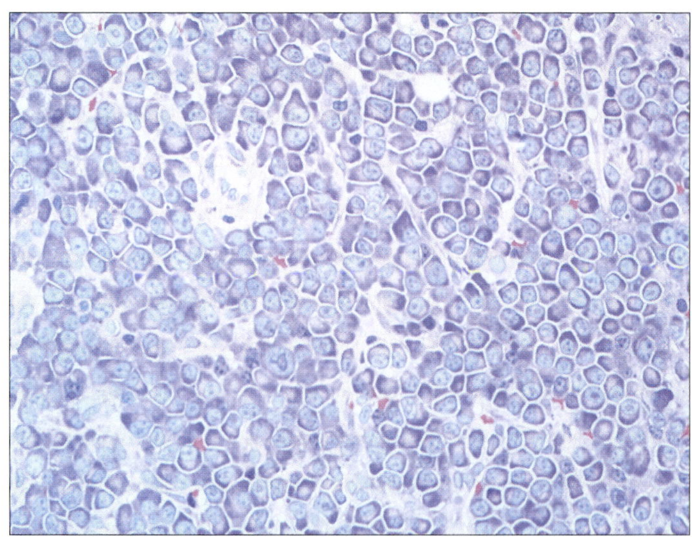

Figure 21.14 Bone marrow trephine biopsy section in multiple myeloma showing sheets of myeloma cells (same case as Figure **21.13**); the Giemsa stain emphasises the cytoplasmic basophilia. Giemsa stain, x 60 objective.

rather than plasma cells (Figure **21.12**). Since a larger amount of tissue is sampled, a trephine biopsy may give strong support to a diagnosis of myeloma when the aspirate is equivocal. Cohesive clumps or sheets of myeloma cells are often present although some patients have only an interstitial infiltrate; cytological abnormalities may be apparent (Figures **21.13**–**21.19**).

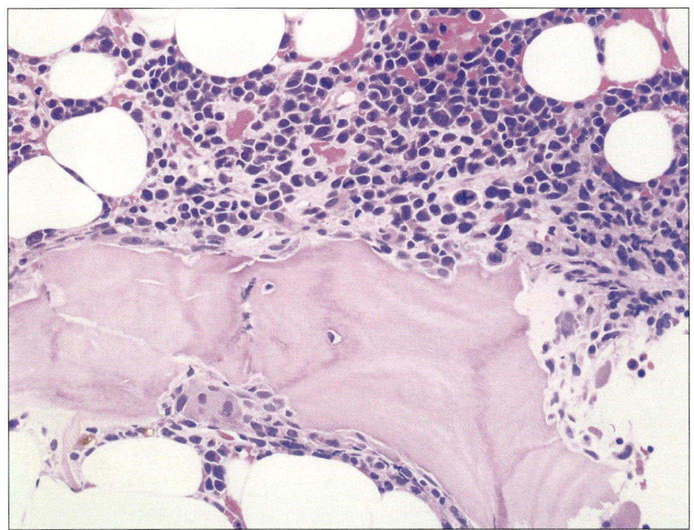

Figure 21.15 Bone marrow trephine biopsy section in multiple myeloma showing bone disease. H&E, x 40 objective.

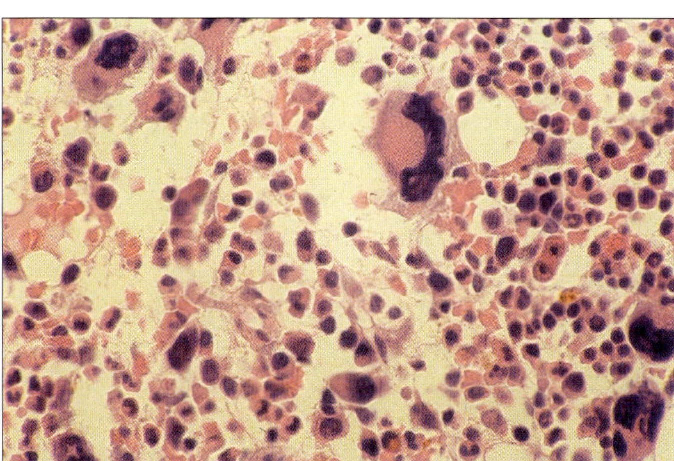

Figure 21.16 Bone marrow trephine biopsy section in multiple myeloma showing small, medium sized, large and giant plasma cells (same case as Figure **21.11**). H&E, x 60 objective.

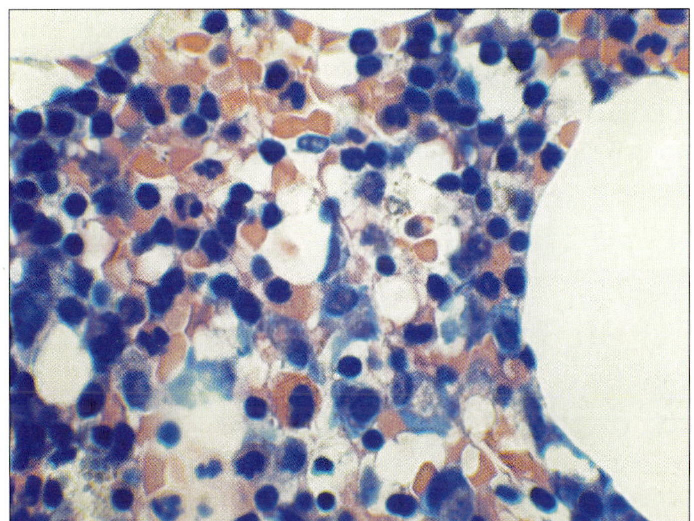

Figure 21.17 Bone marrow trephine biopsy section in multiple myeloma showing an interstitial infiltrate of plasma cells, recognizable by their prominent Golgi zones (same case as Figure **21.7**). Giemsa, x 100 objective.

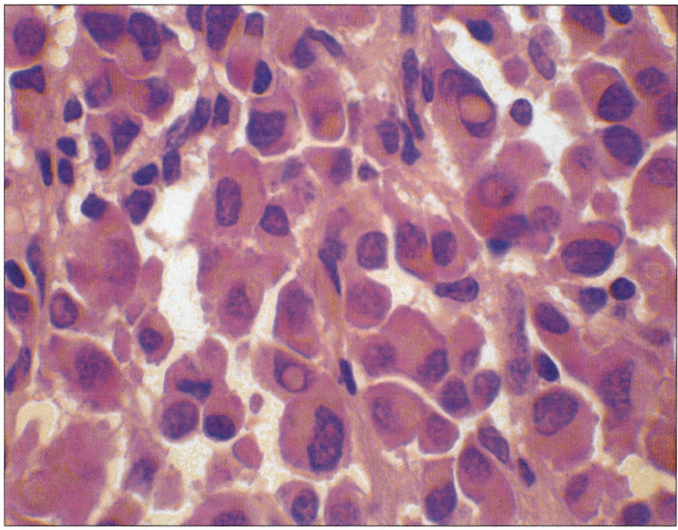

Figure 21.18 Bone marrow trephine biopsy section in multiple myeloma showing Dutcher bodies (apparent intranuclear inclusions that actually represent cytoplasmic invagination). H&E, x 100 objective.

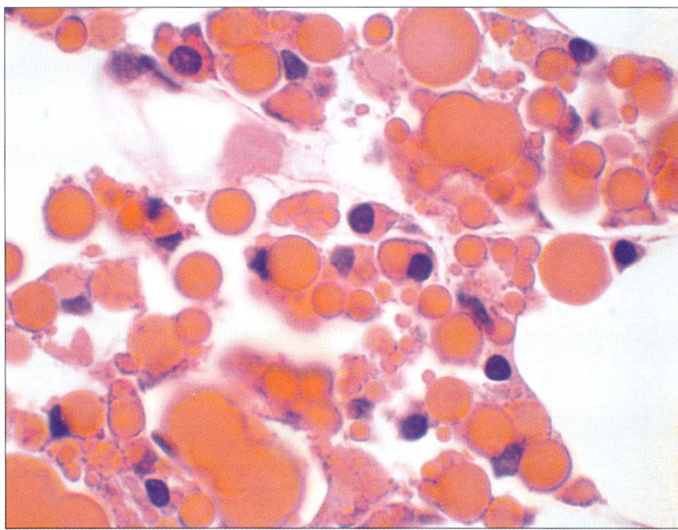

Figure 21.19 Bone marrow trephine biopsy section in multiple myeloma showing Russell bodies, spherical cytoplasmic inclusions. H&E, x 100 objective.

Immunophenotype

Myeloma cells usually express cytoplasmic immunoglobulin or immunoglobulin light chain; even some non-secretory cases have detectable immunoglobulin. The light chain in an individual patient is either kappa (κ) or lambda (λ) (Figures **21.20**–**21.25**) and any immunoglobulin, most often IgG and less often IgA, is also monotypic. Surface membrane immunoglobulin is usually negative but, in contrast to normal plasma cells, is sometimes positive. Myeloma cells usually express CD79a but many other B-lineage associated antigens (e.g. CD19) are usually negative. CD38 and CD138 (Figures **21.26** and **21.27**) are positive and CD56 is usually positive (80% of cases). There may be

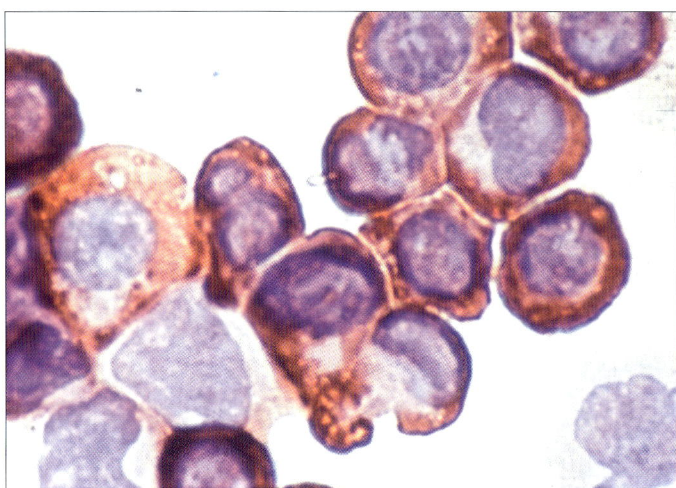

Figure 21.20 Immunocytochemistry showing κ-positive neoplastic cells in plasma cell leukaemia. APAAP technique, x 100 objective.

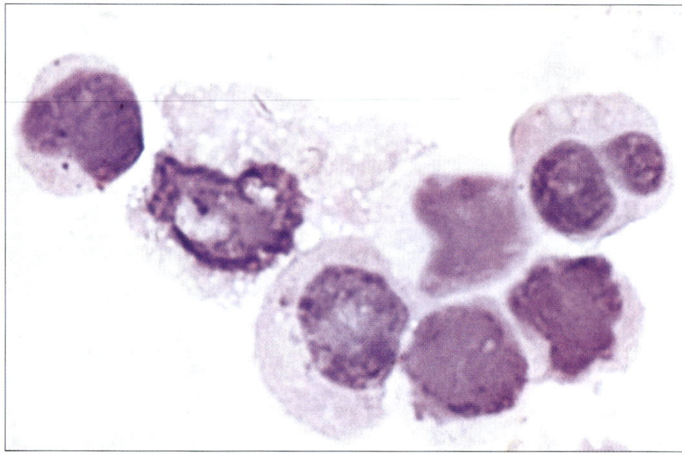

Figure 21.21 Immunocytochemistry showing λ-negative neoplastic cells in plasma cell leukaemia (same case as Figure **21.20**). APAAP technique, x 100 objective.

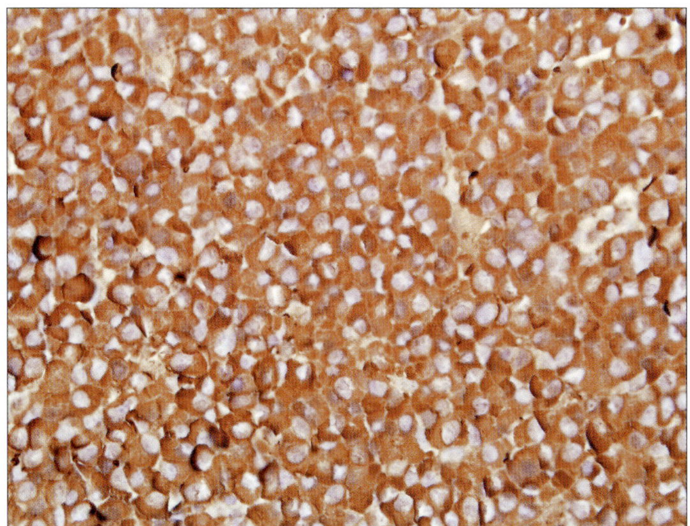

Figure 21.22 Immunohistochemistry showing κ-positive neoplastic cells in multiple myeloma (same case as Figures **21.13** and **21.14**). Immunoperoxidase, x 60 objective.

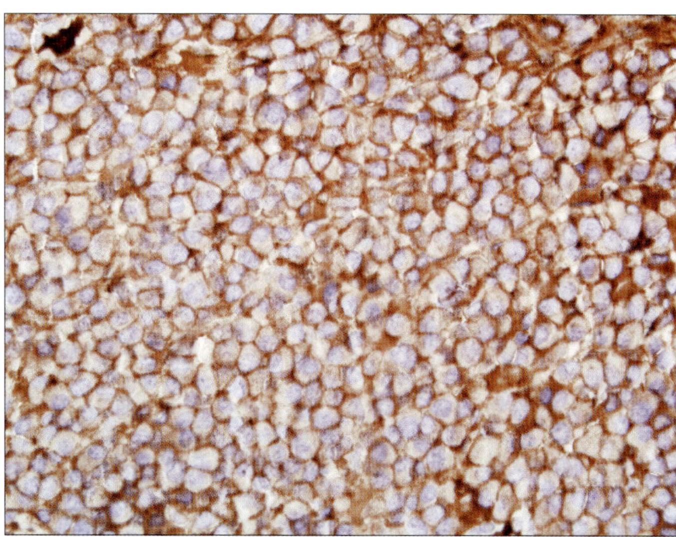

Figure 21.23 Immunohistochemistry showing λ-negative neoplastic cells (but with background staining) in multiple myeloma (same case as Figures **21.13**, **21.14** and **21.22**). Immunoperoxidase, x 60 objective.

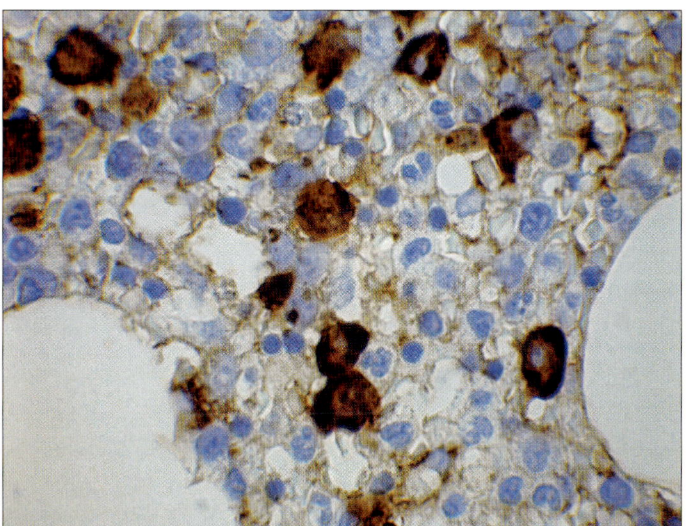

Figure 21.24 Immunohistochemistry showing κ-positive neoplastic cells in multiple myeloma (same case as Figures **21.7** and **21.17**). Immunoperoxidase, x 100 objective.

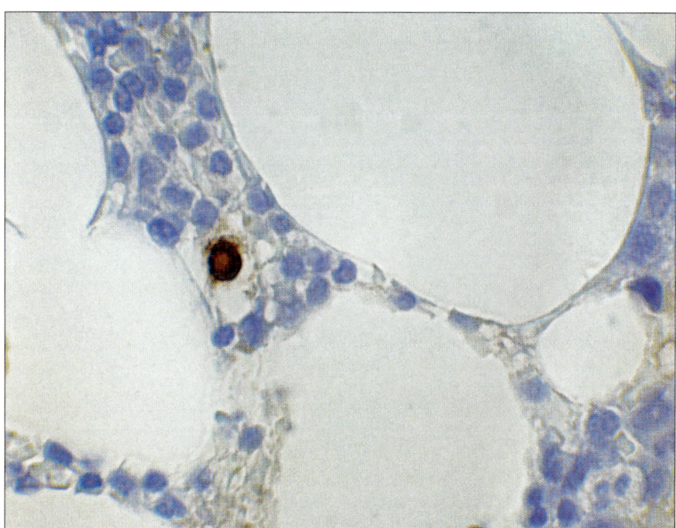

Figure 21.25 Immunohistochemistry showing λ-negative neoplastic cells in multiple myeloma; there is one residual normal plasma cell, which is λ-positive (same case as Figures **21.7**, **21.17** and **21.24**). Immunoperoxidase, x 100 objective.

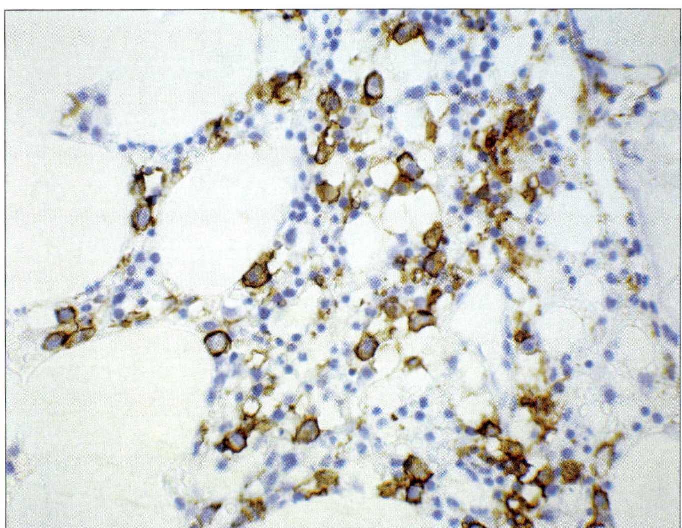

Figure 21.26 Immunohistochemistry showing CD138-positive myeloma cells (same case as Figures **21.7**, **21.17**, **21.24** and **21.25**). Immunoperoxidase, x 60 objective.

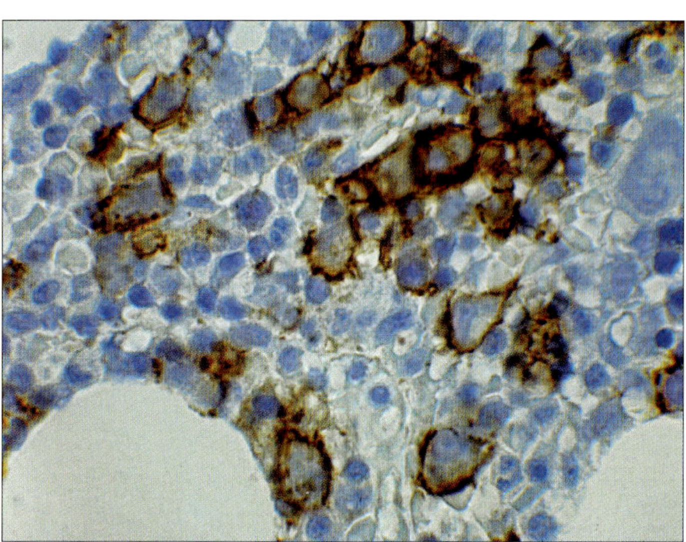

Figure 21.27 Immunohistochemistry showing CD138-positive myeloma cells (same case as Figures **21.7**, **21.17**, **21.24–21.26**). Immunoperoxidase, x 100 objective.

Table 21.1 Immunophenotype of normal plasma cells compared with that of myeloma cells

Marker	*Normal plasma cells*	*Multiple myeloma*
CD19	Positive	Negative
CD20	Negative	Positive in up to about 20% of cases
CD56	Negative	Positive
CD38	Strong	Weak
CD45	Positive	Weak or negative
CD28	Negative	Positive in one-third or more of cases
CD33	Negative	Positive in one-fifth or more of cases
CD117	Negative	Often aberrantly expressed

aberrant expression of myeloid or other antigens, including CD33, CD117, CD57 and CD10. The differences in immunophenotype between myeloma cells and normal plasma cells are summarized in *Table 21.1*.

Immunohistochemistry is valuable in highlighting the presence of plasma cells, particularly when the infiltrate is interstitial. CD38 and CD138 are positive and either κ or λ light chain is detected. Detection of κ or λ light chains may be either by immunohistochemistry or by *in situ* hybridization for detection of κ or λ mRNA. Cyclin D1 is expressed in patients with t(11;14)(q13;q32).

Cytogenetic and molecular genetic abnormalities

Cytogenetic abnormalities can be demonstrated by standard cytogenetic analysis or by fluorescence *in situ* hybridization (FISH). Since the number of myeloma cells in a bone marrow aspirate is very variable, the latter is most effective if performed on myeloma cells purified by fluorescence-activated cell sorting. Frequent cytogenetic abnormalities include hyperdiploidy, hypodiploidy, t(4;14)(p16;q32), t(11;14)(q13;q32), t(14;16)(q32;q22-23) and 13q14 deletion [5, 6].

Diagnosis and differential diagnosis

The differential diagnosis includes reactive plasmacytosis, monoclonal gammopathy of undetermined significance (MGUS) and non-Hodgkin's lymphoma with plasmacytic differentiation, e.g. lymphoplasmacytic lymphoma including Waldenström's macroglobulinaemia. Diagnostic criteria suggested by the WHO are shown in *Table 21.2* [1] and those of the International Myeloma Working Group in *Table 21.3* [3].

Table 21.2 WHO criteria for the diagnosis of multiple myeloma

*Major criteria**	*Minor criteria**
Bone marrow plasmacytosis (> 30% plasma cells)	Bone marrow plasmacytosis of 10–30%
Paraprotein present: serum IgG paraprotein more than 35 g/l or IgA paraprotein more than 20 g/l; urinary Bence–Jones protein more than 1 g/24 hours	Paraprotein present but at lower concentration
Plasmacytoma on biopsy	Lytic bone lesions
	Reduced normal immunoglobulins: IgG < 6 g/l, IgA < 1 g/l, IgM < 0.5 g/l

* One major and two minor criteria or three minor criteria, including the first two listed, must be met

Table 21.3 International Myeloma Working Group criteria for the diagnosis of monoclonal gammopathy of undetermined significance, asymptomatic (smouldering) myeloma and symptomatic multiple myeloma

MGUS	*Asymptomatic (smouldering) myeloma*	*Symptomatic multiple myeloma*
Serum paraprotein less than 30 g/l	Serum paraprotein at least 30 g/l AND/OR	Paraprotein in serum or urine
Bone marrow clonal plasma cells less than 10% and low level infiltration in trephine biopsy specimen	Bone marrow clonal plasma cells at least 10%	Bone marrow clonal plasma cells or plasmacytoma
No evidence of other B-lineage lymphoproliferative disorder		
No related organ or tissue impairment such as bone lesions, light-chain-associated amyloidosis, paraprotein-associated neurological damage, hypercalcaemia, renal impairment, anaemia, symptomatic hyperviscosity, more than two bacterial infections in 12 months	No related organ damage or tissue impairment	Related organ damage or tissue impairment

MGUS, monoclonal gammopathy of undetermined significance

Prognosis

Features indicative of a worse prognosis include anaemia, renal failure, elevated β2-microglobulin, elevated lactate dehydrogenase, elevated C-reactive protein, high plasma cell labelling index, low serum albumin and the presence of hypodiploidy, t(4;14), t(14;16), 13q14 deletion on conventional cytogenetics and 17p13 on FISH analysis [7]. Microarray analysis also gives prognostic information [7].

Treatment

Not all patients require treatment but most patients are symptomatic and treatment is therefore needed [2, 4, 8]. The presence of anaemia, hypercalcaemia, lytic lesions or extramedullary plasmacytoma provides a clear indication for treatment. Asymptomatic patients with 'smouldering myeloma' (criteria for diagnosis of this condition are shown in *Table 21.3*) do not need treatment.

Supportive treatment, including management of hypercalcaemia and renal failure, is important. More active management includes radiotherapy, for focal painful lesions and chemotherapy. Useful chemotherapeutic agents include melphalan, corticosteroids, anthracyclines and nitrosoureas. High-dose chemotherapy with autologous stem cell rescue also has a role in younger fitter patients. The use of drug combinations such as VAD (vincristine, doxorubicin and dexamethasone) and ABCM (doxorubicin, BCNU, cyclophosphamide and melphalan) has declined with the development of newer effective agents such as thalidomide, lenalidomide and the proteasome inhibitor, bortezomib. Bisphosphonates such as clodronate and zoledronate have a role in patients with bone pain and hypercalcaemia and may even have an anti-tumour effect.

References

1. Grogan TM, van Camp B, Kyle RA, Müller-Hermelink HK and Harris NL (2001). Plasma cell neoplasms. *In* Jaffe ES, Harris NL, Stein H and Vardiman JW (Eds). *World Health Organization Classification of Tumours: Pathology and Genetics of Tumours of Haematopoietic and Lymphoid Tissues*, IARC Press, Lyon, pp. 142–156.
2. UK Myeloma Forum Guidelines Working Group (2001). Guidelines on the diagnosis and management of multiple myeloma. *Br J Haematol*, **115**, 522–540.
3. The International Myeloma Working Group (2003). Criteria for the classification of monoclonal gammopathies, multiple myeloma and related disorders: a report of the International Myeloma Working Group. *Br J Haematol*, **121**, 749–757.
4. Kyle RA and Rajkumar SV (2004). Multiple myeloma. *New Engl J Med*, **351**, 1860–1873.
5. Kuehl WM and Bergsagel PL (2002). Multiple myeloma: evolving genetic events and host interactions. *Nat Rev Cancer*, **2**, 175–187.
6. Boersma-Vreugdenhil GR, Peeters T and Bast BJEG (2003). Translocation of the IgH locus is nearly ubiquitous in multiple myeloma as detected by immuno-FISH. *Blood*, **101**, 1653.
7. Stewart AK and Fonseca R (2005). Prognostic and therapeutic significance of myeloma genetics and gene expression profiling. *J Clin Oncol*, **23**, 6339–6344.
8. Singhal S, Mehta J, Desikan R, Ayers D, Roberson P, Eddlemon P *et al.* (1999). Antitumor activity of thalidomide in refractory multiple myeloma. *New Engl J Med*, **341**, 1565–1571.

Chapter 22

Monoclonal gammopathy of undetermined significance (MGUS)

Monoclonal gammopathy of undetermined significance (MGUS) is a common condition, occurring in 3% of individuals over the age of 70 years. It is characterized by the presence of a paraprotein secreted by a neoplastic but clinically benign clone of plasma cells. Over a period of years or even decades, multiple myeloma, light-chain-associated amyloidosis, chronic lymphocytic leukaemia or non-Hodgkin's lymphoma develops in a proportion of individuals with MGUS [1, 2]. In others there is no apparent progression.

Clinical features

There are no clinical features, the diagnosis being an incidental one when serum protein electrophoresis is performed in an individual who does not have signs or symptoms attributable to a lymphoid neoplasm.

Haematological and pathological features

The blood count is normal. The blood film may show some increase in rouleaux formation as a result of the presence of the paraprotein. A bone marrow aspirate shows an increase in plasma cells to between 1 and 10%. These may be cytologically normal or may show minor atypical features such as the presence of a nucleolus or less chromatin condensation than in normal plasma cells. On trephine biopsy sections, there is either an interstitial infiltrate of plasma cells or there are small foci. The paraprotein, detectable by serum protein electrophoresis and immune fixation, may be immunoglobulin (Ig) G, IgA or IgM (Figures **22.1** and **22.2**). Its concentration does not exceed 20–30 g/l. The concentration of normal Igs is not reduced. If a Bence–Jones protein is present in the urine it is at a low concentration.

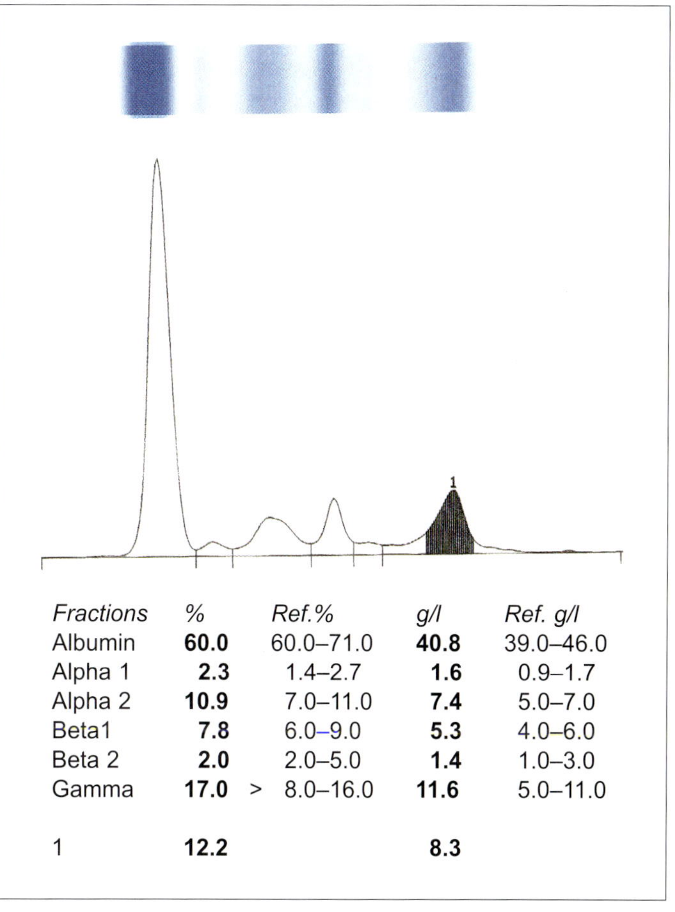

Fractions	*%*		*Ref.%*	*g/l*	*Ref. g/l*
Albumin	**60.0**		60.0–71.0	**40.8**	39.0–46.0
Alpha 1	**2.3**		1.4–2.7	**1.6**	0.9–1.7
Alpha 2	**10.9**		7.0–11.0	**7.4**	5.0–7.0
Beta1	**7.8**		6.0–9.0	**5.3**	4.0–6.0
Beta 2	**2.0**		2.0–5.0	**1.4**	1.0–3.0
Gamma	**17.0**	>	8.0–16.0	**11.6**	5.0–11.0
1	**12.2**			**8.3**	

Figure 22.1 Serum protein electrophoresis in a patient with MGUS showing a paraprotein in the gamma region in a concentration of 8.3 g/l. With thanks to Miss Carol Hughes.

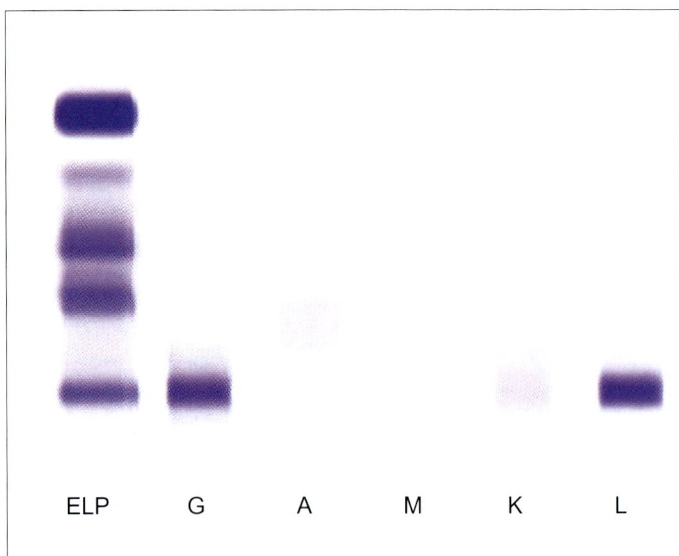

Figure 22.2 Serum protein electrophoresis in a patient with MGUS (left) showing a paraprotein in the gamma region; on immune fixation (right) this is identified as an IgG λ paraprotein. With thanks to Miss Carol Hughes.

Immunophenotype

The clonal plasma cells show light chain restriction of cytoplasmic Ig, i.e. they express either kappa (κ) or lambda (λ) light chains but not both. They express CD79a but do not usually express other pan-B markers. They express CD38 and CD138. They resemble myeloma cells in being CD19 negative but are usually CD56 negative, whereas normal plasma cells are CD19 positive and CD56 negative. In MGUS, polyclonal plasma cells usually co-exist with immunophenotypically aberrant clonal cells, in contrast to multiple myeloma, where only a minority of patients have polyclonal plasma cells detectable by flow cytometry and then only as a low percentage.

Cytogenetic and molecular genetic abnormalities

Fluorescence *in situ* hybridization (FISH) analysis shows, in some patients, the same cytogenetic abnormalities that are observed in multiple myeloma, e.g. t(4;14)(p16;q32), t(11;14)(q13;q32), 13q– or aneuploidy (+3, +7, +9, +11) [3].

Diagnosis and differential diagnosis

The differential diagnosis includes reactive plasmacytosis and multiple myeloma. A diagnosis of reactive plasmacytosis is excluded by the presence of a paraprotein. The distinction from multiple myeloma requires assessment of clinical, radiological and pathological features.

Prognosis

Data from a series of over 1,300 individuals showed that the rate of progression to multiple myeloma or other related condition was about 12% by 10 years, 25% by 20 years and 35% at 25 years [2].

Treatment

Treatment is not indicated.

References

1. Kyle A (1993). 'Benign' monoclonal gammopathy after 20 to 35 years follow-up. *Mayo Clin Proc*, **68**, 26–36.
2. Kyle RA, Therneau TM, Rajkumar SV, Offord JR, Larson DR, Plevak MF and Melton LJ (2002). A long-term study of prognosis in monoclonal gammopathy of undetermined significance. *N Engl J Med*, **346**, 564–569.
3. Fonseca R, Bailey RJ, Ahmann GJ, Rajkumar SV, Hoyer JD, Lust JA *et al.* (2002). Genomic abnormalities in monoclonal gammopathy of undetermined significance. *Blood*, **100**, 1417–1424.

Chapter 23

Other plasma cell neoplasms

There are a number of plasma cell and lymphoplasmacytic neoplasms characterized by specific damaging effects of a paraprotein rather than by the more usual features of a lymphoid neoplasm [1]. Sometimes the haematological and pathological features would lead to a diagnosis of monoclonal gammopathy of undetermined significance (MGUS) if it were not for the effects of the paraprotein. In other patients there is an overt neoplasm at the onset but, in addition, the damaging effects of a paraprotein are apparent. An overt neoplastic condition may emerge some years later in patients in whom none was apparent at onset. The words 'primary' or 'essential' are sometimes used when there is no overt associated neoplasm, e.g. 'primary amyloidosis' or 'essential cryoglobulinaemia'.

Clinical features

The main clinical features are those resulting from the specific effects of the paraprotein in an individual condition [1–7]. These are summarized in *Table 23.1*. Alpha heavy chain disease is a form of MALT lymphoma (see Chapter 9).

Haematological and pathological features

Haematological and pathological features also differ, according to the characteristics of the paraprotein, e.g. red cell agglutinates, polychromasia and a few spherocytes in chronic cold haemagglutinin disease (CHAD), deposition of a cryoglobulin in the case of cryoglobulinaemia or features of hyposplenism when there is amyloid deposition in the spleen. Some patients, e.g. some with CHAD, have lymphocytosis. In the POEMS (**P**olyneuropathy, **O**rganomegaly (hepatomegaly, splenomegaly, lymphadenopathy), **E**ndocrinopathy, **M**-protein and **S**kin changes) syndrome there can be erythrocytosis or thrombocytosis. In some circumstances there is a normocytic normochromic anaemia as a result of renal failure.

A bone marrow aspirate or trephine biopsy usually shows a variable increase of either plasma cells or plasmacytoid lymphocytes, but sometimes no increase is apparent. In patients with amyloidosis, bone marrow trephine biopsy (Figures **23.1**–**23.3**) or, rarely, a bone marrow aspirate (Figure **23.4**), shows amyloid; its nature can be confirmed by a Congo red stain and antisera to light chains also sometimes give positive reactions. Light chain deposition can also be apparent in the walls of bone marrow blood vessels, morphologically resembling amyloid but being Congo red-negative. Its nature can be confirmed by anti-kappa or anti-lambda antisera.

In the POEMS syndrome, lymph nodes may show the features of the plasma cell variant of Castleman's disease.

A serum paraprotein (immunoglobulin [Ig] G, IgA or IgM) or a urinary paraprotein (kappa [κ] or lambda [λ] Bence–Jones protein) may be present. Some paraproteins have the features of a cold agglutinin or a cryoglobulin. Measuring the ratio of free κ to free λ light chains in the serum can be useful in diagnosis in those in whom no serum or urinary paraprotein is detected.

Immunophenotype

Neoplastic cells have the immunophenotypic features of a clonal plasma cell or lymphoplasmacytoid lymphocyte.

Table 23.1 Syndromes resulting from synthesis of a monoclonal paraprotein

Condition	*Type of paraprotein*	*Pathological effects*	*Clinical effects*
Light-chain associated-amyloidosis	Complete immunoglobulin or Bence–Jones protein; 70–80% of paraproteins have λ light chains	Amyloid deposition in many tissues	Heart failure, hepatomegaly, tongue enlargement, malabsorption, peripheral neuropathy, renal failure or nephrotic syndrome
Light-chain- or light- and heavy-chain-deposition disease	About 80% of paraproteins have κ light chains	Light-chain deposition in kidneys	Renal failure or nephrotic syndrome, much less often hepatic, cardiac or adrenal involvement
Cryoglobulinaemia (type I or type II)	Paraprotein that is either a cryoglobulin or forms an immune complex that is a cryoglobulin (in the case of an IgM paraprotein with antibody activity to IgG)	Precipitation of cryoglobulin in blood in cold conditions	Vasculitis, purpura, impaired peripheral circulation
Cold haemagglutinin disease	IgM paraprotein with anti-I activity	Agglutination of red cells by a cold agglutinin in cold conditions	Cold-induced haemolytic anaemia (intravascular haemolysis and haemoglobinuria)
POEMS syndrome	Usually IgGλ or IgAλ		Peripheral neuropathy, hepatomegaly, splenomegaly, lymphadenopathy, endocrine organ failure and skin thickening
Acquired angio-oedema	A cryoglobulin, cold agglutinin or immune complex of an anti-idiotype antibody and the paraprotein to which it is directed	Consumption of C1 esterase inhibitor	Angio-oedema

POEMS, polyneuropathy, organomegaly, endocrinopathy, M-protein, skin changes syndrome; λ, lambda; κ, kappa

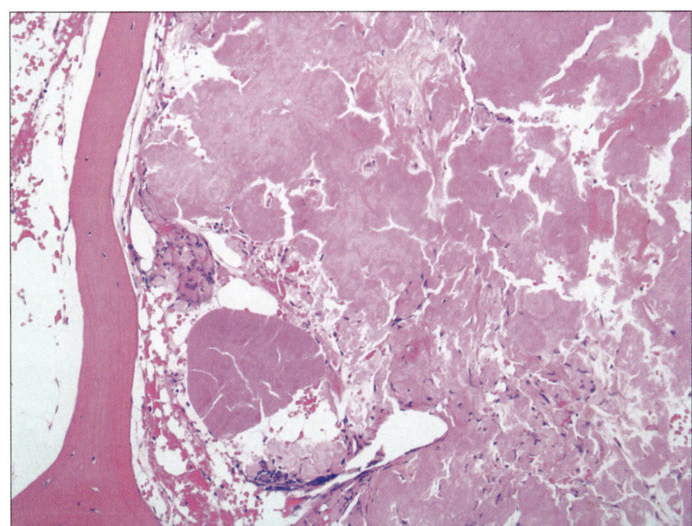

Figure 23.1 Trephine biopsy section showing amyloid deposition. H&E, x 20 objective.

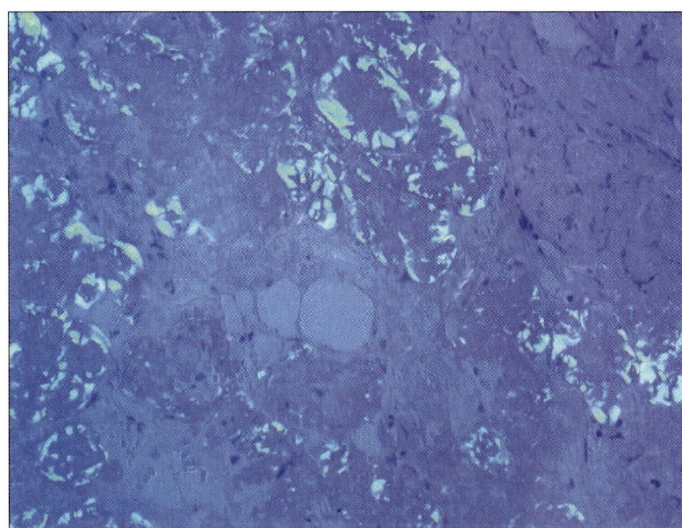

Figure 23.2 Trephine biopsy section showing apple green birefringence of amyloid deposits when the section is examined by polarized light after Congo red staining (same case as Figure **23.1**). Congo red, x 40 objective.

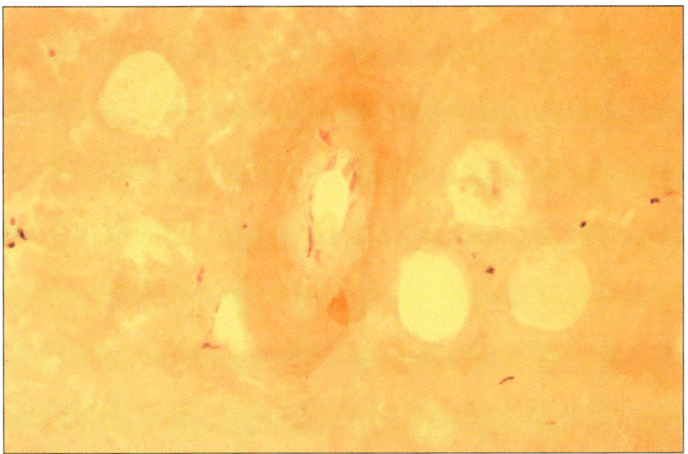

Figure 23.3 Trephine biopsy section showing vascular amyloid deposition. Congo red, x 60 objective.

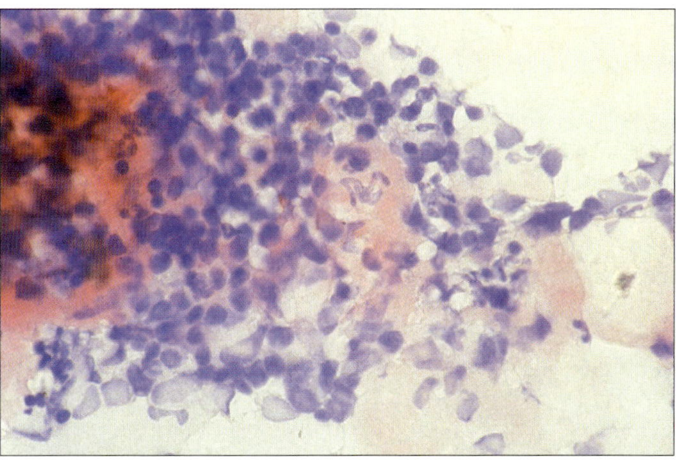

Figure 23.4 Bone marrow aspirate showing amyloid deposition. Romanowsky, x 60 objective.

Cytogenetic and molecular genetic abnormalities

No specific features have been identified.

Diagnosis and differential diagnosis

The differential diagnosis is very broad since tissue effects are very variable.

Prognosis

Prognosis is very variable, in part dependent on the damage caused by the paraprotein and in part on whether or not an overt neoplastic condition is present or later appears. Light-chain-associated amyloidosis usually has a poor prognosis because of the presence of cardiac or renal failure, whereas CHAD and cryoglobulinaemia are compatible with a long survival.

Treatment

Treatment is directed at the neoplastic clone. In addition steps may be taken to ameliorate the symptoms, e.g. by avoiding cold or by administering an androgenic steroid to increase the plasma level of C1 inhibitor.

References

1. Bain BJ, Clark DM, Lampert IA and Wilkins BS (2001). *Bone Marrow Pathology*, Blackwell Publishing, Oxford, pp. 349–357.
2. Kyle RA and Gertz MA (1995). Primary systemic amyloidosis: clinical and laboratory features in 474 cases. *Semin Haematol*, **32**, 45–59.
3. Feiner HD (1988). Pathology of dysproteinemia: light chain amyloidosis, non-amyloid immunoglobulin deposition disease, cryoglobulinemia syndromes and macroglobulinemia of Waldenström. *Hum Pathol*, **11**, 1255–1272.
4. Ferri C, Zignego AL and Pileri SA (2002). Cryoglobulins. *J Clin Pathol*, **55**, 4–13.
5. Bardwick PA, Zvaifler NJ, Gill GN, Newman D, Greenway GD and Resnick DC (1980). Plasma cell dyscrasia with polyneuropathy, organomegaly, endocrinopathy, M-protein, and skin changes: the POEMS syndrome. *Medicine*, **59**, 311–322.
6. Bain BJ, Catovsky D and Ewan PW (1993). Acquired angioedema as the presenting feature of lymphoproliferative disorders of mature B-lymphocytes. *Cancer*, **72**, 3318–3322.
7. Guidelines Working Group of the UK Myeloma Forum on behalf of the British Committee for Standards in Haematology (2004). Guidelines on the diagnosis and management of AL amyloidosis. *Br J Haematol*, **125**, 681–700.

Chapter 24

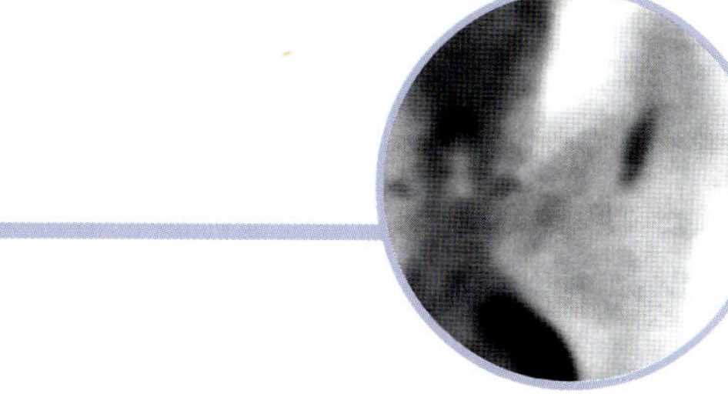

Hodgkin's disease

Hodgkin's disease, in the World Health Organization (WHO) classification known as Hodgkin lymphoma, is a histologically defined disorder. The term encompasses two distinct types of disease, which differ in aetiology, epidemiology, clinical features, pathology and prognosis [1, 2]. They are designated classical Hodgkin's disease (classical HD) and nodular lymphocyte-predominant Hodgkin's disease (NLPHD). It is now known that both types of Hodgkin's disease are B-cell neoplasms but, because of the fairly distinctive features of this condition, subdivision of lymphoma into Hodgkin's disease and non-Hodgkin's lymphoma (NHL) has been maintained. The cell of origin in both cases is a germinal centre B cell. The differences between these two types of Hodgkin's disease are summarized in *Table 24.1*. Histologically Hodgkin's disease is defined by the presence of characteristic neoplastic cells (Reed–Sternberg cells and Hodgkin's cells or their variants) in a setting of inflammatory cells with or without fibrosis. Classical HD is further subdivided into lymphocyte-rich, mixed cellularity, nodular sclerosis (or nodular sclerosing)

Table 24.1 A comparison of features of classical and nodular lymphocyte-predominant Hodgkin's disease (HD)

	Classical HD	*Nodular lymphocyte-predominant HD*
Frequency	95% of cases	5% of cases
Aetiology	Some cases associated with EBV infection	No association with EBV infection
Epidemiology	Double peak of increased incidence in young adults and in old age	Unimodal peak of incidence in young adults
Histology	Reed–Sternberg cells and mononuclear Hodgkin cells	L&H cells (popcorn cells); nodular background
Immunophenotype of neoplastic cells	CD30 positive; CD15 positive in most cases; CD20 expression weak or absent; CD45, CD79a, BCL6, immunoglobulin and epithelial membrane antigen not expressed; J chain negative; PAX5 positive; BOB1 negative; OCT2 variable but more often negative; MUM1 positive; EBV detectable in neoplastic cells in some cases	CD30 and CD15 negative; CD20, CD45, CD79a and BCL6 positive; immunoglobulin usually expressed; epithelial membrane antigen is positive in about half of cases; J chain positive; PAX5 positive; BOB1 positive; OCT2 positive; MUM1 negative; EBV is not detected in neoplastic cells; L&H cells are ringed by CD3-positive and CD57-positive T cells
Nature of relapse	Late relapses very rare; relapse is as classical HD	Late relapses are more common; relapse may be as nodular lymphocyte-predominant HD or as diffuse large B-cell lymphoma

EBV, Epstein–Barr virus; L&H, lymphocytic and histiocytic Reed–Sternberg variants and lymphocyte-depleted subtypes on the basis of the ratio between neoplastic cells and reactive cells, the specific cytological features of the neoplastic cells and the presence or absence of fibrous bands.

Hodgkin's disease commences in a single lymphocyte in a lymph node or other organ and, in the usual case in which disease starts in a lymph node, spreads initially by lymphatics to contiguous lymph nodes. There may also be local invasion and, late in the course of the disease, spreading through the blood stream to distant organs.

Hodgkin's disease is increased in incidence in some families and in individuals who have been exposed to the Epstein–Barr virus (EBV). Incidence is also increased in human immunodeficiency virus (HIV)-positive patients, but not to the same extent as NHL. HIV-related cases are much more likely to be associated with EBV. The epidemiology differs between developed and developing countries, occurring at a younger age in the latter.

Clinical features

Hodgkin's disease most often presents with lymphadenopathy, either localized or generalized. Cervical nodes are those most often involved. Patients with more extensive disease can have systemic symptoms such as fever, night sweats and weight loss (all defined as B symptoms), itch and alcohol-induced cough or pain. Anatomical extent of disease and presence or absence of B symptoms are combined to determine the stage of the disease [3]. Plain radiography (Figure **24.1**), computed tomography (CT) scanning and positron emission tomography (PET) scanning (Figure **24.2**) may reveal disease that is not apparent on clinical examination.

Haematological and pathological features

In patients with localized disease there may be minor or no haematological abnormalities. As disease becomes more extensive there is anaemia, which is initially normocytic and normochromic and later hypochromic and microcytic. The erythrocyte sedimentation rate and rouleaux formation are increased. Sometimes there is neutrophilia, eosinophilia or, occasionally, lymphocytosis. Patients with extensive disease may have abnormal liver function tests, reduced albumin, increased immunoglobulins and increased lactate dehydrogenase.

Lymph node histology in classical Hodgkin's disease shows the presence of Reed–Sternberg cells (Figure **24.3**).

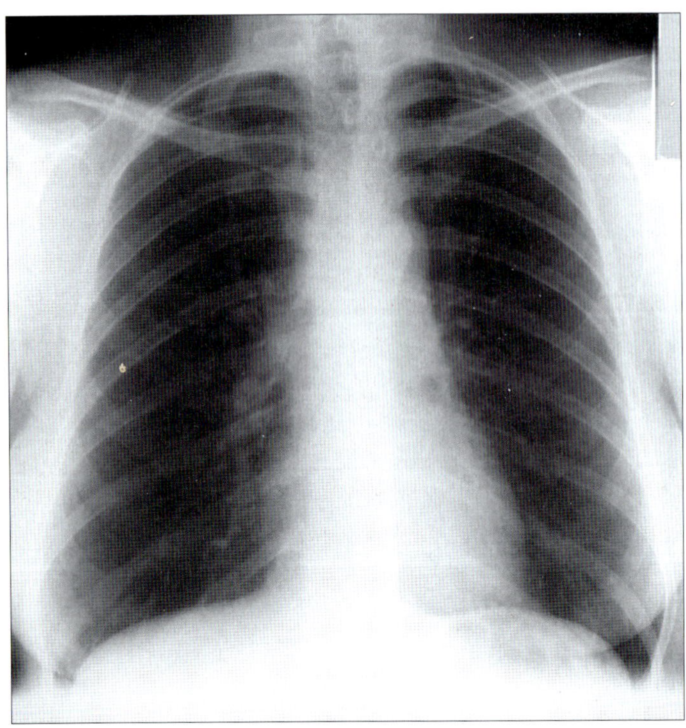

Figure 24.1 Chest radiograph showing mediastinal HD.

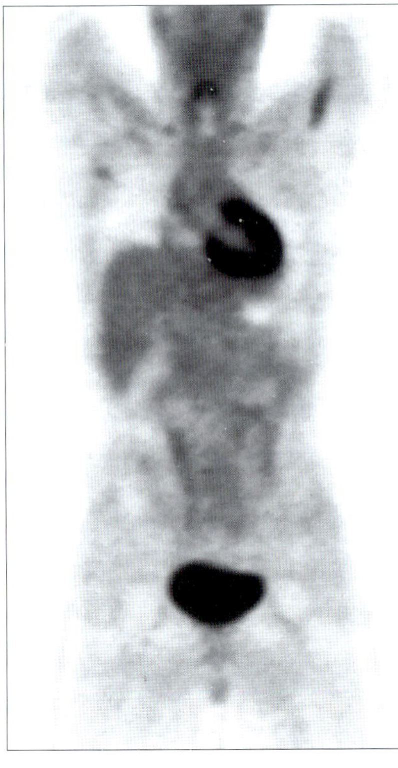

Figure 24.2 ^{18}F-fluorodeoxyglucose PET scan showing left axillary lymphadenopathy. The uptake in the heart and bladder is normal.

These are binucleated or polylobated giant cells with vesicular nuclei and large eosinophilic nucleoli; in the case of binucleated cells there is one nucleolus per nucleus and in polylobated nuclei there are nucleoli in different lobes. In addition to Reed–Sternberg cells, there are mononuclear Hodgkin's cells, which are large cells with a large single nucleus containing a single large eosinophilic nucleolus. In nodular sclerosis HD the neoplastic cells, designated lacunar cells, tend to have more lobated nuclei and less prominent nucleoli and are contained in an artefactual lacuna (Figure **24.4**). The nodules, which are surrounded by dense collagen bands, have B lymphocytes enclosed within a network of CD21-positive follicular dendritic cells. The capsule is thickened. Lymphocyte-rich classical HD can have either a nodular or a diffuse growth pattern whereas in lymphocyte-depleted classical HD the growth pattern is diffuse. In lymphocyte-rich classical HD the neoplastic cells may be infrequent and confined to the mantle zones of reactive follicles. The neoplastic cells of classical HD correspond to transformed post-germinal centre B cells, although phenotypically they lack many B-cell characteristics. Neoplastic cells of all histological subtypes of classical HD share the same immunophenotype, shown in *Table 24.1* [4–7].

In NLPHD, the neoplastic cell differs cytologically and immunophenotypically from the neoplastic cells of classical HD: these cells, designated L&H cells (lymphocytic and histiocytic Reed–Sternberg variants) are large cells with a single large nucleus with small basophilic nucleoli (Figure **24.5**); cytoplasm is scanty; the nuclei are vesicular and highly folded or lobated giving an appearance that leads to an alternative designation as 'popcorn cells'. The lymph node architecture is nodular (Figure **24.6**) or mixed nodular and diffuse with the background cells being lymphocytes, macrophages, epithelioid cells and small lymphocytes (but not neutrophils and eosinophils) in a network of CD21-positive follicular dendritic cells. In both classical and NLPHD the neoplastic cells are B cells, but in the case of classical HD the phenotype is very abnormal so that for many years their B-cell lineage was unrecognized. Neoplastic cells are surrounded by a mixed inflammatory infiltrate of reactive T and B lymphocytes, neutrophils, eosinophils, plasma cells and fibroblasts. The number of neoplastic cells, in relation to the number of inflammatory cells, increases from lymphocyte predominant to mixed cellularity (Figure **24.7**) to lymphocyte depleted. Nodular sclerosis HD is characterized by broad bands of fibrous tissue that divide the node into nodules; the ratio of neoplastic cells to reactive cells is variable.

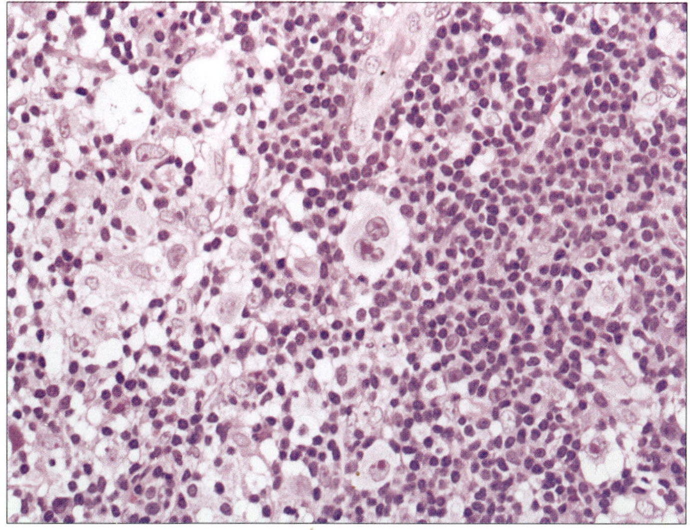

Figure 24.3 A section of a lymph node biopsy showing a binucleated Reed–Sternberg cell with giant eosinophilic nucleoli (centre); there are also mononuclear Hodgkin's cells set in a mixed inflammatory background. H&E, x 60 objective.

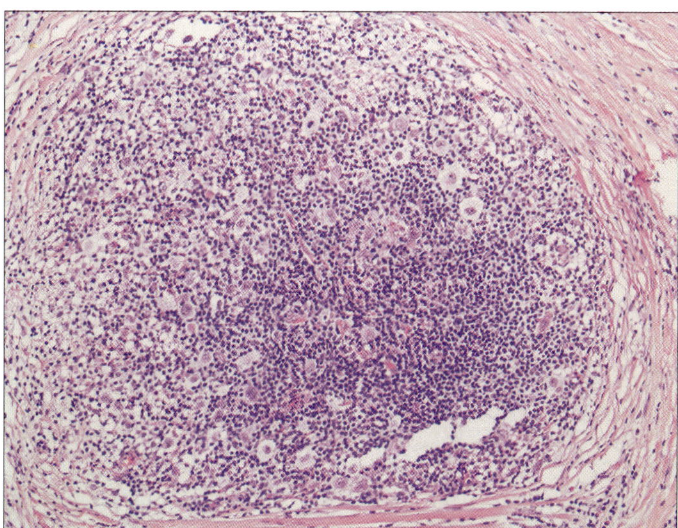

Figure 24.4 A section of a lymph node biopsy in nodular sclerosis HD showing a nodule surrounded by fibrous tissue; lacunar cells are apparent within the nodule and are surrounded by inflammatory cells. H&E, x 20 objective.

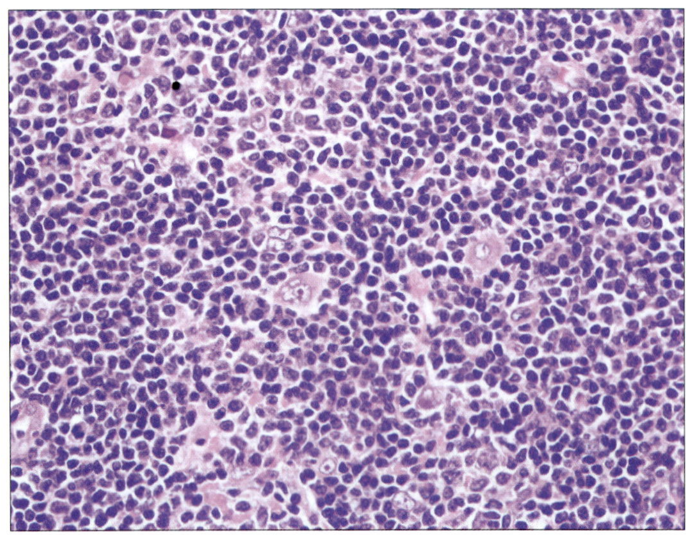

Figure 24.5 A section of a lymph node biopsy in nodular lymphocyte-predominant HD showing L&H cells. H&E, x 60 objective.

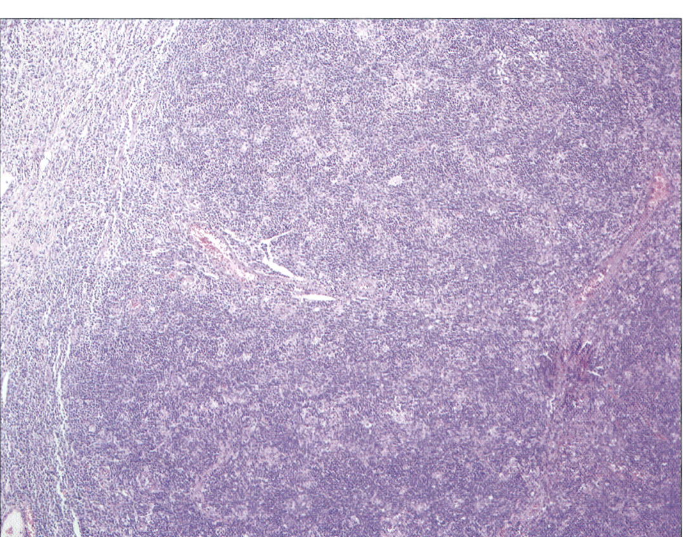

Figure 24.6 A section of a lymph node biopsy in nodular lymphocyte-predominant classical HD showing a nodular pattern. H&E, x 10 objective.

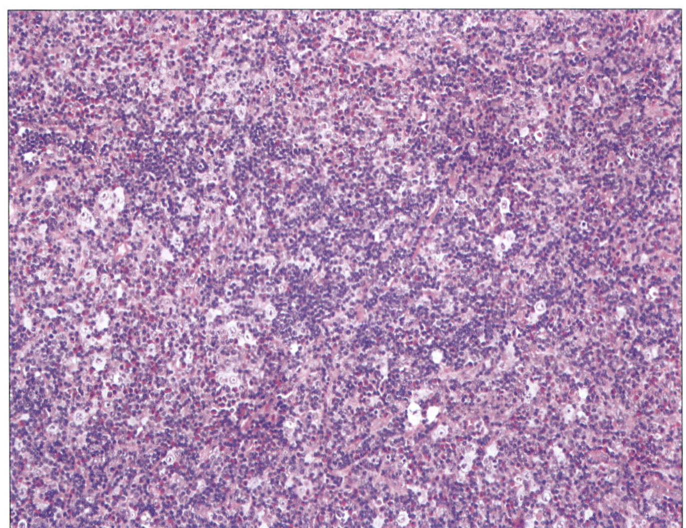

Figure 24.7 A section of a lymph node biopsy in mixed cellularity classical HD showing the expected ratio between neoplastic and reactive cells. H&E, x 20 objective.

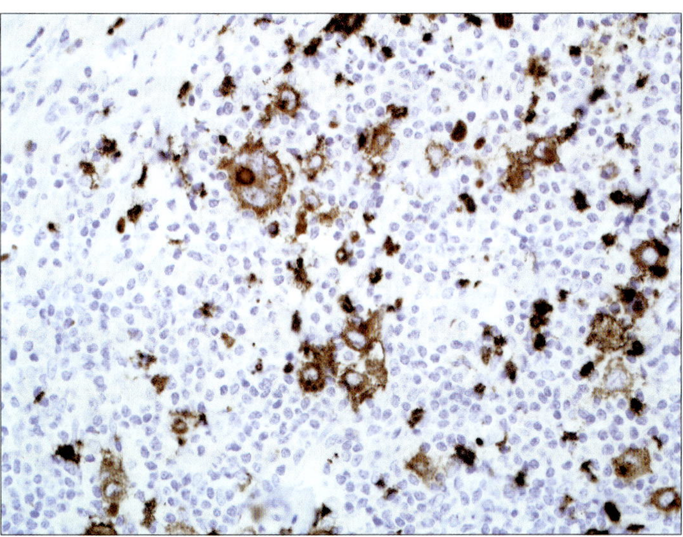

Figure 24.8 A section of a lymph node biopsy in classical HD showing CD15 expression by neoplastic cells. Immunoperoxidase, x 40 objective.

Immunophenotype

The immunophenotype, as determined by immunohistochemistry, is shown in *Table 24.1* and illustrated in Figures **24.8–24.13**.

Cytogenetic and molecular genetic abnormalities

The neoplastic cells in both types of HD are monoclonal [1, 2, 8]. Clonal cytogenetic abnormalities may be present but as the neoplastic cells constitute a low percentage of total cells in the involved tissue they can be difficult to detect. *BCL6* rearrangements are seen in NLPHD.

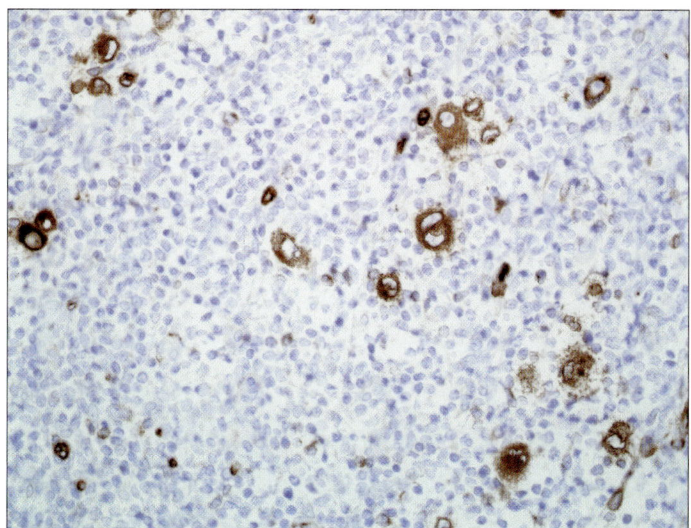

Figure 24.9 A section of a lymph node biopsy in classical HD showing CD30 expression by neoplastic cells; one binucleated Reed–Sternberg cell is apparent. Immunoperoxidase, x 40 objective.

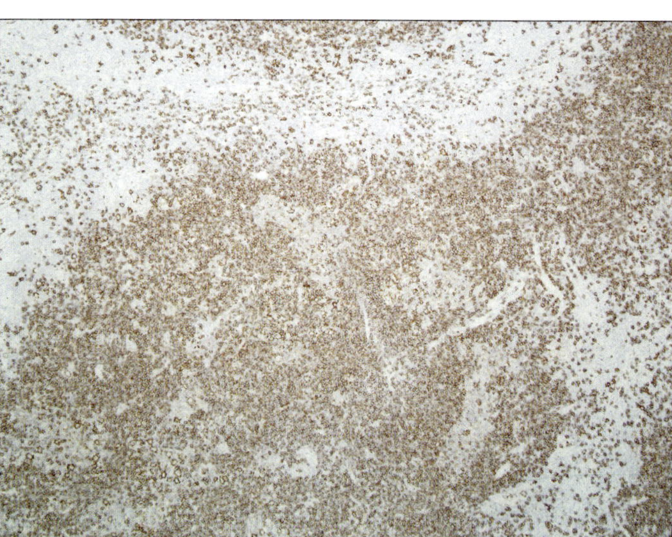

Figure 24.10 A section of a lymph node biopsy in nodular lymphocyte-predominant classical HD showing nodules of CD20-positive cells. Immunoperoxidase, x 10 objective.

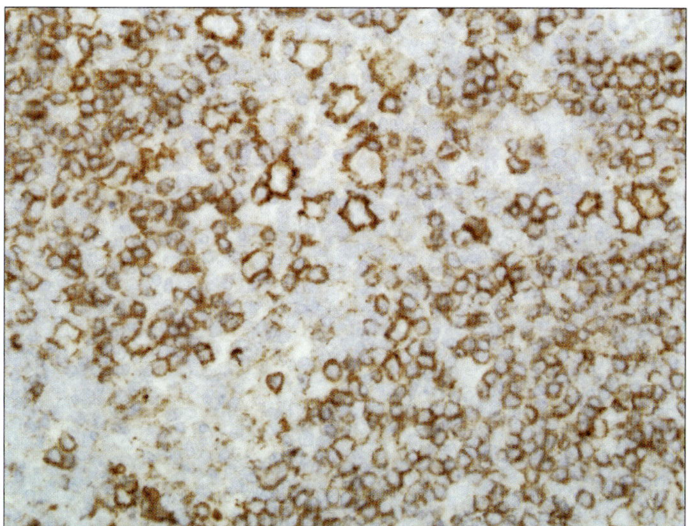

Figure 24.11 A section of a lymph node biopsy in nodular lymphocyte-predominant classical HD showing nodules of CD20-positive cells, both large and small. Immunoperoxidase, x 60 objective.

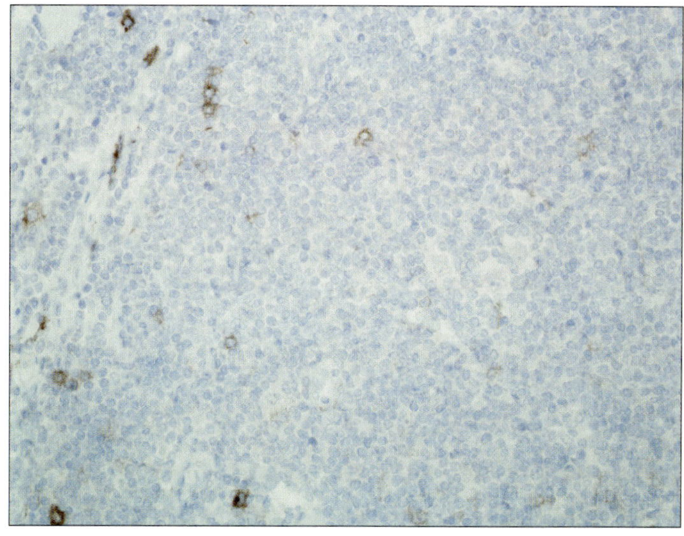

Figure 24.12 A section of a lymph node biopsy in nodular lymphocyte-predominant classical HD showing that neoplastic cells are CD30 negative. Immunoperoxidase, x 40 objective.

Diagnosis and differential diagnosis

The most important differential diagnosis is NHL, particularly T-cell- and histiocyte-rich diffuse large B-cell lymphoma and the anaplastic subtype of diffuse large B-cell lymphoma. Immunohistochemistry is important in distinguishing between these conditions.

Prognosis

Prognosis is generally good with the majority of patients being curable with current therapy. Poor prognostic features include older age, advanced stage and lymphocyte-depleted rather than lymphocyte-predominant histology.

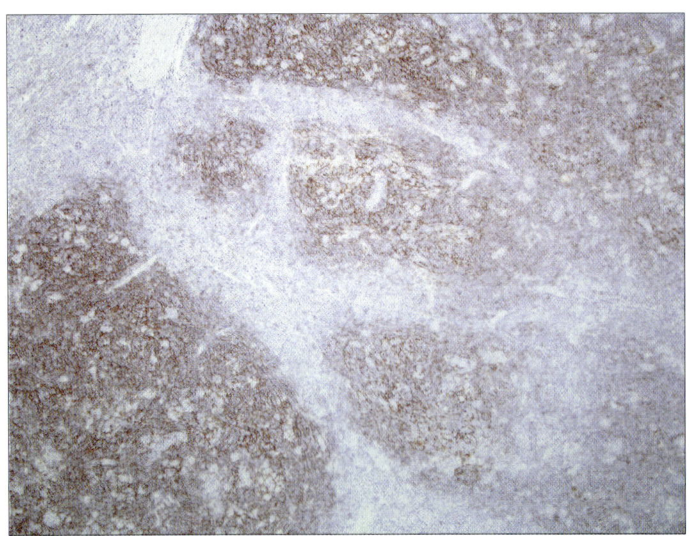

Figure 24.13 A section of a lymph node biopsy in nodular lymphocyte-predominant HD showing the supporting network of CD21-positive follicular dendritic cells. Immunoperoxidase, x 10 objective.

Treatment

Treatment is determined by the extent of disease, and the presence or absence of significant symptoms (B symptoms), being combined to give stages ranging from IA to IVB. Choice of treatment has steadily shifted from radiotherapy towards chemotherapy. Patients with early-stage disease often receive a short course of chemotherapy followed by involved field radiotherapy whereas patients with more advanced disease (stages IIB to IV) are treated by chemotherapy alone. Patients with major mediastinal lymphadenopathy receive chemotherapy, followed by consolidation radiotherapy once the size of the mediastinal mass has decreased.

References

1. Stein H, DelSol G, Pileri S, Said J, Mann R, Poppema S, Swerdlow SH and Jaffe ES (2001). Nodular lymphocyte predominant Hodgkin lymphoma. *In* Jaffe ES, Harris NL, Stein H and Vardiman JW (Eds). *Pathology and Genetics of Tumours of Haematopoietic and Lymphoid Tissues*, IARC Press, Lyon, pp. 240–243.
2. Stein H, DelSol G, Pileri S, Said J, Mann R, Poppema S, Jaffe ES and Swerdlow SH (2001). Classical Hodgkin lymphoma. *In* Jaffe ES, Harris NL, Stein H and Vardiman JW (Eds). *Pathology and Genetics of Tumours of Haematopoietic and Lymphoid Tissues*, IARC Press, Lyon, pp. 244–253.
3. Lister TA, Crowther D, Sutcliffe SB, Glatstein E, Canellos GP, Young RC *et al.* (1989). Report of a committee convened to discuss the evaluation and staging of patients with Hodgkin's disease: Cotswolds meeting. *J Clin Oncol*, **7**, 1630–1636. Erratum in: *J Clin Oncol*, 1990, **8**, 1602.
4. Stein H, Mason DY, Gerdes J, O'Connor N, Wainscoat J, Pallesen G *et al.* (1985). The expression of the Hodgkin's disease associated antigen Ki-1 in reactive and neoplastic lymphoid tissue: evidence that Reed–Sternberg cells and histiocytic malignancies are derived from activated lymphoid cells. *Blood*, **66**, 848–858.
5. Schmid C, Pan L, Diss T and Isaacson PG (1991). Expression of B-cell antigens by Hodgkin's and Reed–Sternberg cells. *Am J Pathol*, **139**, 701–707.
6. Carbone A, Gloghini A, Aldinucci D, Gattei V, Dalla-Favera R and Gaidano G (2002). Expression pattern of MUM1/IRF4 in the spectrum of pathology of Hodgkin's disease. *Br J Haematol*, **11**, 366–372.
7. Garcia-Cosio M, Santon A, Martin P, Camarasa N, Montalban C, Garcia JF and Bellas C (2004). Analysis of transcription factor OCT.1, OCT.2 and BOB.1 expression using tissue arrays in classical Hodgkin's lymphoma. *Mod Pathol*, **17**, 1531–1538.
8. Ohno T, Stribley JA, Wu G, Hinrichs SH, Weisenburger DD and Chan WC (1997). Clonality in nodular lymphocyte predominant Hodgkin's disease. *N Engl J Med*, **337**, 459–465.

Index

Note: page references in *italic* refer to tables or boxes in the text